D0114467

# Occupational Therapy: Work-Related Programs and Assessments

# Occupational Therapy: Work-Related Programs and Assessments

**Karen Jacobs, M.S., OTR**

*Adjunct Clinical Instructor, Boston University, Sargent College, Department of Occupational Therapy, Boston, Massachusetts; Director of Development, Little People's/Learning Prep School, West Newton, Massachusetts*

Line illustrations by Roger Tirrell
*Instructor, Graphic Arts, Learning Prep School*

**Little, Brown and Company**
**Boston/Toronto**

First Edition



Library of Congress Catalog Card No. 84-82436

ISBN 0-316-45547-4

Printed in the United States of America

MV

**To Florence S. Cromwell,**
**mentor and expert**
**in work-related programming**

# Contents

# Foreword

It is an encouraging sign for the profession of occupational therapy that growing numbers of occupational therapists are seeking information about work-related programming [1]. Not only do therapists seek examples of how to develop programs for populations with various work-related needs, but they also evidently wish to affirm, by better responding to the work role needs of their patients, the profession's rightful place in this aspect of rehabilitative care.

Thus it is both timely and fortuitous that the present volume is published with explicit responses to this kind of needs. If we as professionals are to adhere to the basic philosophies of our field [2, 3] and demonstrate solid programming in support of the assertions that occupational therapists are indeed true to those philosophies in their treatment activities, we must begin the active exchange of ideas about treatment needs in these program areas, study models of existing programs and strategies, and develop more active programs.

This text provides descriptions of many current programs that indicate the existence of a rich mosaic of work-related activity in the profession. The author of this book, a most enthusiastic and vocal believer and doer in work-related programming, has gathered an impressive collection of writing from a wide range of authors. Examining this menu should provide concrete ideas and assistance to practitioners regardless of their special interests and needs. This text may well stimulate others to publish and share, through presentations and discussions, additional models that will further enrich the field's image of itself for such activity. The message is that there is still much to be done, but we have a good start.

As one who has championed the role of occupational therapy in this arena for more than 30 years, I greet this addition to our literature with pleasure.

Florence S. Cromwell, M.A., OTR, F.A.O.T.A.

## References


1. The American Occupational Therapy Association. *Memorandum Requesting Support of Application for New Special Interest Section in Work-Related Programs.* Rockville, Md.: AOTA, 1984.
2. Cromwell, Florence S. Vocational Readiness Programming in Occupational Therapy: Its Roots, Course and Prognosis. In *Final Report, AOTA Competency-Based Curriculum in Vocational Readiness.* Rockville, Md.: AOTA, 1984.
3. Kielhofner, G. "Occupation," Chapter 3 in H. L. Hopkins and H. D. Smith, *Willard and Spackman's Occupational Therapy* (6th ed.). Philadelphia: Lippincott, 1983.

# Preface

Work is at the heart of the philosophy and practice of occupational therapy. In its broadest sense, work, as productive activity, is the concern in almost all therapy.

*Occupational Therapy: Work-Related Programs and Assessments* comprehensively examines the topic of work: historically, conceptually, and programmatically, throughout the life span, across various disabilities and facilities. This book is meant to fill a void in the occupational therapy literature. For some time there has been a need for a textbook on this subject, specifically designed for occupational therapists.

Chapter 1 traces the historical perspective of occupational therapy's role in work-related programming from our founding years, outlining the way the foundations were laid for present programs.

Chapter 2 formulates a conceptual framework with which the occupational therapist can develop work-related programs and assessments. Use of the term *work-related*, rather than prevocational and/or vocational rehabilitation, is suggested because it prevents us from becoming confused with other professions, and because it is in itself a more encompassing term. In this chapter, as throughout the text, stress is placed on the need to initiate work-related programming at an early age with special needs children.

Chapter 3 offers an overview of the present state of the art of standard and standardized work-related evaluations. The remainder of Chapter 3 is devoted to an in-depth presentation of the Jacobs Prevocational Skills Assessment (JPSA), which was developed to evaluate a learning-disabled adolescent population. Although a standard evaluation, it is viable as a useful screening tool because it can be adapted to individual client needs. The JSPA is presented in its entirety, including graphic illustrations. It is hoped that therapists will find this a practical instrument and reproduce it in photocopies for their own clinical use. Please note that some of the graphic illustrations must be enlarged for ease of use and for conformity to the standard feature of the assessment materials (for complete size listings, refer to the "shopping list" section of Chapter 3).

To facilitate a better understanding of the JPSA, its part of Chapter 3 is arranged in five sections.

The section on the development of the JPSA describes the way the JPSA evolved, as a guide for other therapists, who may someday find themselves faced with the task of developing their own assessment. The rationale for selecting specific work-related skill areas, tasks, and recording media is explored.

The next section of Chapter 3 describes the test elements. The recording medium, a single-page checklist-style profile sheet, was devised to facilitate recording data and to make the raw data accessible for further analysis, as were the JPSA manual, which includes for each of 15 tasks its purpose, materials, set-up of materials, and instructions for the therapist and/or client/student, and the 15 tasks composing the JSPA. There are numerous photographs and graphic illustrations throughout to facilitate comprehension.

The following section of Chapter 3 consists of a "shopping list" of all the items needed to construct your own JPSA. All the graphic illustrations, including the profile sheet itself, are provided throughout the chapter. Please carefully refer to this "shopping list" when constructing your own assessment, to be sure the materials are kept in a standard form.

The penultimate section of Chapter 3 contains two case studies to exemplify the ease of assessment implementation, data recording, and write-up of results. (One of these case study sample evaluation reports is followed in greater depth in Chapter 4. Individual client case studies, which add clarity to the textbook content, are interwoven throughout Chapters 4 and 5.)

The final section of Chapter 3 is the chapter Appendix, containing the complete JPSA manual ready for photocopying (it is recommended that the photocopied manual later be spiralbound for ease of use).

I invite therapists who use the JPSA to share their experience with me. I am particularly interested in adaptations you may make for the needs of your individual clients. I envision that eventually a network can be established to allow users a forum for exchange.

Chapters 4 and 5 describe work-related programming throughout the life span, from childhood/adolescence to adulthood. I have endeavored to provide comprehensive coverage of this topic by presenting case studies of programs by experts in this area throughout the United States and, to a limited extent, in Canada and Australia. In many instances, individual client case studies are presented for each program. Assessments that have been found useful in some of these programs are highlighted.

Chapter 4 begins with an overview of the need for work-related programming for children. It stresses that the initiation of programming for the special needs child must begin at an early age to facilitate incorporation of these basic skills into their repertoire of behaviors.

Four facilities are described regarding their care of children/adolescents with various developmental disabilities, i.e., the learning-disabled, the mentally retarded, and those with physical disabilities. The Little People's/Learning Prep School has been examined in particular detail as an example of the range of possibilities available for creative work-related program development. In addition, the sample evaluation report on "Stacey," introduced in Chapter 3, continues to reflect the results of the JPSA and the implementation of those results in therapy. In this chapter the use of community as a resource for program development and maintenance is a recurring theme.

Chapter 5 has been divided into four sections.

The first section opens with a brief overview of work-related programming and assessments for adults with psychosocial problems. It continues to explore six programs, including individual client case studies, from a variety of facilities: a Veterans Administration hospital, a community mental health center, hospitals, and correctional institutions. Special attention has been given to describing correctional institutions, in that the field of correction appears to be one that offers increasing opportunity to therapists.

The second section begins with an overview of work-related programming and assessments for adults with neurophysiologic dysfunction. Nine programs are described, incorporating individual client case studies. Hospitals, a rehabilitation center, private practice, and a state school are the settings covered. This section contains a brief survey of the topic of work capacity evaluation and work tolerance screening. Innovative modalities such as microcomputers and drivers' training are highlighted. In addition, a list of agencies selling adaptive equipment has been compiled.

The third section of Chapter 5 considers industry programs. Therapists are finding an increasing demand for their services in industry; and this section offers two examples of the roles therapists can play in industry.

The fourth section focuses on a geriatric program. Although this topic is briefly explored, this section points out that work as a productive activity can continue to be an important part of a retiree's life, as exemplified in the Jewish Rehabilitation Center (JRC) for Aged of the North Shore in Massachusetts. At the JRC, residents participate in an on-site sheltered workshop.

Chapter 6 asks: What is the future outlook for therapists in work-related programming? I believe we should be quite optimistic! Today's therapists are challenged with the role they can play in work-related programming. As trends in employment shift, the therapist must keep pace in treatment and rally to meet the changing needs of our client/patients.

In laypeople's terms, the Appendix to the whole text examines the role of the microcomputer in work-related programs in order to provide the therapist exposure to this additional modality in treatment.

Collectively, the text provides the therapist with a detailed set of guidelines for developing and implementing work-related programs and assessments. The content serves as a resource and reference to be utilized whenever any work-related program is being planned and the subject is being addressed in the classroom.

The task of concluding this text was a difficult one, due to the dynamic nature of this area of practice and the seemingly endless innovative grassroots programs that could be shared. Since this area is expanding so quickly, I urge therapists who read this book to be in touch with me about their programs, so that we can exchange material and have an ongoing update.

K. J.

# Acknowledgments

Appreciation is due everyone who helped in the preparation of this textbook. I would like to express my gratitude to all by listing them by specific chapters.

Chapter 1 was developed in part from information provided by Florence Cromwell and Edwinna M. Marshall. The first draft of Chapter 1 was critiqued by Florence Cromwell and Thelma Hook. Deborah Newman reviewed the first drafts of Chapters 1 through 3.

Occupational therapists at the Little People's/Learning Prep School both of the present (Kathy Pepicelli, Irene Clague, Nancy Mazonson, Wynne Leekoff) and of the past (Debbie Viens, Sara Sicilano, Stacey Schrope-Szklut, Linda Gow, Joan Schiff) contributed to the metamorphosis of the Jacobs Prevocational Skills Assessment presented in Chapter 3. Special thanks to Walter Loan, who posed for photographs, and to Nancy Mazonson, who posed for photographs and also contributed case studies to Chapters 3 and 4. Full acknowledgment must be given to graphic artist and friend Roger Tirrell for his tireless efforts in preparing the illustrations for the Jacobs Prevocational Skills Assessment.

I thank the following individuals for their assistance in the section in Chapter 4 on the Little People's/Learning Prep School: the Director of the school, Nancy Rosoff, for her support of this endeavor; the administrators; the staff; and the students who participated via photographs and the exchange of information. Much of what I have learned about work-related programming came from direct work with all these people. Appreciation to others involved with Chapter 4: Sherry Olin and Mary Haldy, for their contribution of information on the Margaret Walters School; Kathleen Reynolds-Lynch, for the information sent me on the Riley Hospital for Children; and Terry Lyons, who shared information on the Handicapped Employment Training Assistance Unit in Australia.

For the first section of Chapter 5 the following individuals kindly shared information on their programs: Lauren Kirson for the New York Veterans Administration Medical Center program; both Donna Gatti and Francis Palmer for McLean Hospital's Thrift Shop; the McLean Hospital Thrift Shop staff who posed for photographs, and Matthew Gold, who took the pictures; Suzanne Poirier for the Solomon Carter Fuller Mental Health Center; Robin Klein for information on the Clifton T. Perkins Hospital; Robert Schneider for the Calgary General Hospital section, including the photographs; and Sandra Palmer, who provided information on the Washington State Special Offenders Center.

For assistance on the second section in Chapter 5, on programming for adults with neurophysiologic problems, I acknowledge the assistance of the following individuals: Ralph Colangelo, Karen Haggarty-Weake, and Holly T. Ehle, for the information and photographs on Braintree Hospital's Comprehensive Driver Education Program; Karen Lindau, Sara Hargreaves, Carolyn Long, and administrators of the Liberty Mutual Medical Service Center, who provided information, posed for photographs, and contributed the historic photograph of their center for Chapter one: Rhonda Auricht, Pam Dean, and Robert Cox, for their information on the Western Domiciliary Care and Rehabilitation Service of Queen Elizabeth Hospital—Alfreda Rehabilitation Unit; Dorie Milner, who kindly shared both information and photographs on the Institute of Rehabilitation Medicine, New York University Medical Center; Linda Ogden-Dempster and Leonard Matheson, for the information on work capacity evaluation, which came out of an invaluable workshop that they presented; Karen Schultz, for both photographs and information on Downey Community Hospital and Hand Rehabilitation Specialists; Thelma Hook, for writing the section on hand therapy and Rehabilitation Associates; Carolyn Austin and John Basile, who provided information on Walter E. Fernald State School; and friend Shana Krell, for sharing her work at United Cerebral Palsy Day Habilitation Center.

Grateful acknowledgment for information on United Hospitals is due Barbara Johnson for the third section, on industry programs, in Chapter 5.

I thank the Activity Department of the Jewish Rehabilitation Center of the North Shore, directed by Virginia Bradley, for sharing its sheltered workshop program at the conclusion of Chapter 5.

Nancy Wall, my mentor in microcomputers, co-authored the Appendix on microcomputers in work-related programs.

My publisher, Little, Brown and Company, has my appreciation for its assistance. Specifically, I would like to thank Barbara Ward, who supported the concept of this text, and Katharine Tsioulcas, who with her patience made it a reality. Many thanks are extended to others at Little, Brown: Louis Bruno, Lisa O'Brien, Mary Gordon, Dorothy Scott, and Diana Gibney.

Last, and most important, thanks to my family and friends who have tolerated me over the three years it has taken to complete this book: my husband, Matthew Gold, for his logical thinking, and my children, Laela and Joshua; my parents, Ruth and Lawrence Jacobs; my sister Lisa and my brother Jon and their families; my Nanie, who continues to be an inspiration to me; my grandmother, Pearl Demsky, and my grandfather, Al Filler; and my friends Gayle Thompson, Louise Dunn, and Natalie and Martin Goodman.

K. J.

# Occupational Therapy: Work-Related Programs and Assessments

# 1. History of Work-Related Programs in Occupational Therapy

Within the profession of occupational therapy a renewed interest has developed in the area of prevocational and vocational programming and assessment. This movement can be substantiated by noting the recent appearance of this topic in various forums. For example, the American Occupational Therapy Association (AOTA) in 1980 published an official position paper entitled "The Role of Occupational Therapy in the Vocational Rehabilitation Process" [1], which presented the following description of that role:

> Occupational therapy is based upon the fundamental belief that engagement in purposeful activity (occupation), including both the interpersonal and environmental dimensions, may prevent or remediate dysfunction and elicit maximum performance in the work role adaptation.
>
> The principles of occupational therapy practice, as they relate to the vocational process, are applied through the provision of a planned and orderly sequence of services designed to prepare the individual for vocational evaluation, training and eventual employment or the highest degree of independent function. . . . The treatment process involves the use of selected activities, assistive devices, and educational techniques to restore the client to the highest level of independent function. . . . The specific aims of the occupational therapy treatment are to assist the individual to recover or to develop competence in the physical, psychological, social and economic aspects of daily living and to provide opportunities to learn those skills needed for adaptation in educational, work, home and community environments.

Further evidence of renewed interest in prevocational and vocational programs comes from the occupational therapy literature. In recent years the *American Journal of Occupational Therapy* has featured four articles on this topic: "The School Therapist and Vocational Education" [9], "The Role of Occupational Therapy in Vocational Evaluation" [25, 26], "To Market, To Market" [27], and "Factors Affecting Return to Work After Hand Injury" [3]. The *Canadian Journal of Occupational Therapy* continues to have a steady flow of work-related articles [7, 24, 29, 35, 36].

Several major projects have recently been started in this area. In 1982 AOTA initiated a three-year project, funded through the Office of Special Education and Rehabilitation Services, U.S. Department of Health and Human Services, called "Occupational Therapist's Role in Vocational Readiness for Handicapped Students." The project is designed to result in a curriculum for occupational therapists working in the area of vocational readiness for handicapped students. In the same year the American Occupational Therapy Foundation

Partnership in Research Program sponsored a study by an Indiana University research team of clinicians and academicians of prevocational evaluation practices of occupational therapists. The results of this study are not available at this writing but will be disseminated via lectures and an article in the *American Journal of Occupational Therapy.*

The 1982 national conference in Philadelphia witnessed an increased number of presentations on the topic, and the Metropolitan New York District of the New York State Occupational Therapy Association in 1983 offered a two-day conference entitled "Occupational Therapy: Approaches to Clinical Issues in Prevocational Settings." In addition, individual therapists throughout the country have been working to reestablish a prevocational and vocational special interest group in the professional organization. At present an informal network has been established with a newsletter circulated to its members.

Such periods of renewed interest in and enthusiasm for the area of prevocational and vocational programming are not unusual for the profession. The following brief historic overview is presented so that the reader can appreciate more fully the scope and importance of current interest.

For the sake of brevity, this history will begin in the decade of the founding of the profession, 1910 to 1920. This was a time of "watchful . . . custodial conservative treatment and long-term caring for people" [13]. It was a time of reactivation of moral treatment* for the mentally ill and of the use of reconstruction aides, who concerned themselves with the return to work of disabled Great War soldiers [48]. Eleanor Clarke Slagle, earlier a social worker, became one of the first known advocates of occupational therapy as a means of treating the wounded. By the close of the war, thousands of soldiers had received some form of "occupation therapy" [28].

The time was right for the emergence of the profession. As noted by Woodside [48], "The war, a severe polio epidemic in 1916, industrial accidents and the widening use of the automobile all contributed to the need for new methods of treating residual disabilities." The concept of employing crafts to reactivate the minds and motivation of these disabled persons paved the way for the entrance of the occupational therapy profession into vocational training and rehabilitation [38].

In Canada the Military Hospitals' Commission established schools for vocational training in convalescent hospitals and offered instruction in activities that would aid patients to prepare for work [47].

In 1920 the Vocational Rehabilitation Act (Smith-Fess Act, Public Law 66-236) was passed. This landmark legislation defined rehabilitation as "return to remunerative employment," with the provision of funds on a matching basis to states for helping disabled persons. The Act allowed solely for "train-

*Moral treatment came into existence in the early nineteenth century with the development of psychiatric programs such as that of McLean Hospital in Belmont, Massachusetts. According to Sanbourne Bockoven [5], "The history of moral treatment in America is not only synonymous with but is the history of occupational therapy before it acquired its twentieth-century name."

ing in existing schools, industry and commercial establishments, or by a tutor." Medical service was covered only "if needed to determine eligibility for help." Since the training was carried out by state vocational education departments, there were many opportunities for occupational therapists in centers such as sheltered and curative workshops to participate in prevocational programming [49]. *At this time former psychiatric patients were ineligible for benefits derived from the Act. The founders of the AOTA were instrumental in enlisting the assistance of veterans' groups and physicians' associations in campaigning for legislative changes. Public Law 236 gave the profession the ideal opportunity to introduce work-related programming tailored to disabled persons. At this point "our founders were quite committed to look at the total day and future of the individual, not just his current pathology" [13]. Concurrently, other important contributions were made by George Edward Barton, William Rush Dunton, Jr., and Eleanor Clarke Slagle.

Barton became the advocate of occupation therapy who, after suffering tuberculosis and stroke, organized Consolation House in Clifton Springs, New York, as a vocational bureau and community-based activity workshop for ill and disabled persons. "By means of occupations, people could be retrained or adjusted to gainful employment [the philosophy of which was] to give that sort [of activity] which will be preliminary to and dovetailed with the real vocational education which is to begin as soon as the patient is able to go farther along" [28].

Dunton, "the Father of Occupational Therapy," was involved in the use of occupational therapy with psychiatric patients at Sheppard and Enoch Pratt Hospital, Baltimore. He insisted on total workday planning for patients and was primarily concerned to develop and maintain work habits [14].

Slagle made "habit training" the centerpiece of her methods of treatment, which were based on the use of a wide sample of daily occupations. This type of rehabilitation program, which included preindustrial and vocational work, attempted to create a balance of work, rest, and play for psychiatric patients [28].

In Canada another founder of AOTA, T. B. Kidner, who came from an industrial background, was concerned about returning the disabled to work through activity [13, 39].

According to Cromwell [13], the profession received a strong message from its founders "that the occupational therapy profession, small as it was at the time, was devoted to the belief that productivity was possible to prevent the breakdown of skills, habits and attitudes."

During the 1930s therapists were still feeling the impact of World War I and the Vocational Rehabilitation Act. This was the time of "curative workshops," which were specifically aimed at the injured industrial worker and

*The Rehabilitation Service Administration (U.S. Department of Health, Education and Welfare) evolved from this legislation. At present the agency serves the psychiatrically and developmentally disabled and, to a more limited degree, the physically disabled. As a result of 1978 amendments, a large proportion of clients served are severely handicapped [25].

which utilized work-related activity as the treatment. Occupational therapists were instrumental in the organization and development of such workshops in Philadelphia, Milwaukee, and St. Louis. The Pre-vocational Unit at the Institute for the Crippled and Disabled (ICD) founded in New York City in 1936 may be viewed as the forerunner of present prevocational programs. For this program the institute modified evaluation techniques used for applicants to industry and trade schools to evaluate and train the disabled [28].

Similar trends were apparent in Europe and Canada, also because of the need to reeducate the disabled. In 1938 the Occupational Therapy Workshop of the Canadian Workmen's Compensation Board was opened. Its goal was to shorten the convalescent period of injured workmen, thus cutting costs of compensation, through a concentrated program of occupational, recreational, and physical therapy. In this workshop tasks specifically related to the patient's former job were utilized as treatment. For example, patients built brick walls, painted buildings, laid railroad ties, and repaired plumbing [31, 42]. Numerous articles in the *Canadian Journal of Occupational Therapy* during the early 1940s also reflected local interest in this area [31, 42, 44, 47].

West [47] notes that during the world wars occupational therapy as a profession grew tremendously as a result of its role in work adjustment of soldiers. World War II allowed disabled soldiers and workers to emerge as a major force in the United States because of the scarcity of able-bodied workers in an expanding industrial economy. Many industries modified work environments to accommodate disabled workers.

Passage of the Vocational Rehabilitation Amendments (Barden-La Follette Act) of 1943 (Public Law 78-113), for which AOTA founders had actively campaigned in the 1920s, was another landmark. For the first time developmentally and psychiatrically disabled persons were made eligible for rehabilitation services. With this legislation the need for vocational training for those who had *never* been employed was recognized.

Despite all the pioneering efforts that show continuing and active involvement in work-related treatment, the early postwar period saw a noticeable move by the occupational therapy profession away from prevocational rehabilitation activities. According to West [47], this trend may have resulted from heavy case loads, poor training of professional personnel, and the high cost of facilities. In addition, according to Cromwell [13], "Occupational therapists were looking for more scientific approaches and beginning to reject 'occupation' alone. Occupational therapists choose more often to be identified with the medical model than with a social or vocational model." This period, however, saw the rise of many military and veterans' hospitals. Therapists in these centers developed the army model of rehabilitation and used activities adapted from hospitals and industry as treatment. Occupational therapists also gradually turned from work-related activities to the development of adaptive tools and devices for clients with various orthopedic and neurologic injuries [13].

During this same period Liberty Mutual became the first insurance company

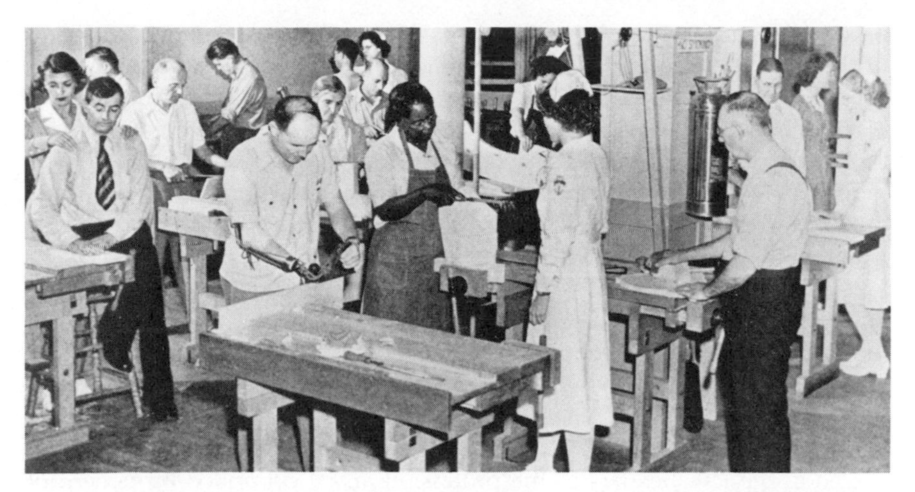

*Fig. 1-1. The occupational therapy at the Liberty Mutual rehabilitation center, late 1940s. (Photo courtesy of Liberty Mutual Insurance Companies, Boston, Massachusetts.)*

to establish rehabilitation workshops. These workshops, located in Boston and Chicago, provided rehabilitation services to disabled workers with the intent of returning them to their jobs as quickly as possible. In San Francisco Carlotta Wells and Signe Brunstrum established a program using intensive work-oriented treatment at the May T. Mornson Center, which served persons with many kinds of physical and psychological illnesses [13].

Declining professional interest in work-related programming was somewhat bolstered in 1954 with the adoption of amendments to the Vocational Rehabilitation Act. As a result of this legislation, prevocational units were established within rehabilitation facilities. Occupational therapists assumed a major responsibility in the development of principles of prevocational exploration [1, 8]. The Department of Physical and Rehabilitation Medicine at New York University Medical Center established possibly the largest prevocational exploration unit in the world at the time [16].

In 1955 AOTA held an institute "to reassess professional education and practice as related to rehabilitation" [47]. In the following year the association held another institute with the specific purpose of addressing the concept, purposes, methods, values, and rationale of prevocational programming, as well as prevocational techniques and media [23, 39].

As noted by Reed and Sanderson [39], "Prevocational exploration and training became the glamor area of practice in the late fifties and early sixties." There even emerged within AOTA a prevocational specialty group. Interest in this group has come and gone through the years.

The content of the *American Journal of Occupational Therapy* between 1957 and 1961 reflects the increased interest in this area with a total of 11 work-related articles [46, 47]. An example is Rosenburg and Wellerson's explanation of the differences between the prevocational and vocational evaluation programs at the ICD [41]. Aims of prevocational programming for physically disabled populations at the ICD included the development of three aspects of the individual: work habits; work tolerance; and coordination, production, and speed. In the ICD program clients were exposed to activities such as clerical and sales tasks, upholstery refinishing, power press operation, industrial leather manufacturing, and assembly and packaging tasks. Task selection was based on the client's interest and work history, and the average length of programming was between 2 weeks and 6 months [41]. The TOWER (Testing, Orientation, and Work Evaluation in Rehabilitation) system, an outgrowth of early programs developed at ICD, continues today to be a much-used evaluation instrument [28]. Many occupational therapists received training in the use of this instrument and were subsequently employed as vocational evaluators in rehabilitation centers serving patients with many kinds of disabilities.

One of the later leaders in the profession and a continued proponent of work-related programming is Florence Cromwell [10–13]. Her many articles, lectures, and research reports and her manual on prevocational evaluation continue to be valid references for today's therapist. Cromwell herself remains an inspirational role model and resource person for those committed to contributions by occupational therapy in work-related programs. In her 1962 presentation [11] to the Third International Congress of the World Federation of Occupational Therapists, she reiterated the profession's commitment: "Work Adjustment is and has always been a function of occupational therapy."

The 1960 Iowa Conference on Prevocational Activities was another effort to clarify the role and structural framework of prevocational programs in occupational therapy [34]. The questions addressed in 1960 [37] are similar to those being asked today:

1. What progress has been made in more sharply defining the term pre-vocational?
2. Can we obtain agreement on working definitions for the following terms:
   a. work adjustment
   b. work conditioning
   c. pre-vocational unit
   d. job sampling
3. What are the characteristics of a good vocational evaluation system? . . .

I. What is the scope of pre-vocational activities?
II. What contribution . . . [do] . . . the following personnel [make] to the prevocational process? . . .

According to West [47], despite the increase in publications on and interest in work-related programming, the literature was "extremely limited in terms of our total professional picture." Reed and Sanderson [39] note that "no specific issue diminished the interest in prevocational practice, but as health care swung toward acute and short term care there simply was not time to provide prevocational exploration and training." On the international scene, however, there remained a greater focus on work-related treatment [22], and, according to Cromwell [13], "Our colleagues in other countries really left us behind."

Curative workshops were beginning to turn from restoration and work-related treatment to straight vocational counseling. Much of the work performed by the occupational therapist was being passed by default to the emerging work evaluators. The University of Wisconsin–Stout, with strong federal support, established the Stout Vocational Rehabilitation Institute. A division of the institute, the Materials Development Center (MDC) [45], is presently "the national central source for the collection, development, and dissemination of information and materials in the areas of vocational evaluation, work adjustment, and rehabilitation facility management and operations. The goal of MDC is to improve the performance of rehabilitation facilities serving the handicapped, resulting in the increased economic independence for disabled persons."

In the early 1960s Mary Reilly suggested the need for the profession to increase its knowledge of the work–play continuum as an appropriate base for occupational therapy. This continuum has subsequently been designated *occupational behavior.* Reilly's understanding of occupational behavior is built on the premise that "the play of childhood . . . contains a critical ability to transmit the adaptive skills necessary for complex work technology and urban living of today" [40]. She stresses the importance of "examining the various life roles of the population relative to community adaptation, to identify the various skills that support these roles, and to create an environment in treatment where the relevant behavior could be evoked and practiced" [40]. Much of what Reilly suggests is reminiscent of Slagle's habit training.

Articles published in the *American Journal of Occupational Therapy* after 1966 express concern about the sparsity of literature related to work-related programming, particularly in the treatment of psychiatric populations. Ethridge [19] noted that over a period of years literature discussing prevocational evaluation was totally concerned with the assessment of physically handicapped patients, with almost no mention of the psychiatrically disabled. Two notable exceptions were articles by Llorens and colleagues [30] and Fidler [20].

Beginning in the late 1960s and 1970s more interest in the psychiatrically disabled developed. Articles by Clark and Lerner [6], Ethridge [19], Diasio and Jones [17], Distefano and Pryer [18], Deacon and associates [15], and Solberg and Chueh [43] all relate to the psychiatric population and emphasize evaluation checklists. Theoretical articles by various therapists appeared at the same time. Bailey [2] identified work habits—attitudes toward work, punctuality, regular attendance, appearance, speed of work, manual dexterity, concentration, cleanliness, and social skills—and traced them to theories of childhood and vocational development. In Reed and Sanderson [39] Maurer defined skills important to vocational development: identifying with a worker, learning about work and its varieties, getting along with peers, developing basic habits of industry, developing a self-concept and translating it into occupational terms, and learning to work with and adjust to authority (see Table 2-1).

The impetus for establishing occupational therapy services in schools was provided by the enactment of Public Law 94-142, the Education of All Handicapped Children Act of 1975, which mandates the opportunity for appropriate education for every child. Public Law 93-112, Section 504, the Rehabilitation Act of 1973, also has played an important role in the provision of services to children [9]. Occupational therapy has been readily recognized as a valuable service within the educational system. The occupational therapist has become a vital member of teams developing and providing appropriate educational and health care programs for special needs students [9].

Gilfoyle and Hays [21] believe that occupational therapy will be important in student career development in the near future:

> . . . An increase in the number of handicapped children can be predicted for secondary schools and/or vocational training programs centers administered by public school programs as impact of Federal legislation will provide more appropriate education for the adolescent age group. Occupational therapy must play a vital role with educational programs of career development and prevocational training for handicapped students.

According to Cromwell [14], "Vocational educators in the school system who are beginning to get handicapped youngsters in labs and classes have indicated a real need for help. They need to know how to adapt settings, materials and methods, to manage these persons with different ways of functioning. What more perfect place for the occupational therapist to consult and aid in the development of these programs?"

## References

1. Ad Hoc Committee of the Commission on Practice. The role of occupational therapy in the vocational rehabilitation process: Official Position Paper. *Am. J. Occup. Ther.* 34:881, 1980.
2. Bailey, D. Vocational theories and work habits related to childhood development. *Am. J. Occup. Ther.* 25:298, 1971.
3. Bear-Lehman, J. Factors affecting return to work after hand injury. *Am. J. Occup. Ther.* 37:189, 1983.
4. Bing, R. K. Eleanor Clarke Slagle Lectureship—1981—Occupational therapy revisited: a paraphrastic journey. *Am. J. Occup. Ther.* 35:499, 1981.
5. Bockoven, J. S. Occupational therapy—a historical perspective: legacy of moral treatment—1800s to 1910. *Am. J. Occup. Ther.* 25:223, 1971.
6. Clark, B., and Lerner, G. E. Occupational therapists participate in prevocational screening. *Am. J. Occup. Ther.* 20:91, 1966.
7. Clements, L., and Dixon, M. A model of occupational therapy in back education. *Can. J. Occup. Ther.* 46:161, 1979.
8. Combs, M. H., Nadler, E. B., and Thomas, C. W. Vocational exploration—Methodological problems and a suggested approach. *Am. J. Occup. Ther.* 22:64, 1958.
9. Creighton, C. The school therapist and vocational education. *Am. J. Occup. Ther.* 33:373, 1979.

10. Cromwell, F. S. A procedure for prevocational evaluation. *Am.J. Occup. Ther.* 13:1, 1959.
11. Cromwell, F. S. Looking ahead in work evaluation: Work adjustment as a function of occupational therapy. In *Proceedings of the Third International Congress of the World Federation of Occupational Therapists*, Dubuque, Iowa: Wm. C. Brown, 1964. Vol. 5, p. 16.
12. Cromwell, F. S. *Occupational Therapist's Manual for Basic Assessment—Primary Prevocational Evaluation.* Altadena, California: Fair Oakes Printing Company, 1976.
13. Cromwell, F. S. The world of industry: arena for OT skills. Presented at the National Occupational Therapy Association Conference, Philadelphia, May 1982.
14. Cromwell, F. S. Personal communication, 1983.
15. Deacon, S., Dunning, R. E., and Dease, R. Jobs: a job clinic for psychotic clients in remission. *Am. J. Occup. Ther.* 28:144, 1974.
16. Department of Physical Medicine and Rehabilitation. *Pre-Vocational Therapy Demonstration in a General Hospital and a Rehabilitation Center* (SP-234). Report to the National Advisory Council on Vocational Rehabilitation, U.S. Department of Health, Education and Welfare. New York: New York University Medical Center, 1960.
17. Diasio, K., and Jones, M. S. Prevocational services for young adult psychiatric patients. *Hosp. Community Psychiatry* 21:217, 1970.
18. Distefano, M. K., and Pryer, M. W. Vocational evaluation and successful placement of psychiatric clients in a vocational rehabilitation program. *Am. J. Occup. Ther.* 24:205, 1970.
19. Ethridge, D. A. Prevocational assessment of rehabilitation potential of psychiatric patients. *Am. J. Occup. Ther.* 22:161, 1968.
20. Fidler, G. S. A second look at work as a primary force in rehabilitation and treatment. *Am. J. Occup. Ther.* 20:72, 1966.
21. Gilfoyle, E., and Hays, C. Occupational therapy roles and functions in the education of the school-based handicapped student. *Am. J. Occup. Ther.* 33:565, 1979.
22. Goode, D. G. The role of occupational therapy in work adjustment: Work adjustment as a function of occupational therapy. In *Proceedings of the Third International Congress of the World Federation of Occupational Therapists*, Dubuque, Iowa: Wm. C. Brown, 1964. Vol. 5, p. 99.
23. Granofsky, J. *A Manual for Occupational Therapists on Prevocational Exploration.* Dubuque, Iowa: Wm. C. Brown, 1959.
24. Green, A., Gould, L., Mailer, M., Otto, K., and Henderson, R. Task groups: how they work in one vocational assessment unit. *Can. J. Occup. Ther.* 45:61, 1978.
25. Hightower-Vandamm, M. Nationally Speaking: The role of occupational therapy in vocational evaluation, Part 1. *Am. J. Occup. Ther.* 35:563, 1981.
26. Hightower-Vandamm, M. Nationally Speaking: The role of occupational therapy in vocational evaluation, Part 2. *Am. J. Occup. Ther.* 35:631, 1981.
27. Hightower-Vandamm, M. Nationally Speaking: To market, to market. *Am. J. Occup. Ther.* 36:293, 1982.
28. Hopkins, H. L., and Smith, H. D. *Willard and Spackman's Occupational Therapy* (6th ed.). Philadelphia: Lippincott, 1983.
29. Lewchuk, S. The occupational therapist in industry—a developing challenge. *Can. J. Occup. Ther.* 47:159, 1980.
30. Llorens, L. S., Levy, R., and Rubin, E. Z. Work adjustment program—a pre-vocational experience. *Am. J. Occup. Ther.* 28:15, 1964.
31. Lomey, M. B. Rehabilitation under the workmen's compensation act. *Can. J. Occup. Ther.* 8:25, 1941.
32. Maurer, P. A. Prevocational activities and evaluation for the child and adolescent. *Phys. Ther.* 48:771, 1968.
33. Maurer, P. A. Antecedents of work behavior. *Am. J. Occup. Ther.* 25:295, 1971.

34. Moed, M. B. Procedures and practices in prevocational evaluation: a review of current programs. In J. E. Muthard (Ed.), *Proceedings of the Iowa Conference on Prevocational Activities.* Washington, D.C.: Office of Vocational Rehabilitation, U.S. Department of Health, Education and Welfare, 1960.
35. Monfette, L. Vocational counselling and the alienated worker. *Can. J. Occup. Ther.* 46:57, 1979.
36. Murphy, M. Developments in a rehabilitation service for psychiatric patients. *Can. J. Occup. Ther.* 47:15, 1980.
37. Muthard, J. E. (Ed.) *Proceedings of the Iowa Conference of Prevocational Activities.* Washington, D.C.: Office of Vocational Rehabilitation, U.S. Department of Health, Education and Welfare, 1960.
38. O'Donnell, D. T. A descriptive study of the frequency and nature of the application of pre-vocational activity in occupational therapy settings in the state of Maryland. University of Maryland Master's thesis, 1983.
39. Reed, K., and Sanderson, S. R. *Concepts of Occupational Therapy* (2nd ed.). Baltimore: Williams & Wilkins, 1983.
40. Reilly, M. Occupational therapy can be one of the great ideas of 20th century medicine. *Am. J. Occup. Ther.* 16:1, 1962.
41. Rosenburg, B., and Wellerson, T. A structured prevocational program. *Am. J. Occup. Ther.* 14:57, 1960.
42. Smith, H. V. Workmen's compensation board, occupational therapy workshop. *Can. J. Occup. Ther.* 7:26, 1940.
43. Solberg, N. A., and Chueh, W. Performance in occupational therapy as a predictor of successful prevocational training. *Can. J. Occup. Ther.* 30:481, 1976.
44. Storms, H. D. Occupational therapy in the treatment of industrial casualties. *Can. J. Occup. Ther.* 10:40, 1943.
45. Stout Vocational Rehabilitation Institute Catalog. Menomonie, Wisconsin: University of Wisconsin, 1983.
46. Wegg, L. S. Eleanor Clarke Slagle Lecture—The essentials of work evaluation. *Am. J. Occup. Ther.* 14:65, 1960.
47. West, W. L. The role of occupational therapy in work adjustment: Work adjustment as a function of occupational therapy. In *Proceedings of the Third International Congress of the World Federation of Occupational Therapists.* Dubuque, Iowa: Wm. C. Brown, 1964. Vol. 5, p. 1.
48. Woodside, H. H. Occupational therapy—a historical perspective: the development of occupational therapy—1910–1929. *Am. J. Occup. Ther.* 25:226, 1971.
49. Cromwell, Florence S. Vocational readiness programming in occupational therapy: Its roots, course, and prognosis. In *Competency-Based Curriculum in Vocational Readiness.* Baltimore, Md.: American Occupational Therapy Association, 1984.

# 2. Conceptual Framework

Throughout this book I will use the term *work-related* as synonymous with *prevocational* and *vocational*. Although *prevocational* and *vocational* are easily differentiated, the differences become blurred when one observes existing programs. *Prevocational skills* can be defined as the antecedents to job skill development, that is, skills, behaviors, and habits developed from infancy onward: establishment of eye contact, cooperative behavior, task focus, motivation, reliability, independence. According to Ogden [7], *prevocational programming* "refers to occupational therapy evaluation/treatment that is work-oriented and provides the individual who has an impediment to work performance with an opportunity to engage in simulated work experience on a trial basis." On the other hand, vocational skills are more specifically related to job skill development, for example, learning the skill of operating a carpenter's lathe or a chef's steam kettle.

*Work-related* was selected with the intent of eliminating the confusion associated with *prevocational* and *vocational* in the literature and in clinical settings. *Prevocational*, or *prevoc* (as it is more commonly called), has a negative or derogatory connotation among many therapists. In addition, these terms are derived from other professions; *work-related* is occupational therapy terminology.

Work-related programming requires a holistic approach to the needs of the person—social, psychological, physical, and academic—in his or her development of a work role, irrespective of whether the person is "normal" or has a dysfunction. *Work* includes all forms of productive activity, regardless of whether they are reimbursed. According to Gary Kielhofner [3]:

> Productive activities are those that provide a service or commodity needed by another or that add new abilities, ideas, knowledge, artistic objects, or performances to the cultural tradition. The productive activity of work thus maintains and advances society. When an activity is considered to be one's work, it is generally organized into a major life role. Life roles are positions in life recognized by the social environment and by the role incumbent. Thus, activities engaged in to fulfill one's duties as a student, housewife, volunteer, serious hobbyist, or amateur, and that are part of one's identity, can be considered work.

According to this definition, work is not limited to adulthood but is relevant throughout the life span, from school age to retirement. In the transition from childhood to adulthood, a person undergoes an important process of occupational choice: exploration, tentative choice, and realistic final choice. Maurer [5, 6] has suggested that we learn how to work through a sequential

*Table 2-1. Developmental Tasks in Prevocational Development*

| *Age (years)* | *Task* | *Sample Activities* |
|---|---|---|
| 5–10 | Identification with a worker | Role modeling in play and fantasy<br>Imitation of workers |
| ?–adolescence | Learning about work | Observing the environment |
| ?–adolescence | Getting along with peers | Interaction with others in play and work |
| 10–15 | Formation of basic habits | Organization of time and behavior<br>Part-time jobs<br>School work<br>Chores |
| ?–18 | Self-concept elaboration, including | Reactions of significant others |
| 11–12 | Interests | Identifying likes and dislikes |
| 13–14 | Capacities | Awareness of what person does well |
| 15–16 | Values | Selecting what is important in life |
| ?–adolescence | Relation to authority | Obeying mother<br>Obeying other adults, teachers<br>Adjusting to supervision |

Source: From P. A. Maurer, in K. Reed and G. Sanderson, Concepts of Occupational Therapy (2nd ed.). Baltimore: Williams & Wilkins, 1983.

process that begins in childhood (Table 2-1). She notes that the rate of learning and the age of achievement of various stages may vary among individuals.

Because occupational choice is a dynamic process, programming must begin at an early age with the introduction of activities to foster career awareness and exploration of vocational capabilities and interests. Although such awareness and exploration must be reinforced with normal children, it is particularly critical for programming to be presented developmentally and initiated at an early age for special needs children. The reasons for this are their limited exposure (or lack of exposure) to the world of work, and limited career expectations for them on the part of parents and society. In addition, as noted by Lynch and colleagues [4], "Training materials and work performance requirements should increasingly approximate actual industrial demands and training should move from the school to the actual work site as soon as possible." Lynch and associates have proposed a constellation of activities that can be considered as in a developmental sequence for work-related programming (Table 2-2).

Traditionally, the occupational therapist has been faced with clients who are either unsuccessful at work or unable to work for a variety of reasons or who have never had the opportunity to acquire work-related skills. Such clients may include an upper-extremity amputee from a recent industrial accident; a stockboy with an acquired chronic back injury who now perceives himself as unable ever to return to work; a computer analyst who, after severe head trauma, has limited cognitive and physical functioning; a secretary who has become severely depressed and is unable to hold her office job; and an institutionalized mentally retarded adolescent who has never been exposed to appropriate work behaviors and skills.

*Table 2-2. Activities for Work-Related Programming by Developmental Stage*

| *Age (years)* | *Activity* |
|---|---|
| 3–7 | Elevating parents' expectation of child's vocational potential |
| | Sorting (large cue difference) |
| | Stacking |
| | Attending behavior |
| | Simple direction following |
| 7–12 | Working alone |
| | Working in small groups |
| | Higher rates of attending |
| | Sorting (small cue differences) |
| | Small assembly (hand and simple tool) |
| | Switching task upon command |
| | Starting to work on time |
| | Remaining at activity site until given permission to move |
| 12–18 | High rates of production on assigned tasks |
| | High rates of attention on high- and low-interest tasks |
| | Low error rates |
| | High rate of switch-task compliance |
| | Starting to work on time |
| | Returning from breaks promptly |
| | Remaining at work station |
| | Signaling supervisor when encountering difficulties |
| | Working alone |
| | Working in groups |
| | Working quietly |
| | Recognizing work defects |
| | Correcting work defects |
| | Using common tools |
| | Hand tools |
| | Power tools |
| | Work site safety behavior |
| | Head protection |
| | Uniform use |
| | Eye protection |
| | Recognition of and response to work site warning signs |

Source: From K. F. Lynch, W. E. Kiernan, and J. A. Stark (Eds.), *Prevocational and Vocational Education for Special Needs Youth: A Blueprint for the 1980s.* Baltimore: Paul H. Brookes, 1982.

Functionally, these persons' disabilities can be viewed in two major categories: (1) a lack of work skills, habits, and behaviors; and (2) neurophysiologic impairments. The importance of the former category is emphasized by the fact that most unemployed workers have lost their jobs because of problems with interpersonal relationships, that is, trouble getting along with co-workers and supervisors, rather than because of inadequate skills.

As therapists we can provide "the client with a series of learning experiences that will enable [him or her] to make appropriate vocational decisions and develop work habits necessary for eventual employment" [1].

In program development I have found that many commonalities exist across the various client populations and clinical settings. When developing a work-related program for any population in any setting, the therapist must first obtain information on the client for appropriate treatment planning. This can be done by performing a work-related evaluation. Historically, occupational therapists have often been involved in some type of assessment to measure work-related behaviors and skills. According to the 1980 official position paper by the American Occupational Therapy Association on the role of occupational therapy in vocational rehabilitation [1], the goal of work-related evaluation is

> . . . to assess and predict work behavior and vocational potential through the application of practical, reality-based assessment techniques. The objectives include: testing and evaluating work abilities related to a specific job task; assessing the client's learning abilities and retention of skills; evaluating physical, psychological, and social factors such as work tolerance, habits, and interpersonal qualities. Testing objectives are met through the use of carefully selected media that simulate or closely resemble actual job-related requirements.

In reviewing the "state of the art" of assessments, one finds them in a variety of standardized and nonstandardized forms: interest inventories, such as the California Preference Inventory, the Kuder, and the Strong-Campbell; work samples, such as the TOWER battery and the Singer system; checklists; and situational assessments. The majority of these assessments are expensive, time-consuming, and cumbersome; they require additional training to administer and are not easily adaptable to various populations. For example, Harris [2] notes that formal, standardized tests measure aptitudes and skill levels and define expectations; however, because of their complexity these tasks are not easily adapted to the brain-injured patient. Harris finds that informal testing is more valuable in the treatment of these patients. Such informal tests consist of tasks that include instructions, a time limit, multiple steps, and defined outcome criteria. The therapist must observe the patient's approach to the task, his or her task focus, the manner in which the patient formulates a plan, and its execution. These tasks must make demands on the appropriate systems of attention, memory, and planning [2].

I found that the available standardized and nonstandardized evaluations were also inappropriate for use with a learning-disabled adolescent population. For this reason I had to devise an appropriate instrument to ascertain these students' level of functioning with respect to work-related skills and behaviors before program development. I set specific criteria for the tasks that would make up this assessment: (1) limited task duration, (2) adaptability of each task to the specific student's needs, (3) a range of complexity within individual tasks and among tasks, (4) a strong relationship to components of work, (5) a high interest level for preadolescents and adolescents, (6) a reward built into some tasks, (7) compactness of task elements, (8) limited cost of test elements (most would be available in an occupational therapy department), (9) ease of administration (minimal special training required), and (10) a simple method of recording results.

The resulting evaluation I called the Jacobs Prevocational Skills Assessment (JPSA). In clinical use since 1979, it has been found to be a useful instrument for formulating a work-related program based on a student's specific needs. The JPSA is presented in its entirety in Chapter 3.

From the information gathered in the assessment, the therapist can begin to plan an appropriate work-related program. In this development stage many factors must be taken into account: (1) What are the patient's interests? (2) What are his or her aspirations and interests regarding future employment? (3) Are the patient's job goals realistic? (4) What is the extent of the patient's job experience? (5) What type of work is available to the patient, particularly in his or her local community? Does the patient have the necessary skills to do this kind of work? (6) What type of budget do you have in developing and operating the program? (7) Do you have access to equipment and supplies? (8) How much physical space will you have for the program? (9) Do you have the support of the administration and staff of your facility?

After these questions have been answered, the key word to keep in mind in setting up the program is *resourcefulness.* Look to your own in-house resources for areas of simulated job experiences for your client. Check to see if you have access to a business office, food preparation area, or maintenance or laundry service; then make arrangements to use this area, equipment, or supplies. When appropriate, ascertain whether you can obtain support from the supervisors and workers for eventual work placement of your clients. In addition, contact your local community businesses—for example, copy shops, hardware stores, restaurants—for donations of supplies and equipment.

Programs should cater to the needs of the individual client, yet realistic expectations must be established. Many difficulties arise when a client returns to work or is first placed on a job site and finds that it is very different from the therapy milieu. Any problems should be brought back to the clinic, where the client can receive support and work on problem areas. A good example of this process comes from the Learning Prep School, a vocational work-study program for learning-disabled students. As their job placement coordinator, I placed eight students in the work-study program in the student cafeteria at a local college. After a week on the serving line, the manager told me that, although the students were doing fine, they needed to increase their speed and accuracy. This area of difficulty was brought back to the treatment setting and addressed in simulated job experiences. In addition, the staff therapist devised a plan whereby these issues would be reinforced in both the students' vocational and academic classes.

Throughout this book you will read about work-related programs and assessments. I hope that this sampling will be a catalyst to you in your endeavor to develop programs and assessments suitable to your population.

## References

1. Ad Hoc Committee of the Commission on Practice. The role of occupational therapy in the vocational rehabilitation process: Official Position Paper. *Am. J. Occup. Ther.* 34:881, 1980.

2. Harris, P. The role of occupational therapy in cognitive remediation and prevocational rehabilitation. Presented at New England Rehabilitation Hospital, Woburn, Massachusetts, November, 1983.
3. Kielhofner, G. "Occupation," Chapter 3 in H. L. Hopkins, and H. D. Smith, *Willard and Spackman's Occupational Therapy* (6th ed.). Philadelphia: Lippincott, 1983. P. 31.
4. Lynch, K. F., Kiernan, W. E., and Stark, J. A. (Eds.). *Prevocational and Vocational Education for Special Needs Youth: A Blueprint for the 1980s.* Baltimore: Paul H. Brookes, 1982.
5. Maurer, P. A. Prevocational activities and evaluation for the child and adolescent. *Phys. Ther.* 48:771, 1968.
6. Maurer, P. A. Antecedents of work behavior. *Am. J. Occup. Ther.* 25:295, 1971.
7. Ogden, L. Referral criteria for occupational therapy services (unpublished). In Occupational Therapy Association of California (OTAC) Practice Guidelines (draft), 1983.
8. Reed, K., and Sanderson, S. R. *Concepts of Occupational Therapy* (2nd ed.). Baltimore: Williams & Wilkins, 1983.

# 3. The Jacobs Prevocational Skills Assessment

This chapter presents an in-depth look at the Jacobs Prevocational Skills Assessment (JPSA), which was developed for a learning-disabled adolescent population at the Learning Prep School. The JPSA is composed of 15 tasks designed to assess performance in specific work-related skill areas. The rationale behind the JPSA will be explored in contrast to previously available evaluations. In addition, the assessment in its entirety, including graphics, will be presented. It is my intention to share this instrument with therapists who will find it useful in their clinical practice.

## Standard and Standardized Evaluations

Before proceeding any further, a clear differentiation must be made between standardized and standard evaluations. *Standardization* implies uniformity of procedure in administering and scoring the test and has the advantage of affording comparison of test results with normative or average performance. In addition, validity and reliability have been established [1]. With *standard evaluations* a uniform procedure in administering and scoring the test may be established, but normative data, validity, and reliability have not been determined; therefore results are not comparable.

Examination of the literature on work-related assessments revealed many standard and standardized instruments that have been developed for the normal population or those with a specific disability. At present there are no assessments universally applicable to all populations. This is not surprising, since one would not expect a test developed for a blind, mentally retarded client to be a valid instrument for a cognitively normal right-upper-extremity amputee. For this reason, many occupational therapy departments have developed standard assessments to be used with their specific populations. Examples of these will be presented throughout the text. You will find that the formats differ; however, the skills and behaviors assessed—cooperation, task focus, personal appearance, punctuality—remain fairly constant from assessment to assessment. Therefore, irrespective of disability there are specific behaviors and skills that should be assessed in any work-related evaluation.

In some instances, standard instruments are used as adjuncts to standardized assessments. As noted by Trombly and Scott [8], "Non-standardized tests are also used to observe work habits, physical capacities, and other areas of concern which may not be observed during standardized testing. When craft and shop activities are carefully analyzed, they allow for observation of many of the basic skills common to all work."

*Table 3-1. Work-Related Assessments and Their Sources*

| *Item* | *Source* |
| --- | --- |
| Minnesota Rate of Manipulation Test | Western Psychological Services<br>12035 Wilshire Boulevard<br>Los Angeles, California 90025 |
| Crawford Small Parts Dexterity Text | Psychological Corporation<br>304 E. Forty-fifth Street<br>New York, New York 10017 |
| Farnsworth Dichotomous Test for Color Blindness | Psychological Corporation |
| Bennett Hand-Tool Dexterity Test | Psychological Corporation |
| Pennsylvania Bimanual Work Sample | American Guidance Service, Inc.<br>720 Washington Avenue S.E.<br>Minneapolis, Minnesota 55414 |
| Purdue Pegboard | Science Research Associates<br>259 E. Erie<br>Chicago, Illinois 60611 |
| Moore Eye-Hand Coordination and Color-matching Test | Joseph E. Moore and Associates, Psychologists<br>4406 Jett Road N.W.<br>Atlanta, Georgia 30327 |
| Bennett Mechanical Comprehension Test | Psychological Corporation |
| Graves Design Judgment Test | Psychological Corporation |
| Minnesota Clerical Test | Psychological Corporation |
| Purdue Clerical Adaptability Test | Occupational Research Center<br>Purdue University<br>Lafayette, Indiana 47907 |
| McCarron-Dial Work Evaluation System | Commercial Marketing Enterprises<br>Department MDWES<br>11300 North Central, Suite 105<br>Dallas, Texas 75231 |
| Philadelphia Jewish Employment and Vocational Systems (JEVS) | Vocational Research Institute<br>Jewish Employment and Vocational Services<br>1700 Sansom Street,<br>Ninth Floor<br>Philadelphia, Pennsylvania 19103 |

| Item | Source |
| --- | --- |
| Singer Vocational Evaluation System | Singer Educational Division<br>Career Systems<br>80 Commerce Drive<br>Rochester, New York 14623 |
| Hester Evaluation System | Evaluations Systems, Inc.<br>640 North La Salle Street<br>Suite 698<br>Chicago, Illinois 60610 |
| TOWER (Testing, Orientation, and Work Evaluation in Rehabilitation) | I.C.D. Rehabilitation and Research Center<br>340 East Twenty-fourth Street<br>New York, New York 10010 |
| Valpar Component Work Sample Series | Valpar Corporation<br>3801 East Thirty-fourth Street<br>Tucson, Arizona 85716 |
| Talent Assessment Programs | Talent Assessment Program<br>7015 Colby Avenue<br>Des Moines, Iowa 50311 |
| Wide Range Employement Sample Test (WREST) | Guidance Associates of Delaware, Inc.<br>1526 Gilpin Avenue<br>Wilmington, Delaware 19806 |
| Vocational Information and Evaluation Work Sample (VIEWS) | Vocational Research Institute<br>Jewish Employment and Vocational Services<br>1700 Sansom Street<br>Ninth Floor<br>Philadelphia, Pennsylvania 19103 |
| Comprehensive Occupational Assessment and Training System (COATS) | Prep, Inc.<br>1575 Parkway Avenue<br>Trenton, New Jersey 08628 |
| General Aptitude Test Battery (GATB) | Supt. of Documents<br>U.S. Printing Department<br>Washington, D.C. 20402 |

Many standardized evaluations are available (Table 3-1). These evaluations range in complexity from short but sketchy to diagnostic but cumbersome; most of them lack optimal clinical utility because of these limitations. Most require special training to administer and typically are performed by the vocational counselor or work evaluator; they are also expensive and cumbersome to transport. Hopkins and Smith [4] note, "Most work sample systems are technically inadequate in that validity, reliability and norms are poorly established, if at all."

A closer review of three major evaluations reveals these important limitations:

The *Philadelphia Jewish Employment and Vocational System* is an assessment device for the special needs population. The system contains 28 work samples organized into 10 worker trait groups for reporting and interpretation purposes. According to Hopkins and Smith [4], "A major problem [with the JEVS] is the abstract nature of many of the work samples, which affects the client's ability to relate them to real jobs." The cost of the JEVS is $9,000.

The *Singer Vocational Evaluation System* consists of 25 independent, self-contained work samples that could be used with a wide range of rehabilitation, educational, and manpower populations. According to Hopkins and Smith [4], "The built-in career exploration and occupational information are strong points of this program, but this is often gained at the expense of increased knowledge of the client's potential. Many of the procedures are not clarified in the manual." The cost of this system is $1,000 per sample.

The *TOWER Work Sample Battery* [5] was originally developed by the Institute for the Crippled and Disabled (ICD) for use with physically disabled persons. This system contains 93 work samples arranged into 14 job training areas. Kester [6] notes that this system "applies only to a narrow group of jobs unless the counselor utilizes the DOT [Dictionary of Occupational Titles, 4th ed.; available from the U.S. Dept. of Labor] to broaden the scope. Precise definitions of performance and behavior . . . are the major weaknesses of the system." ICD estimates the cost of the TOWER Work Sample Battery at $5,000.

**Development of the JPSA**

Despite the number of commercially available systems, none fitted my needs. There appeared to be no one evaluation universally applicable to the learning-disabled population because of their diverse visual, perceptual, motor, and language abilities and social, developmental, and academic profiles. For example, one learning-disabled student may be able to follow written directions, while another cannot read beyond a first-grade level but understands verbal instructions with visual demonstrations. Lynch et al. [7] support this realization: "Despite the focus on assessment, vocational assessment for learning disabled students is an area in which little work has been done." For these reasons the JPSA was developed.

It has been six years since the JPSA was developed. During this time it has seen many constructive changes as the result of clinical use. Many of the changes evolved from an effort to key words and tasks more toward "real" work. The revised instrument is presented in this book, along with some background on the instrument's evolution.

The JPSA is a *standard* instrument, with all the aforementioned limitations of this type of test. However, it has proved to be a useful screening tool for obtaining pertinent information for occupational therapy treatment planning and referrals. For example, from assessment results I have been able to suggest academic and vocational programming appropriate to the student's ability. The JPSA was not designed to be applicable to a wide variety of work-related programs with respect to age and disability; however, the general concept may serve as a model for designing a similar instrument, or the JPSA may be adapted to meet the particular needs of a therapist's patients.

## SELECTION OF SKILL AREAS

The basis for the development of any evaluation instrument is observation. A large part of occupational therapy training is directed toward honing this skill as an objective tool. Applying this skill to the preadolescent and adolescent learning-disabled population at the Learning Prep School revealed deficiencies in need of remediation in the following work-related skill areas:

I. Motor coordination
   A. Fine
   B. Gross
II. Eye-hand coordination
III. Conceptual skills
   A. Alphabet recognition and ordering
   B. Number
   C. Number quantity
   D. Money and money concepts
   E. Recognition of the student's own name
   F. Color
IV. Motor planning
V. Figure-ground discrimination
VI. Sorting ability
VII. Matching ability
VIII. Classification ability
IX. Sequencing ability
X. Problem solving
XI. Decision making
XII. Following directions with one, two, three, or more steps
   A. Oral directions
   B. Written directions
   C. Visual directions

XIII. Memory
- A. Auditory
- B. Visual

XIV. Task focus

XV. Work-related behavior

These original categories became the foundation for assessing work-related skills and behaviors. However, in the course of clinical implementation several basic categories were revised or deleted, and others were inserted. These changes facilitated a clearer distinction among areas needing remediation as reasonably independent variables. Certain distinctions were found too impractical for the therapist to make readily. For example, gross motor coordination was dropped as a separate category because its contribution to the overall validity of the assessment did not justify the sacrifice of brevity, another major criterion of the test. Furthermore, areas that represented developmentally sequential skills that would require many independent tasks to test were merged. For instance, the two categories of classification and sequencing became a single category. Additional variables including organizational skills and use of tools were added on the basis of clinical experience. Currently, the following categories are thought to represent the most useful information (definitions have been included for clarity):

1. Fine motor coordination: the ability to perform small movements (grasping, writing) in the most efficient manner
2. Eye-hand coordination: the ability to use eyes and hands together to perform a task
3. Motor planning: the ability to plan new or nonhabitual movements
4. Figure-ground discrimination: the ability to focus on the important aspects of one's visual field and "tune out" the unimportant background
5. Sorting: the ability to select by similar traits
6. Classification and sequencing: the ability to arrange items by class (e.g., all tools) and in an orderly succession
7. Decision making: the ability to consider evidence and reach some conclusion without undue delay
8. Problem solving: the ability to devise an appropriate solution for a new problem (It is my opinion that problem solving is a difficult skill to assess. Placing an individual in a situation that calls for this skill and observing how he or she responds is one method. Throughout the JPSA, such situations have been devised.)
9. Organizational skills: the ability to organize one's approach to and performance of an activity (e.g., the ability to use time and work space appropriately)
10. Use of tools: the ability to use common tools and equipment (e.g., a hammer and nails) appropriately
11. Ability to follow verbal, written, or visual directions
12. Conceptual skills including alphabet recognition and alphabetical ordering, number and number quantity, money and money quantity, reading, functional mathematics, telling time
13. Task focus: the ability to attend to an activity for a period of time
14. Work-related behavior and attitudes such as communication skills, perseverance, motivation, reliability, initiative, good posture, neat personal appearance, memory, positive attitude toward the therapist and other students

## TASK SELECTION

The tasks chosen to assess the student's performance in these skill areas underwent a similar evolution. The following technical factors and theoretical considerations related to the school's population were the initial criteria for inclusion in the assessment:

*Technical Factors*

1. Compactness of task elements
2. Low cost of elements (optimally, those available in an occupational therapy department)
3. Ease of administration (minimal special training required)
4. Brevity

*Theoretical Considerations*

1. Range of complexity level within and among individual tasks
2. Adaptability to physical and cognitive limitations
3. High relation to work
4. High interest level for preadolescents and adolescents
5. Built-in rewards
6. Limited task duration (because of attentional difficulties)
7. Provision for comprehension of written, visual, and verbal instructions

The original tasks were nail inspection, alphabetical ordering, filing by color, hammer and screwdriver activity, envelope stuffing, nut and bolt assembly, sorting and naming money, an activity involving matching and/or body awareness, four increasingly complex mazes, a kitchen activity involving sequencing, classification of food items, leather key ring assembly, and a cooking activity. In general these tasks proved to be reasonably useful. Several improvements have been made, however. These changes resulted from brainstorming with therapists and from using the assessment with a widening range of ages and disabilities.

A calculator was added to increase task complexity and because of the increasing use of calculators in the work environment. The tasks' names and vocabulary were modified to parallel those of the work setting. For example, *nail inspection* became *quality control*, *alphabetical ordering* became *filing*, *cooking activity* became *food preparation*, *cat* became *chef.*

The current tasks are (1) Quality Control, (2) Filing, (3) Carpentry Assembly, (4) Classification, (5) Office Work, (6) Telephone Directory, (7) Factory Work, (8) Environmental Mobility, (9) Money Concepts, (10) Functional Banking, (11) Time Concepts, (12) Work Attitudes, (13) Body Scheme, (14) Leather Assembly, and (15) Food Preparation.

## RECORDING DATA

My criteria for the recording medium were that it be easy to use, that is, entry of data would require minimal disruption of the test procedure, and that the raw data be easily accessible for further analysis. The matrix tabular form (see profile sheet, Fig. 3-1) has proved ideal and has been retained through all the test content changes because of its conciseness.

Date(s)_____ ____________

| Tasks: | Fine Motor Coordination | Eye-Hand Coordination | Motor Planning | Figure-Ground | Sorting | Classification | Sequencing | Decision Making | Problem Solving | Orga |
|---|---|---|---|---|---|---|---|---|---|---|
| Quality Control: 1 | | | | | | | | | | |
| Filing: 2 A. | | | | | | | | | | |
| B. | | | | | | | | | | |
| C. | | | | | | | | | | |
| Carpentry Assembly: 3 | | | | | | | | | | |
| Classification: 4 | | | | | | | | | | |
| Office Work: 5 A. | | | | | | | | | | |
| B. | | | | | | | | | | |
| C. | | | | | | | | | | |
| Telephone Directory: 6 A. | | | | | | | | | | |
| B. | | | | | | | | | | |
| Factory Work: 7 | | | | | | | | | | |
| Environmental Mobility: 8 A. | | | | | | | | | | |
| B. | | | | | | | | | | |
| Money Concepts: 9 A. | | | | | | | | | | |
| B. | | | | | | | | | | |
| C. | | | | | | | | | | |
| D. | | | | | | | | | | |
| Functional Banking: 10 A. | | | | | | | | | | |
| B. | | | | | | | | | | |
| Time Concept: 11 A. | | | | | | | | | | |
| B. | | | | | | | | | | |
| C. | | | | | | | | | | |
| Work Attitudes: 12 A. | | | | | | | | | | |
| B. | | | | | | | | | | |
| Body Scheme: 13 | | | | | | | | | | |
| Leather Assembly: 14 | | | | | | | | | | |
| Food Preparation: 15 | | | | | | | | | | |

*Fig. 3-1. A blank JPSA form for the reader's use.*

Name: ____________________

| Use of Tools | | Ability to Follow Directions | | Memory | | Conceptual Skills | Task Focus | Behavioral Observations | Time |
|---|---|---|---|---|---|---|---|---|---|
| | Visual | Written | Verbal | Auditory | Visual | | | | |
| | | | | | | | | | |
| | | | | | | | | | |
| | | | | | | | | | |
| | | | | | | | | | |
| | | | | | | | | | |
| | | | | | | | | | |
| | | | | | | | | | |
| | | | | | | | | | |
| | | | | | | | | | |
| | | | | | | | | | |
| | | | | | | | | | |
| | | | | | | | | | |
| | | | | | | | | | |
| | | | | | | | | | |
| | | | | | | | | | |
| | | | | | | | | | |
| | | | | | | | | | |
| | | | | | | | | | |
| | | | | | | | | | |
| | | | | | | | | | |
| | | | | | | | | | |
| | | | | | | | | | |
| | | | | | | | | | |
| | | | | | | | | | |
| | | | | | | | | | |
| | | | | | | | | | |
| | | | | | | | | | |
| | | | | | | | | | |

**Test Elements**

On the following pages the JPSA is described. First the profile sheet (scoring form) is discussed, and an illustration (suitable for photocopying) is presented (Fig. 3-1). The manual is then discussed. Its contents are presented in the Appendix at the end of this chapter. Descriptions of the 15 tasks are then given, along with examples of possible modifications. Next the materials necessary for the assessment are listed. Finally, a suggested format for summarizing the results of the assessment is given in the form of two case studies.

PROFILE SHEET

A single-page (8½″ × 11″) checklist-style profile sheet was constructed with the skills in columns across the top of the page and the individual tasks in rows along the side. If a specific skill is required in a task, the box where the skill and task intersect is checked. The placement of these checks was determined by numerous activity analyses of the tasks and was reviewed by the school's occupational therapists (Fig. 3-28).

The therapist uses the profile sheet throughout the testing session to record results. When a specific skill is noted to be limited or absent during a specific task, the check in the corresponding box is circled. For example, if the student awkwardly manipulated tools (e.g., screwdriver, knife, pencil), then the fine motor check would be circled in the appropriate tasks. If a student were easily "stumped" and unable to think of alternative approaches to a problem, the problem solving check would be circled in the corresponding tasks. On completion of the total assessment (after approximately 1–2 hours) a pattern of circled checks will be evident in the columns. Any skill area with two or more circled checks will be an area for remediation in therapy. In the provided Work-related Behavior section, the therapist notes important test behaviors and skills: motivation, perseverance, cooperative behavior, personal appearance, hand dominance. Treatment goals then can be established by integrating the limited or absent skill areas and the observations noted during the testing session. In addition, the therapist notes any modification of task instructions or adaptive equipment utilized.

The *time* required to complete each task is recorded on the profile sheet. A maximum time for task completion is listed (Fig. 3-28), these values determined by testing a population sample of normal adolescents and then doubling their average time for each task. If the student reaches this maximum without completing the task, the therapist terminates the task.

MANUAL

A manual (4″ × 5″) is used by the therapist throughout the testing procedure. The manual contains the general guidelines as well as the purpose, materials, and instructions for each of the 15 tasks. The manual in its entirety is printed as the Appendix to this chapter.

Many of the tasks have been divided into parts of increasing difficulty. If a student is unable to do the first part of a task, the therapist should use his

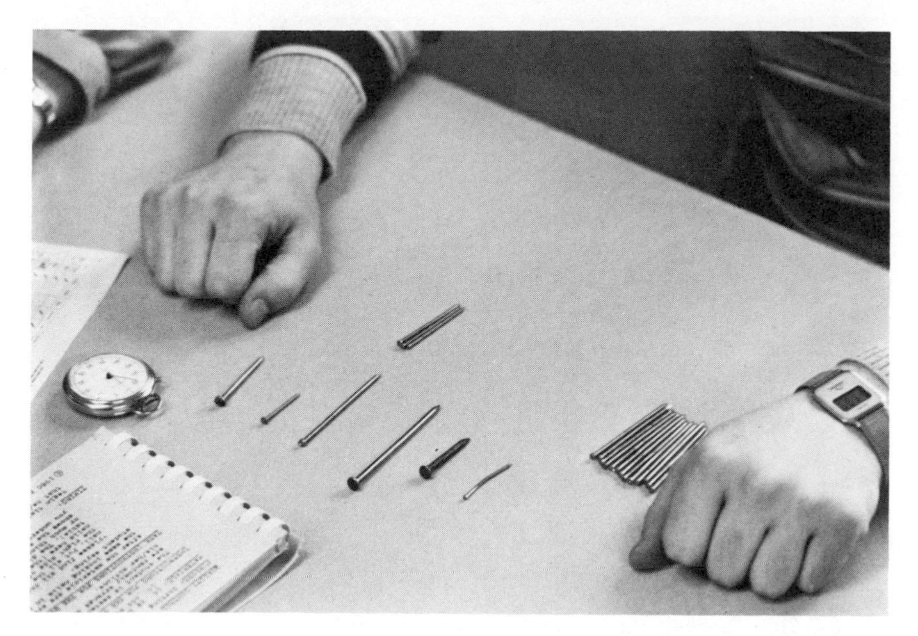

*Fig. 3-2. Task 1, Quality Control. Student inspects nails.*

or her judgment as to whether to proceed with the next part or go on to the next task.

A brief description of each task, examples of task modifications, and graphics are presented below. A list of all materials needed for the assessment follows these descriptions.

TASKS

*1. Quality Control*

Twenty-six nails of various sizes are placed in a random pile on the table. The student is instructed to find all the nails that look the same as the one shown by the therapist (Fig. 3-2).

Modification: For students with poor or absent upper-extremity coordination, the therapist can pick up each nail individually and ask for a verbal or gestural yes or no response as to its sameness to the model nail.

*2. Filing*

In Part A, the therapist places a two-sided instruction card in front of the student to read silently (Fig. 3-3). The instructions have been typed on the card so as to have on the first side an incomplete sentence, which is completed on the second. The instruction card is removed, and the student is given a packet of 26 cards (Fig. 3-4), each bearing one word for each letter of the alphabet. The student is to alphabetize the cards and place them once again in a packet.

Modification: An alphabet can be provided as a guide for this part.

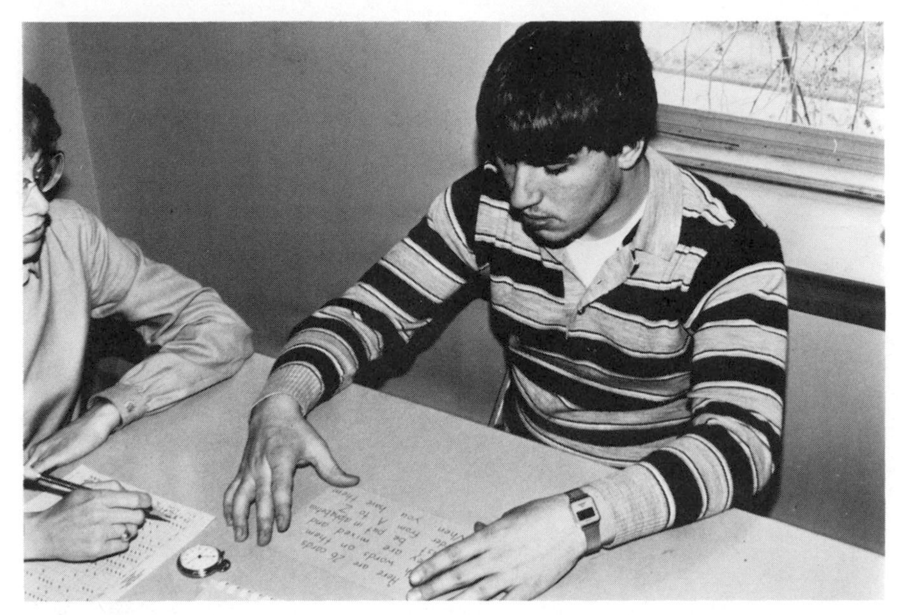

*Fig. 3-3. Task 2, Filing, Part A. Student examines the instruction card before starting to alphabetize 26 cards.*

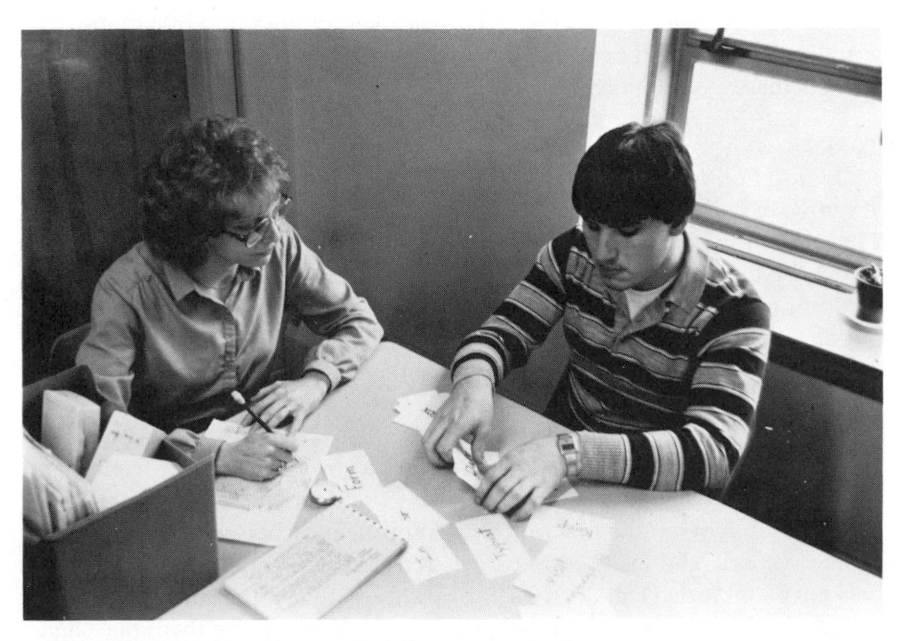


*Fig. 3-4. Task 2, Filing, Part A. Alphabetizing 26 cards.*

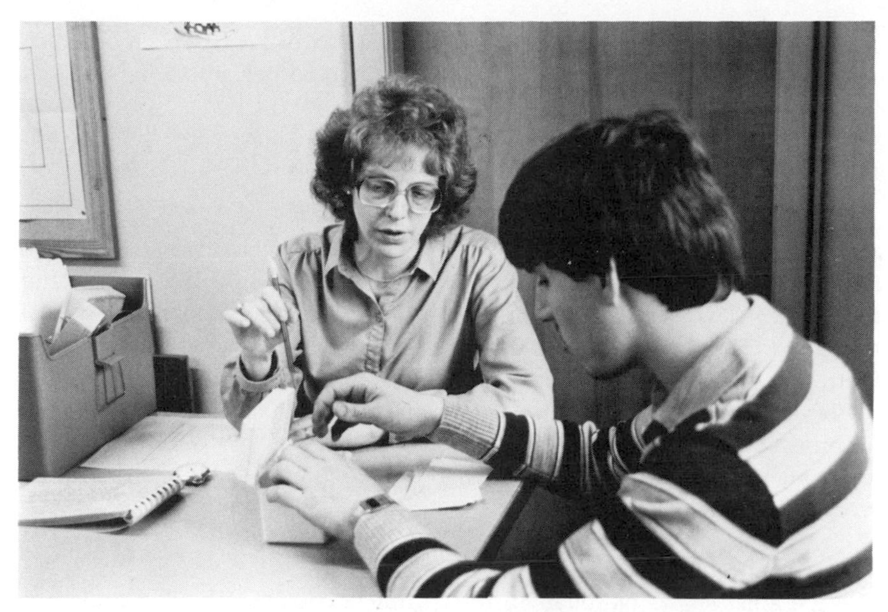

*Fig. 3-5. Task 2, Filing, Part B. Student places 13 alphabetized cards in a file box.*

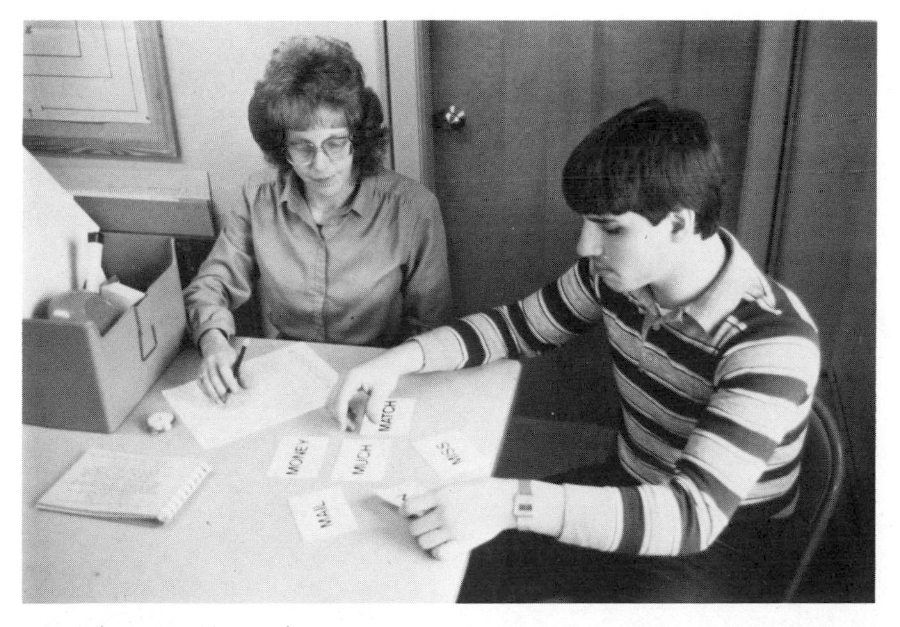


*Fig. 3-6. Task 2, Filing, Part C. Student alphabetizes six words starting with the same letter.*

In Part B, the student is instructed to alphabetize 13 cards, each of which bears a last name and first initial in the left-hand corner, into a file box that contains *A* to *Z* separation cards (Fig. 3-5).

In Part C, the student is instructed to alphabetize six cards with words starting with the same letter (e.g., money, match) (Fig. 3-6).

*3. Carpentry Assembly*

A wooden board with two nails and three screws (one blade-head and two Phillips Screw) three-quarters of the way into the wood is placed in front of the subject. Two screwdrivers and a hammer are placed on either side of the board. The therapist instructs the student to name the tools and to use them to put the nails and screws all the way into the board. The second step of the task involves having the student position a nail independently and hammer it into the wood (Fig. 3-7).

Modifications: Clamp the wooden board to the table. Use an adaptive screwdriver. Build up the handles on the tools.

*4. Classification*

The therapist shows optionally a restaurant kitchen sketch. The student is presented with 17 pictures of items related or not related to a restaurant kitchen and is instructed to find all the items that belong in the restaurant kitchen (Fig. 3-8). The therapist then optionally asks questions about the pictures, for example, "Name the items shown."

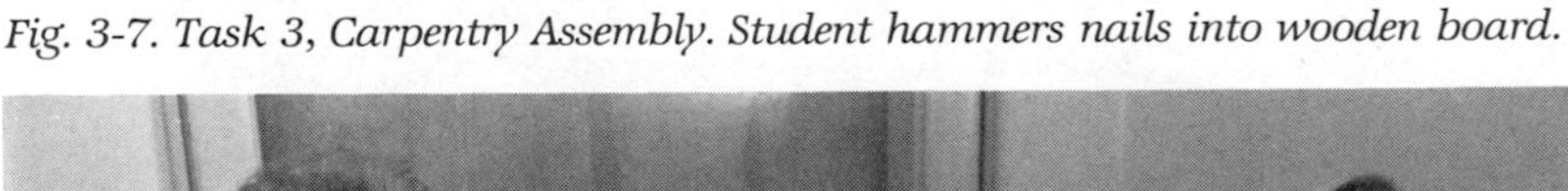

*Fig. 3-7. Task 3, Carpentry Assembly. Student hammers nails into wooden board.*

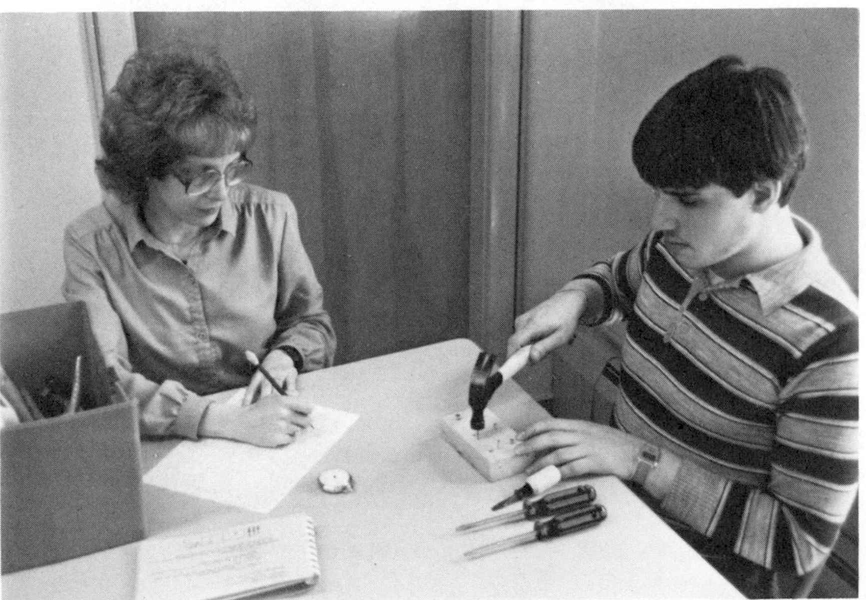

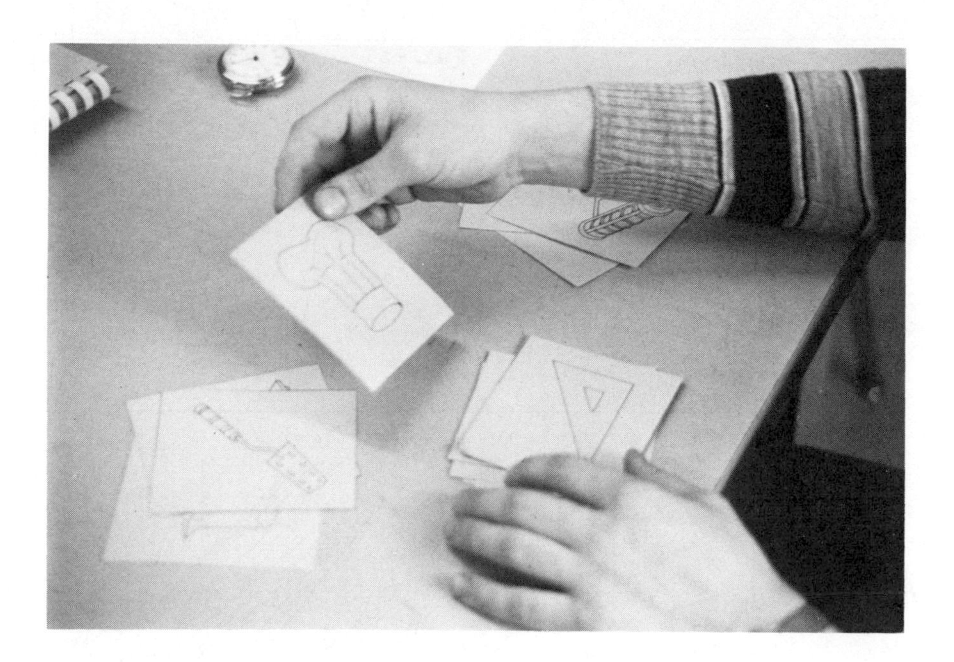

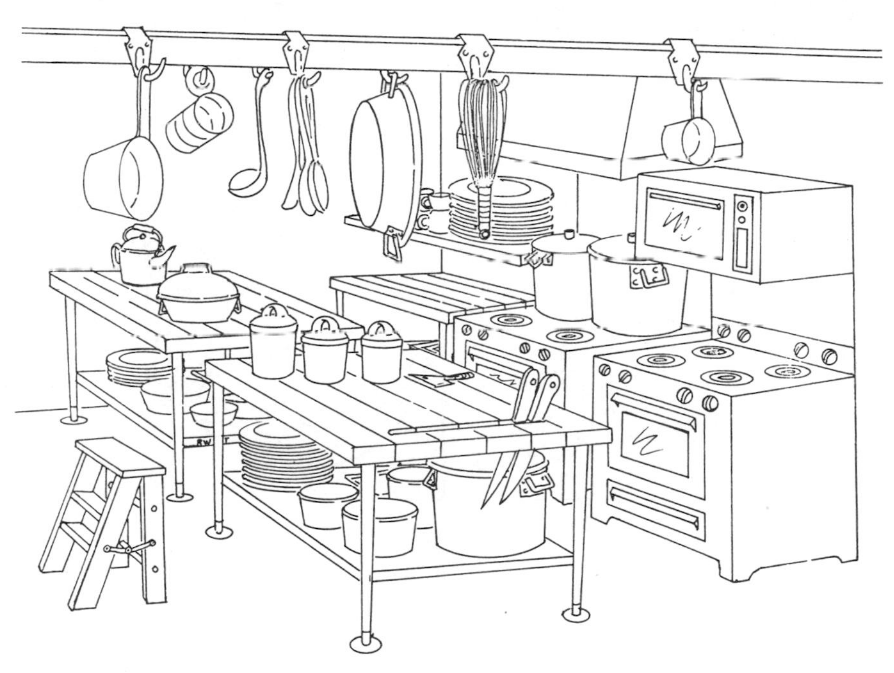

*Fig. 3-8. Task 4, Classification. Student finds all the items that belong in a restaurant kitchen. The first drawing (for optional use) shows a restaurant kitchen; the second and third drawings show 12 items that might be found in a restaurant kitchen; the fourth and fifth drawings show five non-kitchen items.*

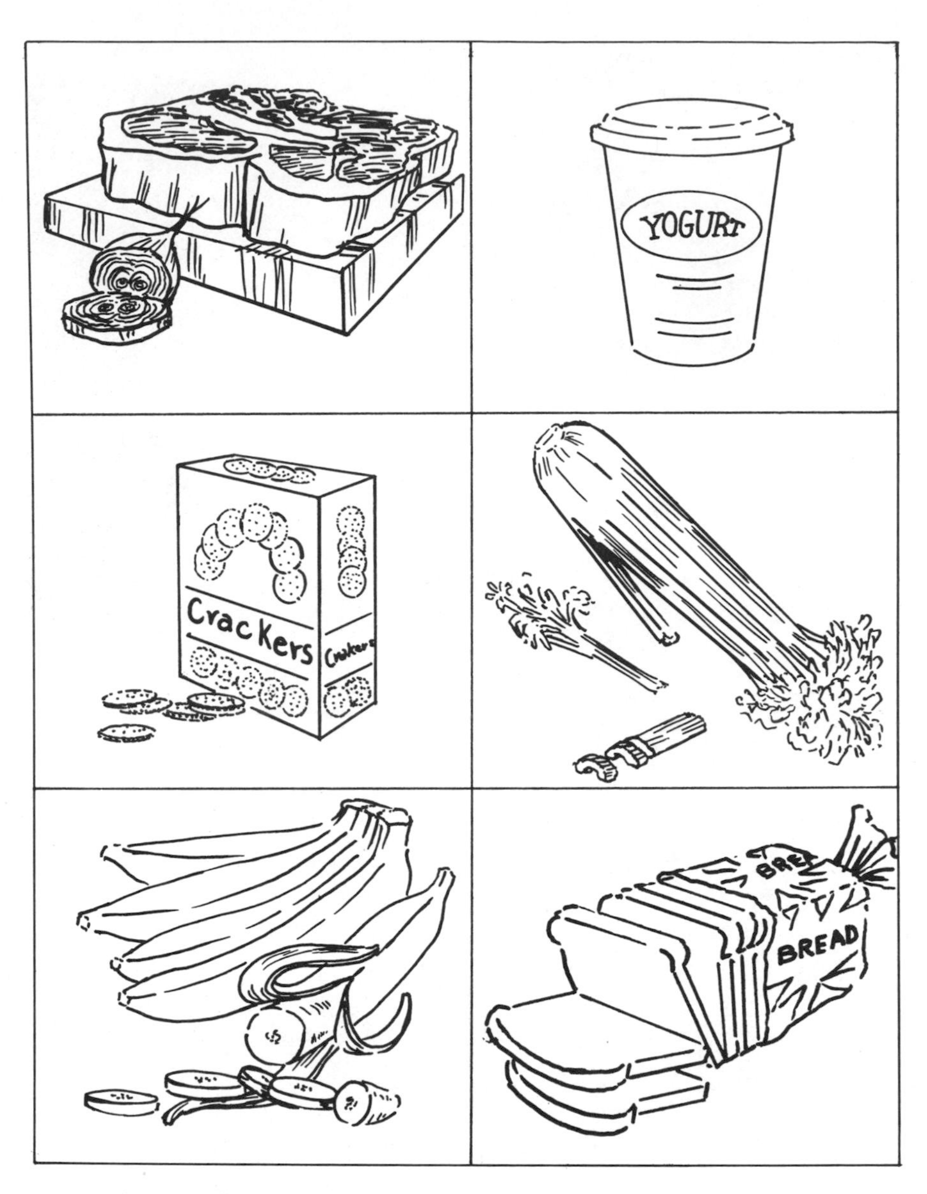


*Fig. 3-8 (continued)*

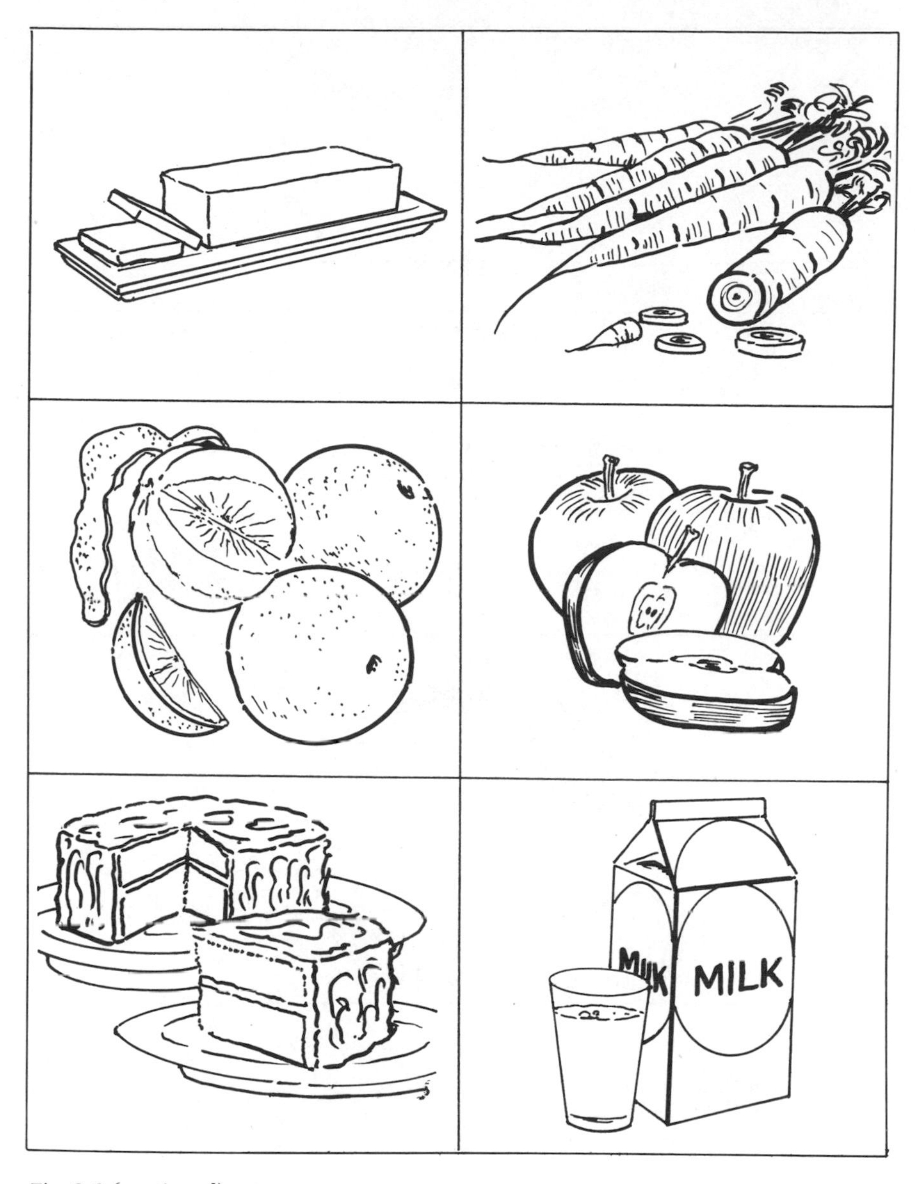


*Fig. 3-8 (continued)*

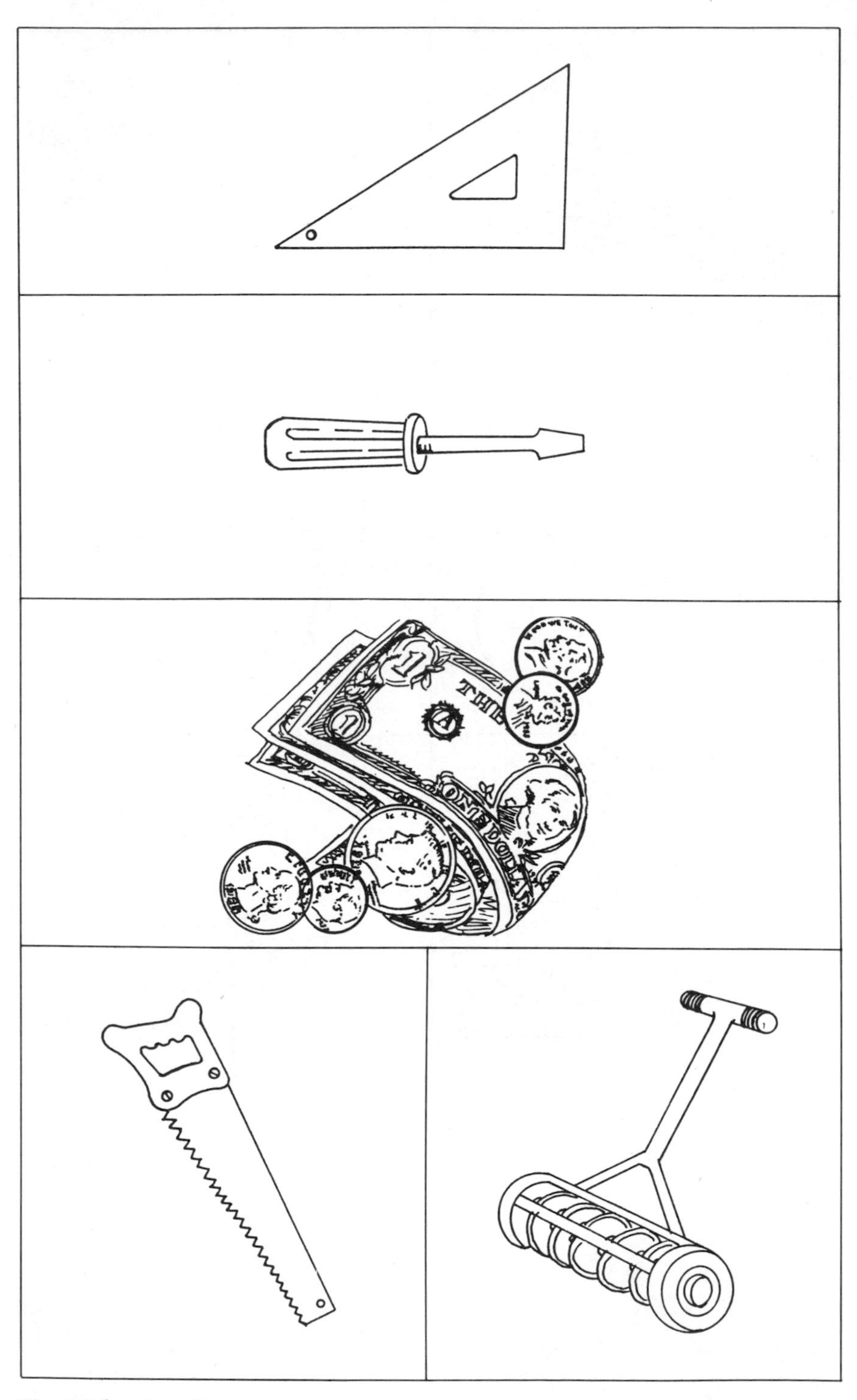

*Fig. 3-8 (continued)*

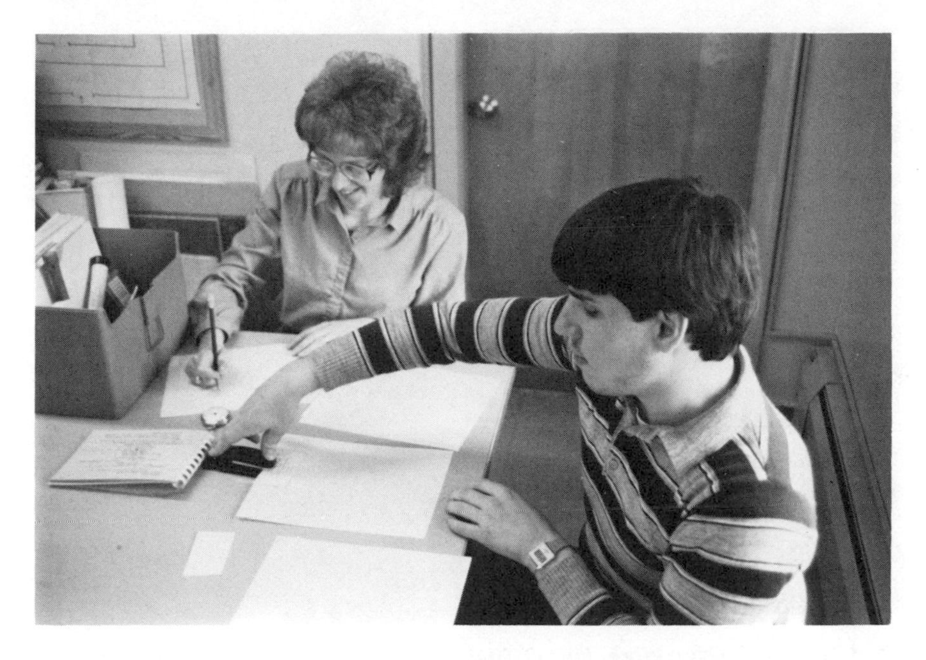

*Fig. 3-9. Task 5, Office Work, Part A. Student staples business cards to sheets of paper.*

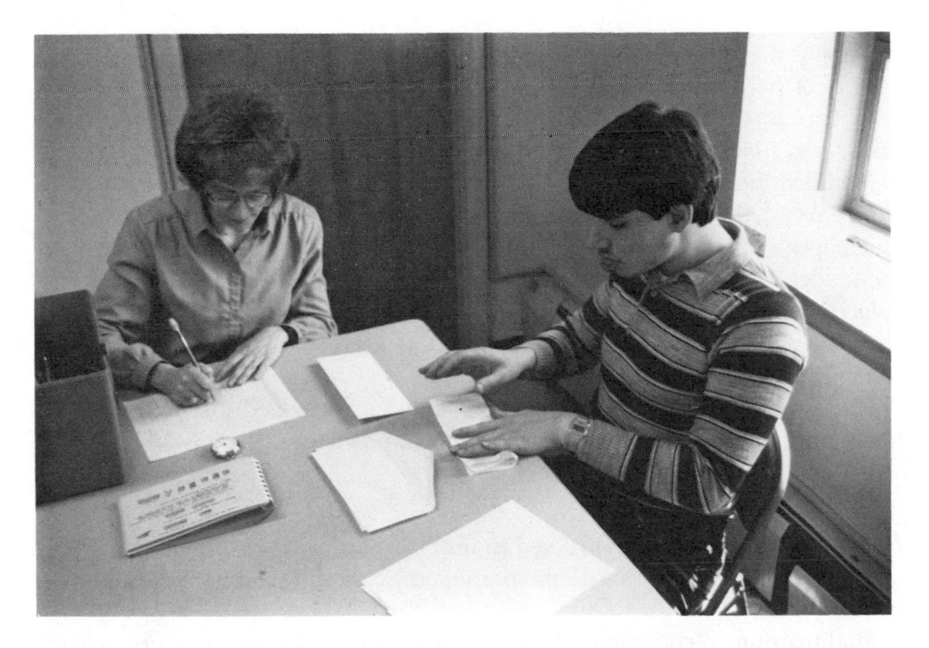

*Fig. 3-10. Task 5, Office Work, Part B. Student folds stapled sheets and places them in envelopes.*

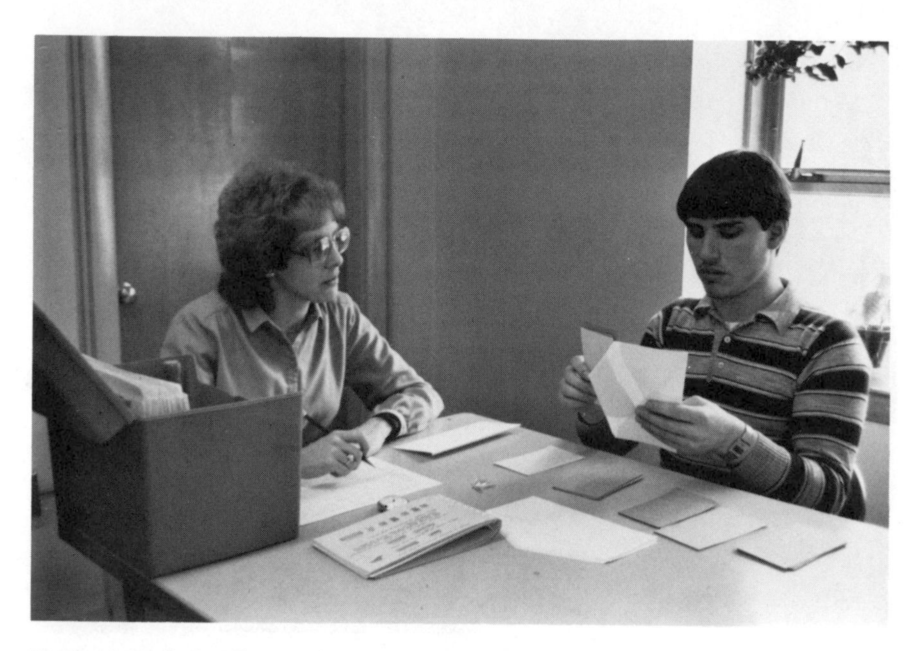

*Fig. 3-11. Task 5, Office Work, Part C. Student follows written directions to collate colored paper and places the resulting piles in envelopes.*

*5. Office Work*

In Part A, the student is to staple business cards in a designated position on a sheet of paper (Fig. 3-9).

In Part B, the student is instructed to fold the sheets from Part A into thirds and place them in individual envelopes (Fig. 3-10).

Modification: Draw lines on the paper to indicate where to fold.

In Part C, the stuffed envelopes remain, and five piles of colored paper and paper clips are arranged on the table. Written directions are given to the student to read silently. The instructions tell the student to collate the colored paper, paper clip the resulting piles, and place them in the envelopes. Extra paper and paper clips have been deliberately added to test problem solving ability (Fig. 3-11).

Modification: Use larger paper clips. Use a color-coded instruction card, for example, with the word *green* written in green ink.

*6. Telephone Directory*

In Part A, the student is instructed to find the name of a company in a small telephone directory and write the name, address, and telephone number on a card (Fig. 3-12).

Modification: Write one address on a separate sheet for the student who is unable to use the directory.

In Part B, the directory is removed and the student is instructed to address a blank envelope from the information on the card from Part A. In addition

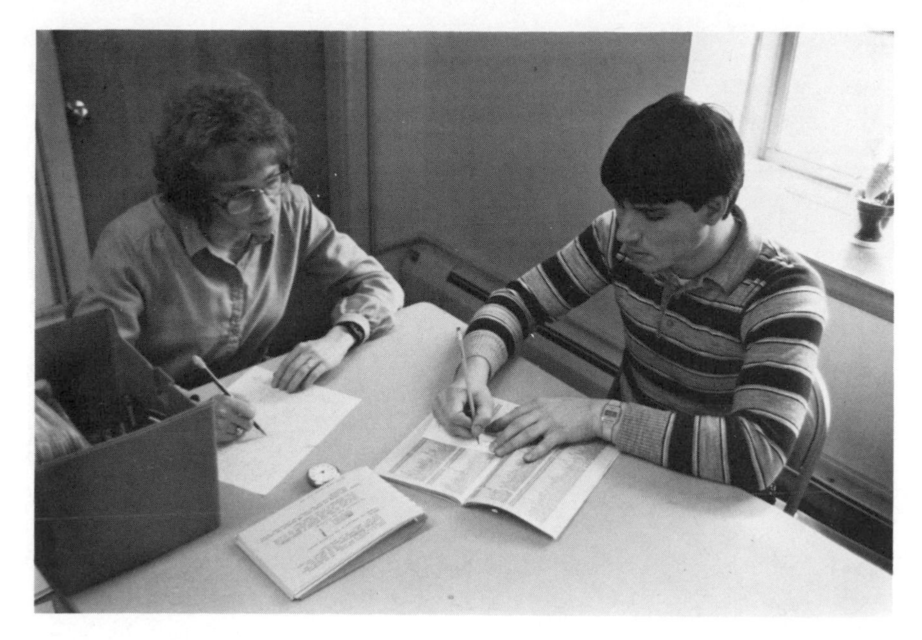

*Fig. 3-12. Task 6, Telephone Directory, Part A. Student uses the directory to locate an address.*

the student is asked to put his or her return address and a stamp on the envelope.

Modification: Present two envelopes addressed incorrectly and have the student indicate what is missing, for example, zip code, return address.

*7. Factory Work*

The student is presented with a wooden board containing six flat-head bolts in various sizes arranged in two rows. Two nuts are screwed onto the shank of each bolt until the end of the shank is flush with the nut. The two smallest bolts have been purposely given three nuts each to observe how the student responds to the task instruction of removing *all* the nuts from the bolts. The student is verbally instructed to remove all the nuts from the bolts and to place them in the cup provided. When this is completed, the student is instructed to put all the nuts back onto the bolts (Fig. 3-13).

Modifications: Clamp the board to the table. Use a modified version of the board containing a single row of the larger bolts, or instruct the student to remove the nuts only from the row of large bolts.

*8. Environmental Mobility*

In Part A, an opened street map of Washington, D.C., covered with a sheet of clear plastic of the same dimensions, is placed on the table. The therapist instructs the student to use a marking pen to mark the streets from the train station to the White House and from the White House to the Jefferson Memorial.

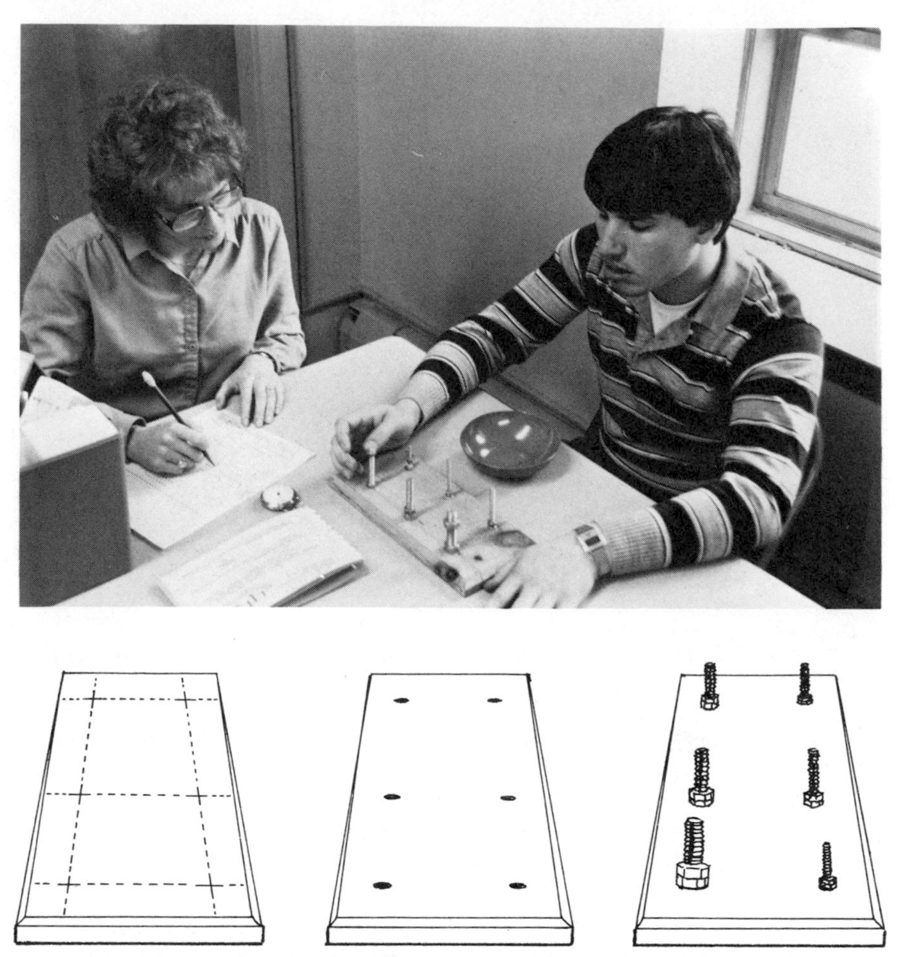

*Fig. 3-13. Task 7, Factory Work. Student removes all nuts from bolts and then replaces them.*

Modification: Simplify the instructions, for example, "Follow the streets from the White House to the Jefferson Memorial."

In Part B, after all the materials from Part A have been removed, the student is presented a card with directions and is instructed to follow them to perform a simple errand, for example, to fetch an envelope from the therapist's mailbox (Fig. 3-14). Devise your own directions and have a colleague follow them before using them in the assessment. This should eliminate any confusion.

*9. Money Concepts*

In Part A, the student is asked to identify four coins and a dollar bill.

Modification: For nonverbal students, the therapist can point to each coin and ask, "Is this a penny?" and so on.

In Part B, the student is presented with four sets of coins of various denominations and is asked to state the value of each set (Fig. 3-15).

Modification: For the nonverbal student, write out answers, including the correct ones, on a card, and ask the student to point to the correct answer.

In Part C, a cash register receipt is placed on the table with a specified assortment of money. The therapist instructs the student to find the total on the receipt and read it aloud and then find the corresponding amount of money on the table (Fig. 3-16).

*Fig. 3-14. Task 8, Environmental Mobility, Part B. Therapist instructs student to follow written directions to perform a simple errand.*

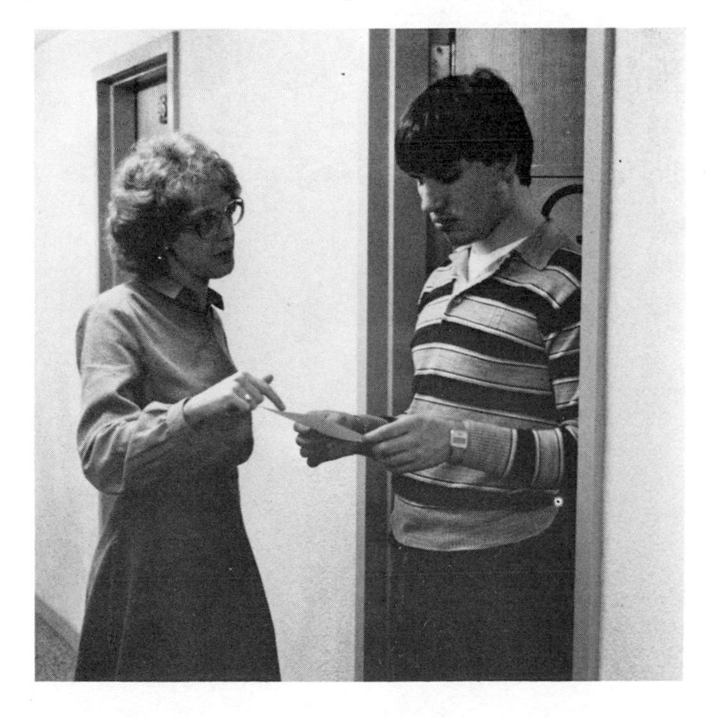

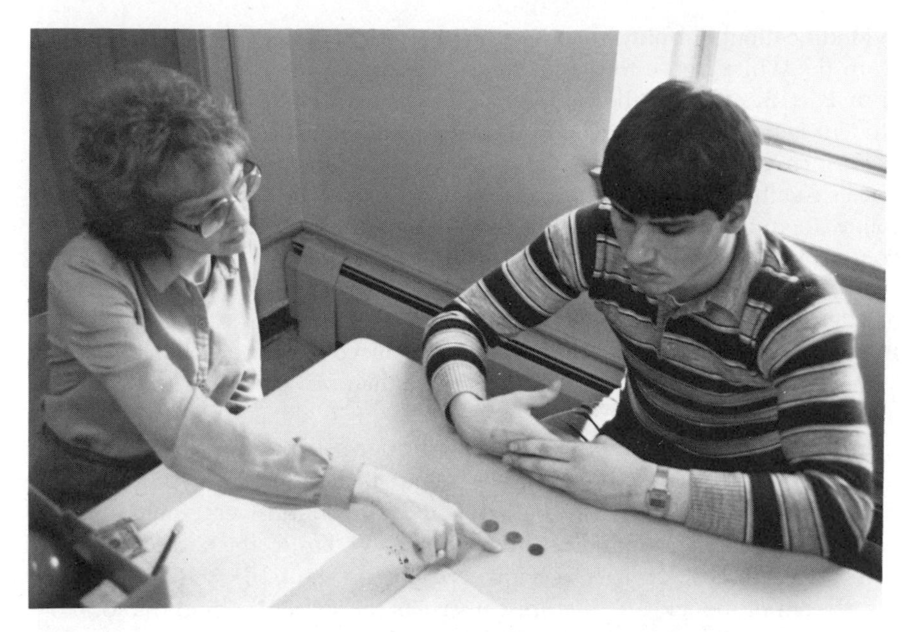

*Fig. 3-15. Task 9, Money Concepts, Part B. Student identifies different coins.*

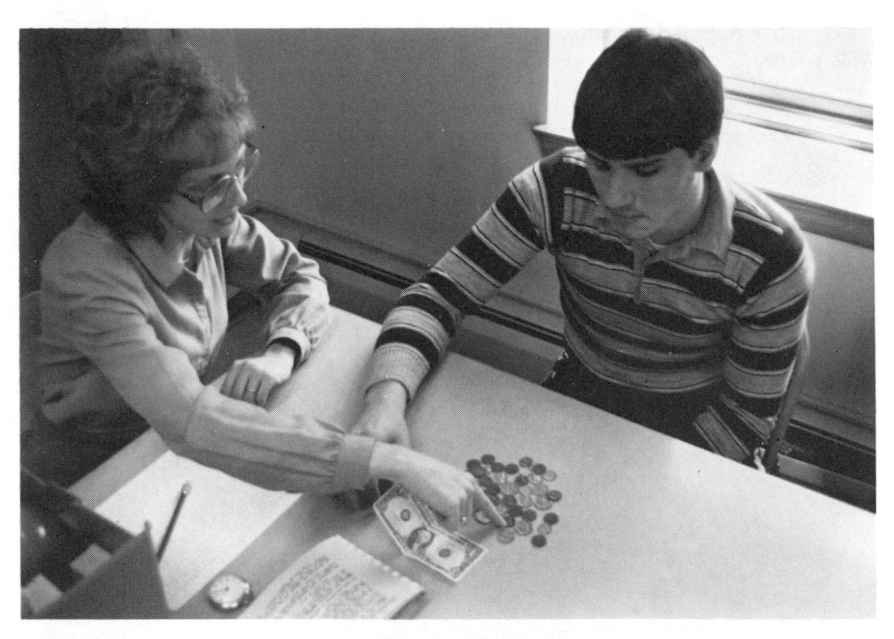

*Fig. 3-16. Task 9, Money Concepts, Part C. Student finds the amount of money on the table that corresponds to that from the cash register receipt.*

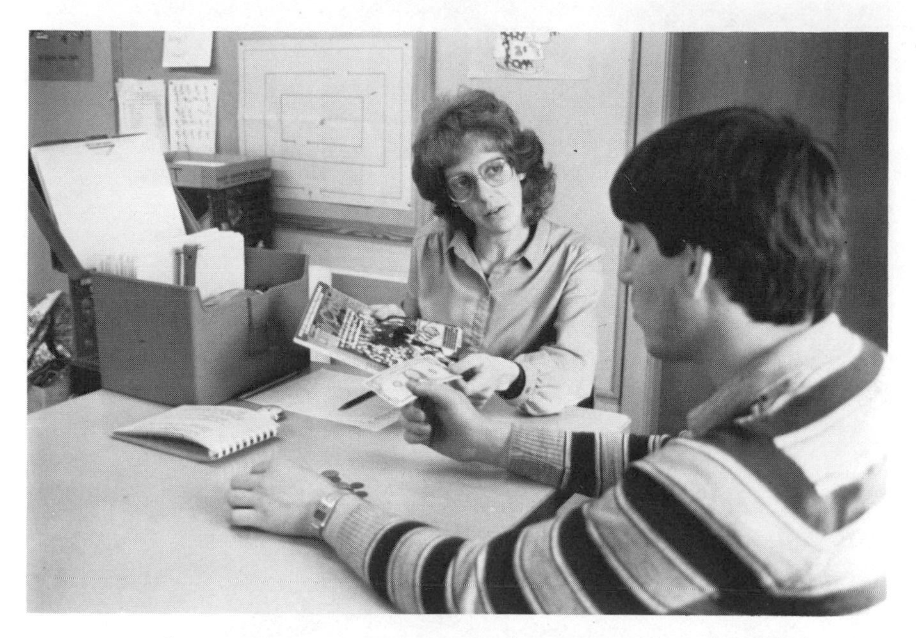

*Fig. 3-17. Task 9, Money Concepts, Part D. Student presents therapist with the correct amount of change after purchase of a magazine.*

In Part D, there is a brief simulation. The money from Part C remains on the table. The therapist pretends to purchase an inexpensive magazine (priced under a dollar) from the student. The therapist hands the student a dollar bill and asks for the appropriate change. The solution should be calculated mentally (Fig. 3-17).

*10. Functional Banking*

In Part A, an enlarged bank check is presented, and the student must write out the answers to a set of questions pertaining to the check—the amount of the check, the date, the account number (Fig. 3-18).

In Part B, the student is instructed to use a calculator to find the balance in the checking account after the check is paid (Fig. 3-19).

Modification: For students with fine motor difficulties, Sharp* makes an excellent solar-cell calculator, model QS-2125, with large keys and an angled base. This calculator can be useful in the clinic as well. It lists at $59.50.

*Sharp Electronics Corporation, 10 Sharp Plaza, Paramus, New Jersey 07652.

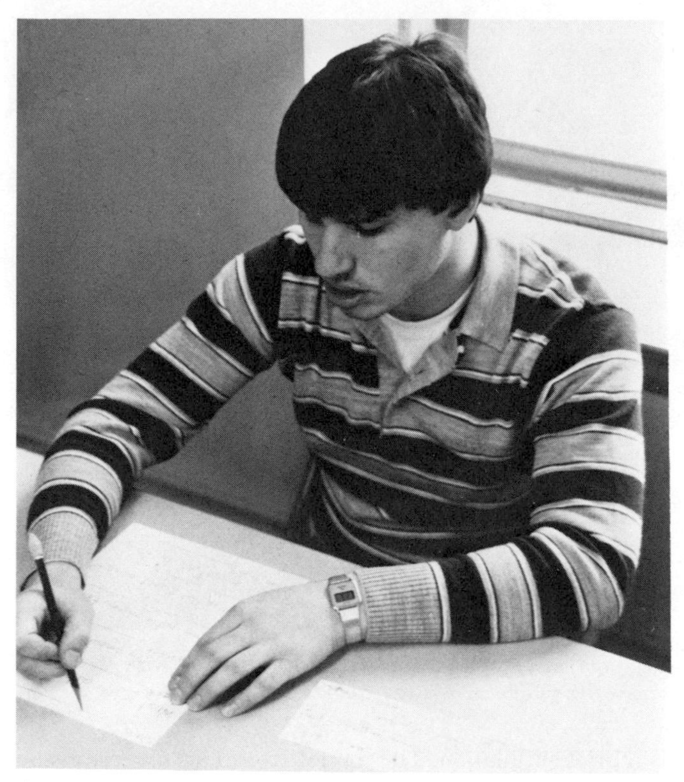

*A*

NO. 175 $ 3.99
Jan. 2 19 83
PAY TO: Learning Prep School
FOR: books

| | $ | ¢ |
|---|---|---|
| OLD BALANCE | 15 | 95 |
| (+)DEPOSIT (-)CHARGE | | |
| NEW BALANCE | | |
| AMOUNT OF CHECK | 3 | 99 |
| FINAL BALANCE | | |

KAREN JACOB-GOLD
ANY STREET
YOUR TOWN, USA 53660

NUMBER
175

Jan. 2 19 83

PAY TO THE ORDER OF Learning Prep School $ 3. 99/100
three 99/100 DOLLARS

YOUR TOWN BANK, USA

MEMO books
537 - 211

Karen Jacob-Gold

*B*

*Fig. 3-18. Task 10, Functional Banking, Part A. A: Student answers questions about a bank check. B: Sample check.*

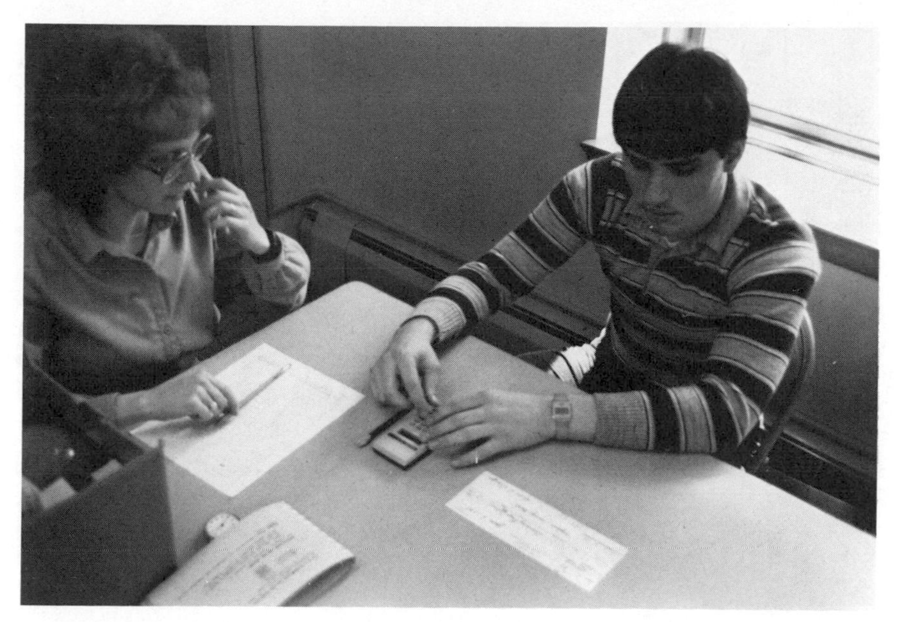

*Fig. 3-19. Task 10, Functional Banking, Part B. Using a calculator, student finds the balance in a checking account.*

*11. Time Concepts*

In Part A, the student is presented three pictures of a clock face, each showing a different time. The therapist instructs the student to read each time (Fig. 3-20).

In Part B, two pictures of clocks are presented together, and the student is asked to decide which clock has the later time.

In Part C, a picture of a digital clock reading 12:40 is placed on the table, and the student is asked what time it will be in 30 minutes.

*12. Work Attitudes*

This task is concerned with the student's work attitude and decision-making ability.

In Part A, the therapist randomly places before the student five cards, each depicting a step in a sequence of purchasing a meal at a fast-food shop. The student is asked to place the cards in correct order (Fig. 3-21).

Modification: Present a three-card sequence.

In Part B, the task is a totally verbal one, which requires the student to devise solutions to three small vignettes relating to work. For example, "You are working at the grill at McDonald's when a fire starts. What do you do?"

Modification: To adapt for a nonverbal student, print up a card with several solutions to each vignette for the student to choose from.

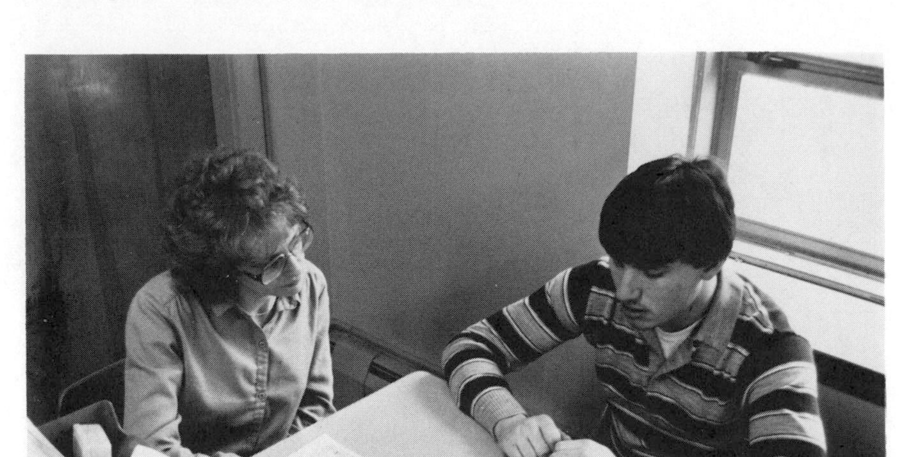

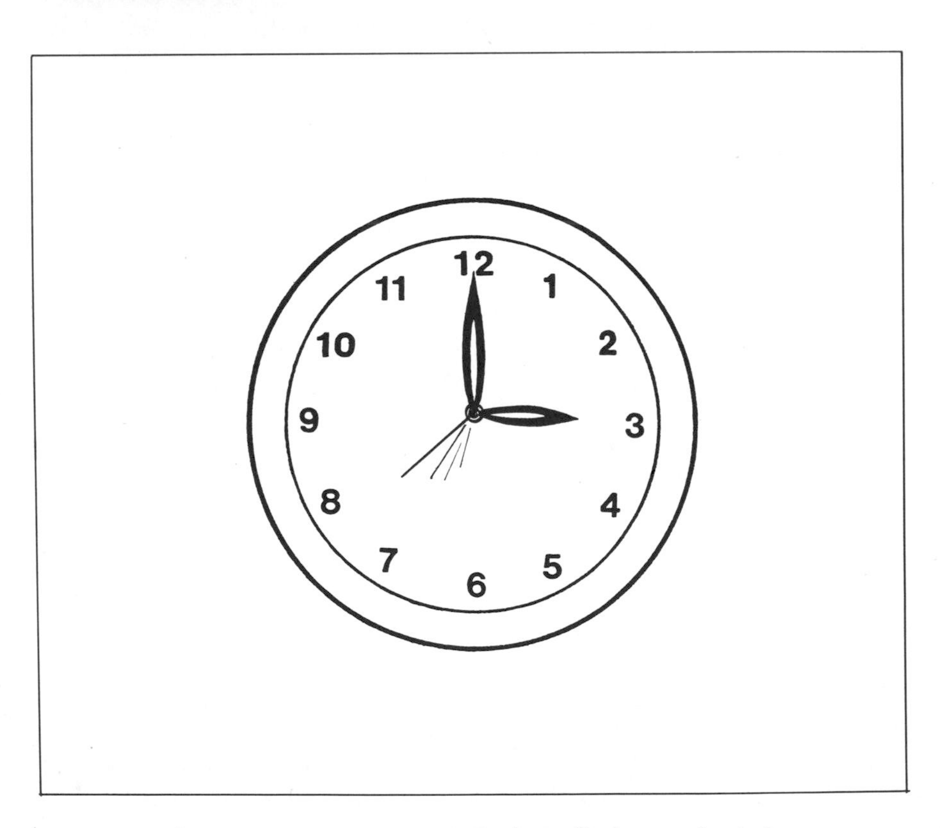


*Fig. 3-20. Task 11, Time Concepts, Part A. Student tells time on the clock.*

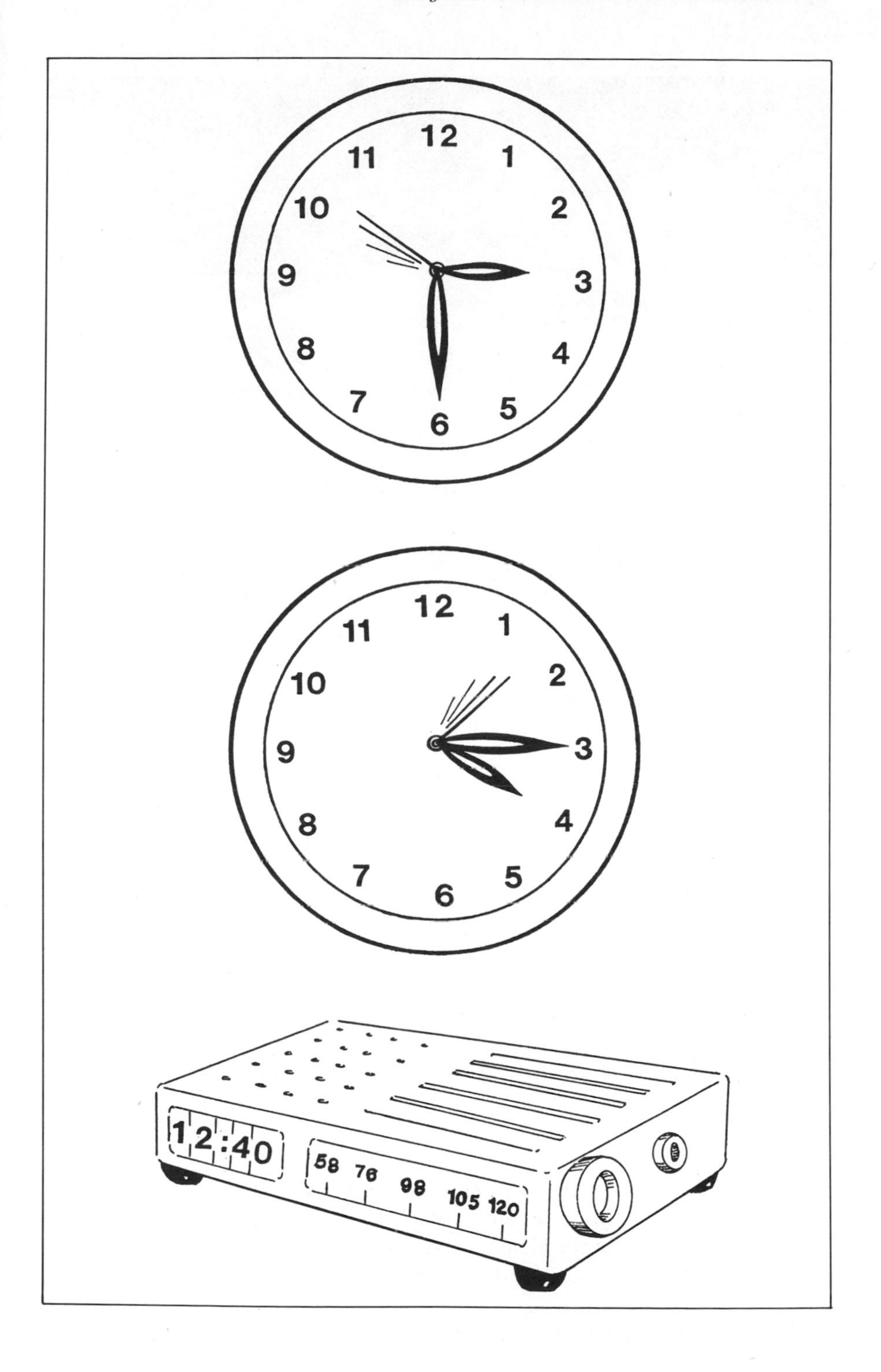
12:40
58 76 98 105 120

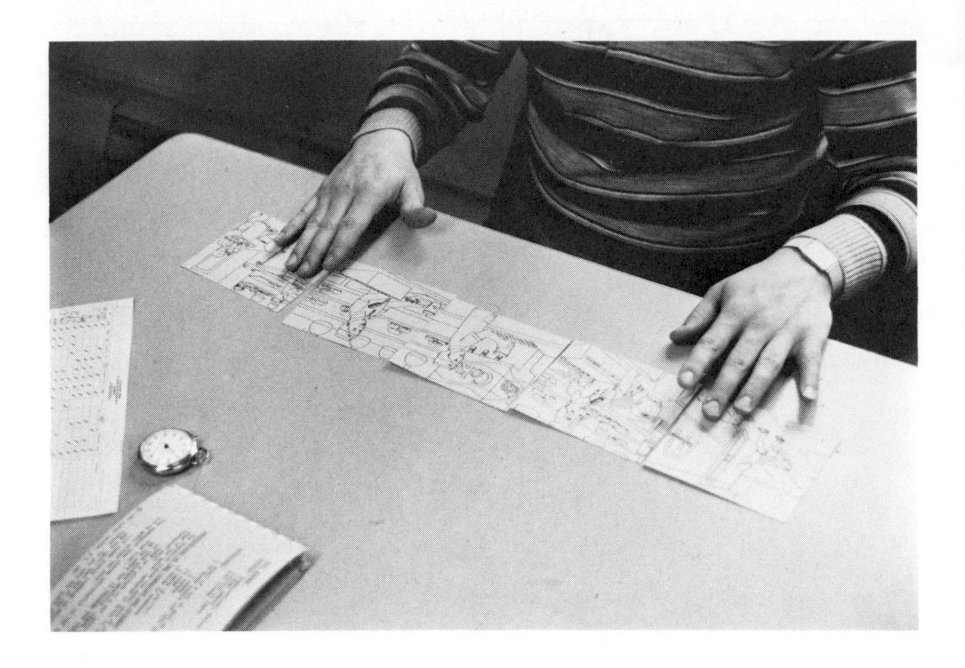

*13. Body Scheme*
The student is shown a drawing of a teenaged boy for 15 seconds. Upon its removal, five identical drawings that have been cut up (i.e., five heads, ten arms, etc.) are presented. The student reassembles the parts (Fig. 3-22).

*14. Leather Assembly*
The therapist demonstrates the construction of a simple leather key ring and instructs the student to make a similar one (Fig. 3-23). A reward feature has been integrated into this task: The student is allowed to keep the key ring. (Through the years of test use, I have found that this task provides the foundation for spin-off activities in treatment, such as the purpose of keys. This is the first experience some students have with keys!) Since the main purpose of this task is to reward the student, the therapist should assist the student if he or she is having difficulty.

Modifications: Increase the size of the rivets. Eliminate the extra sets of rivets.

*15. Food Preparation*
The student is requested to follow five visual instructions to make honey butter (Fig. 3-24). This is an enjoyable final activity for the testing session and gives the therapist the chance to speak informally with the student. The option of eating the honey butter on crackers is provided as another form of positive reward.

Modification: Use adaptive equipment, for example, stabilize bowl.

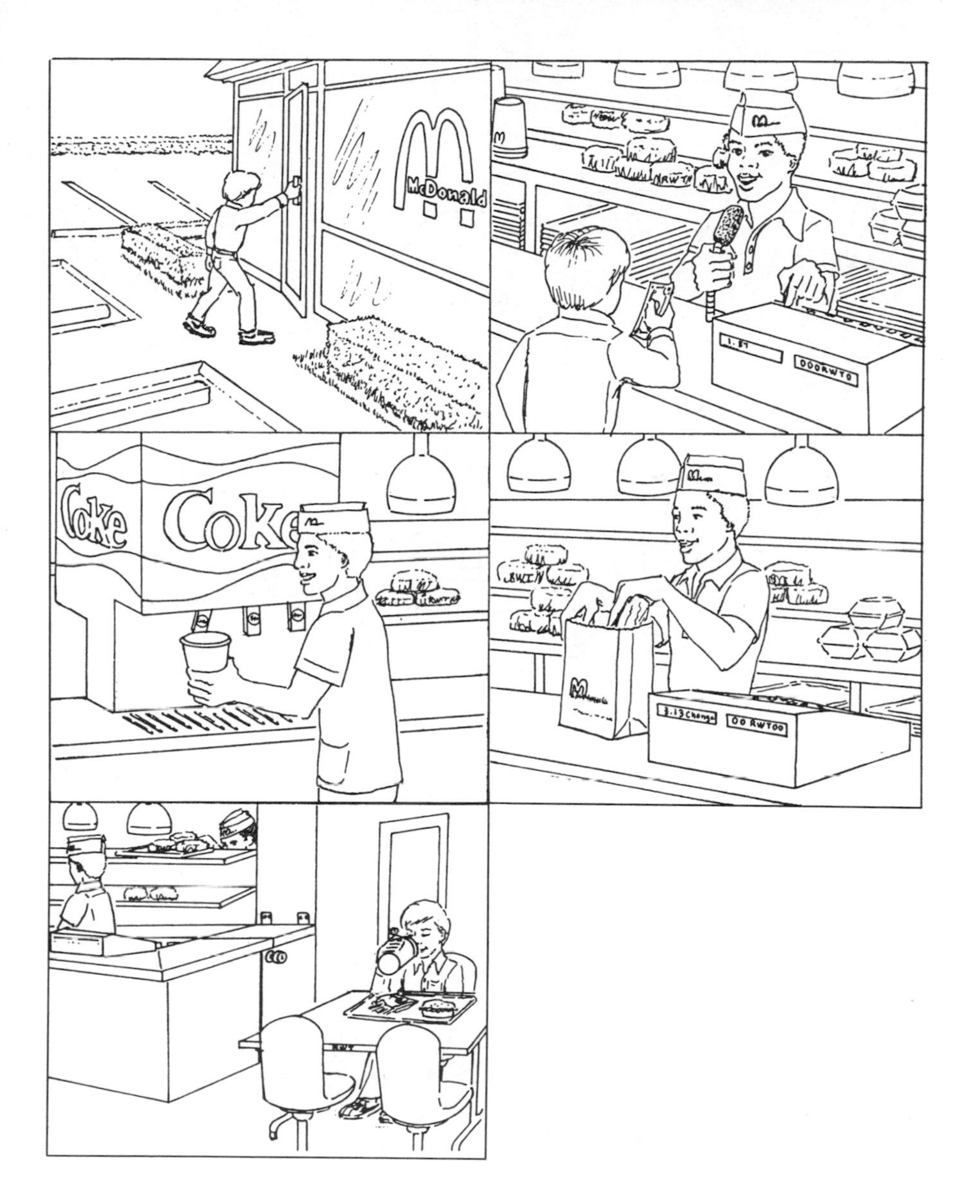


*Fig. 3-21. Task 12, Work Attitudes, Part A. Student arranges in sequence five cards illustrating purchase of a meal at a fast-food shop.*

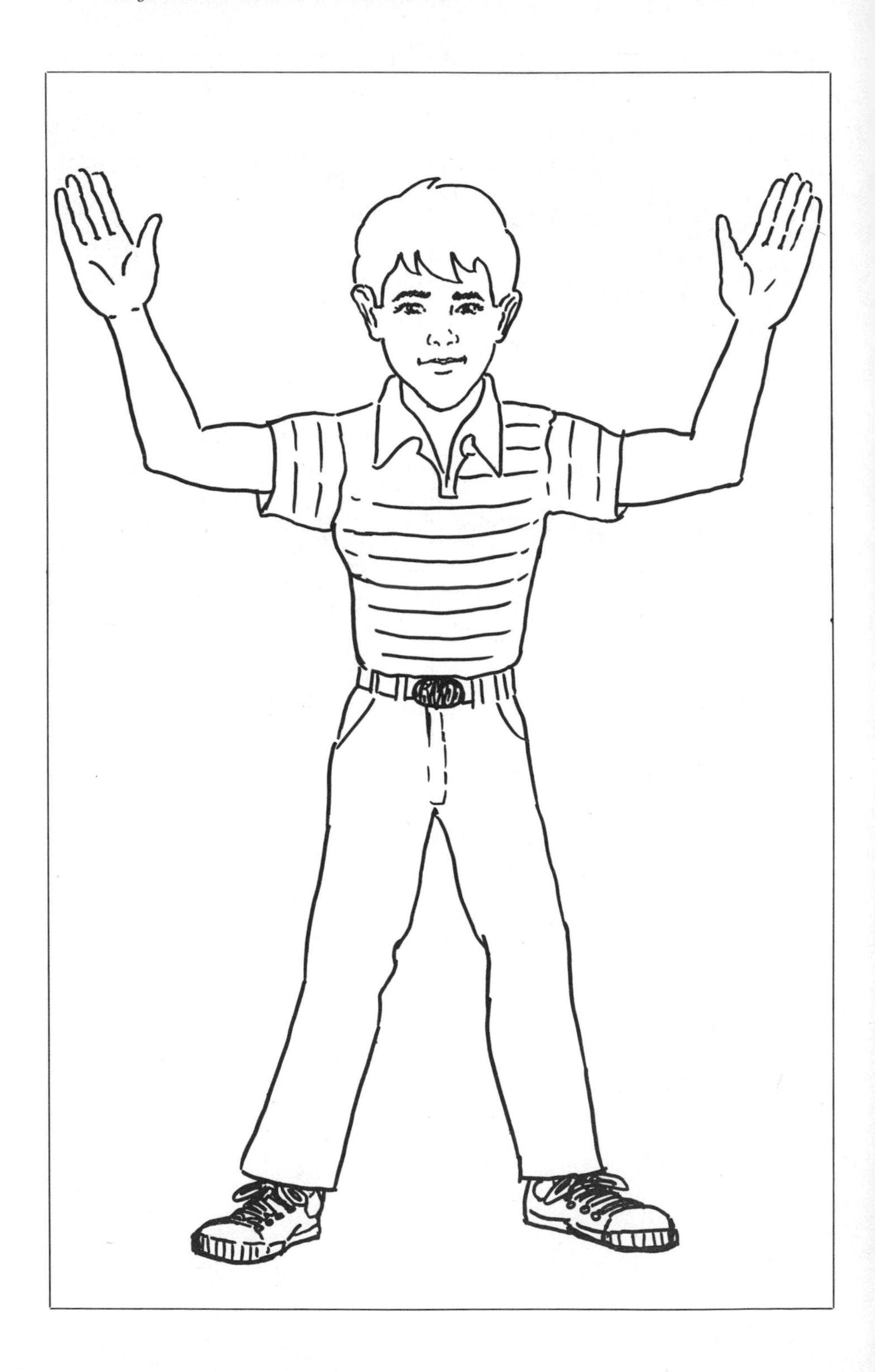

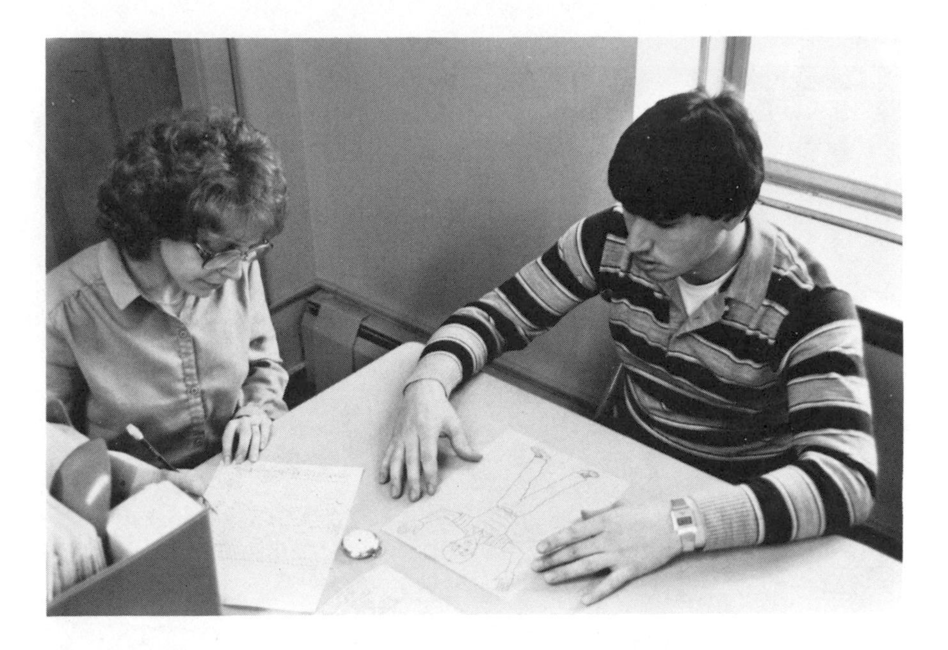

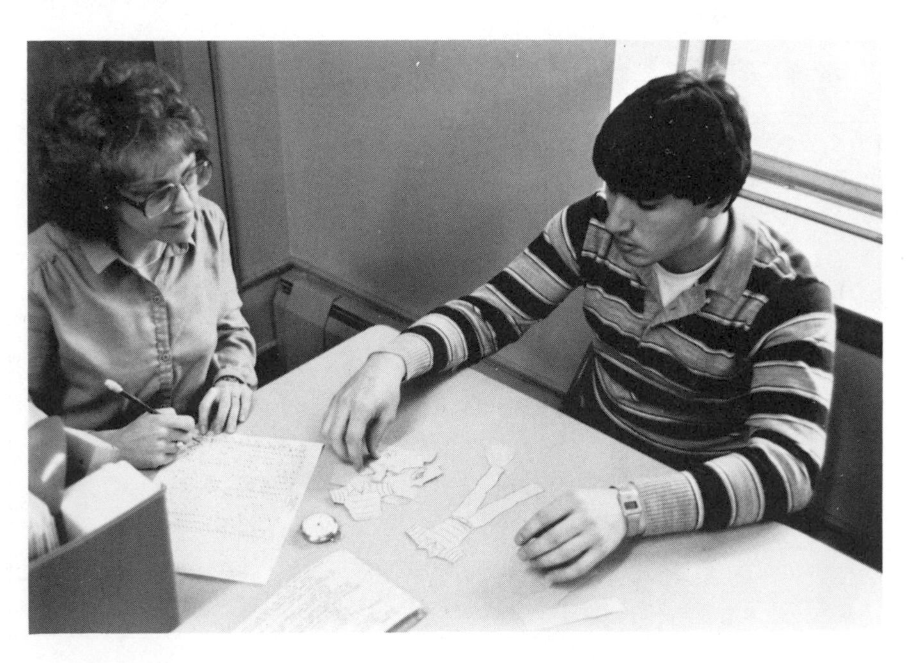

*Fig. 3-22. Task 13, Body Scheme. Student is presented with an intact drawing of a boy, which is removed, and is then given a cut-up version of the same drawing to put together correctly. The drawing used in this task is to be photocopied—one copy to remain intact, the five other copies to be cut up into parts for reassembly.*

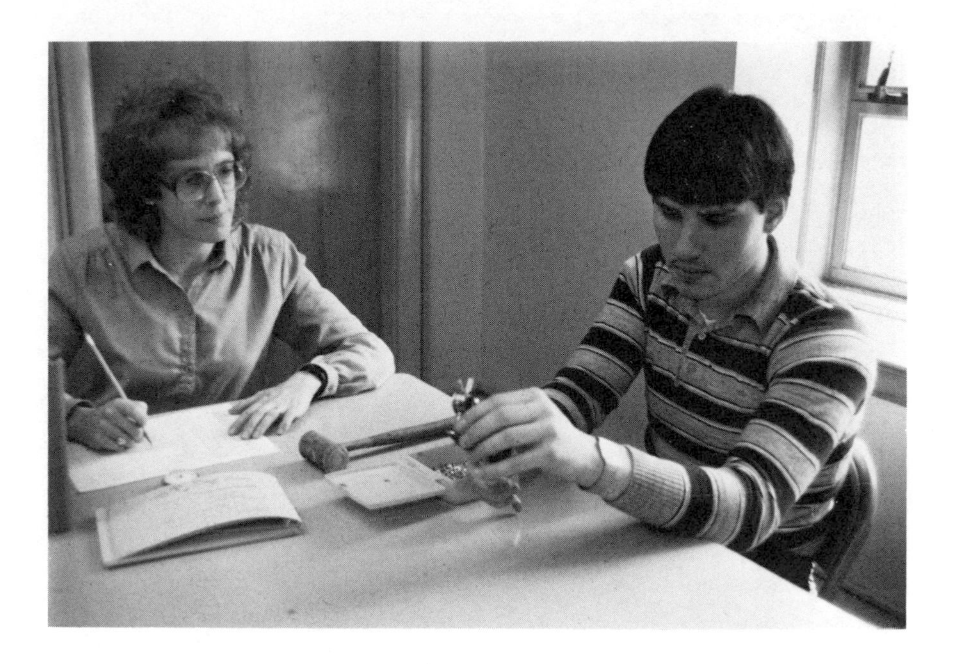

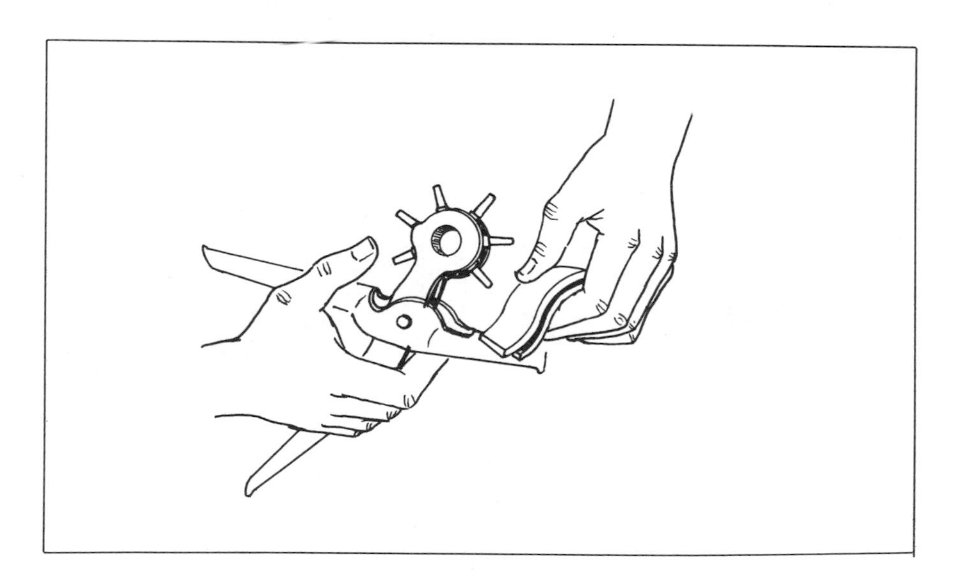

*Fig. 3-23. Task 14, Leather Assembly. Following the instructional drawings shown here, the therapist demonstrates to the student how to make a simple leather key ring. Immediately following this demonstration, the student makes a leather key ring.*

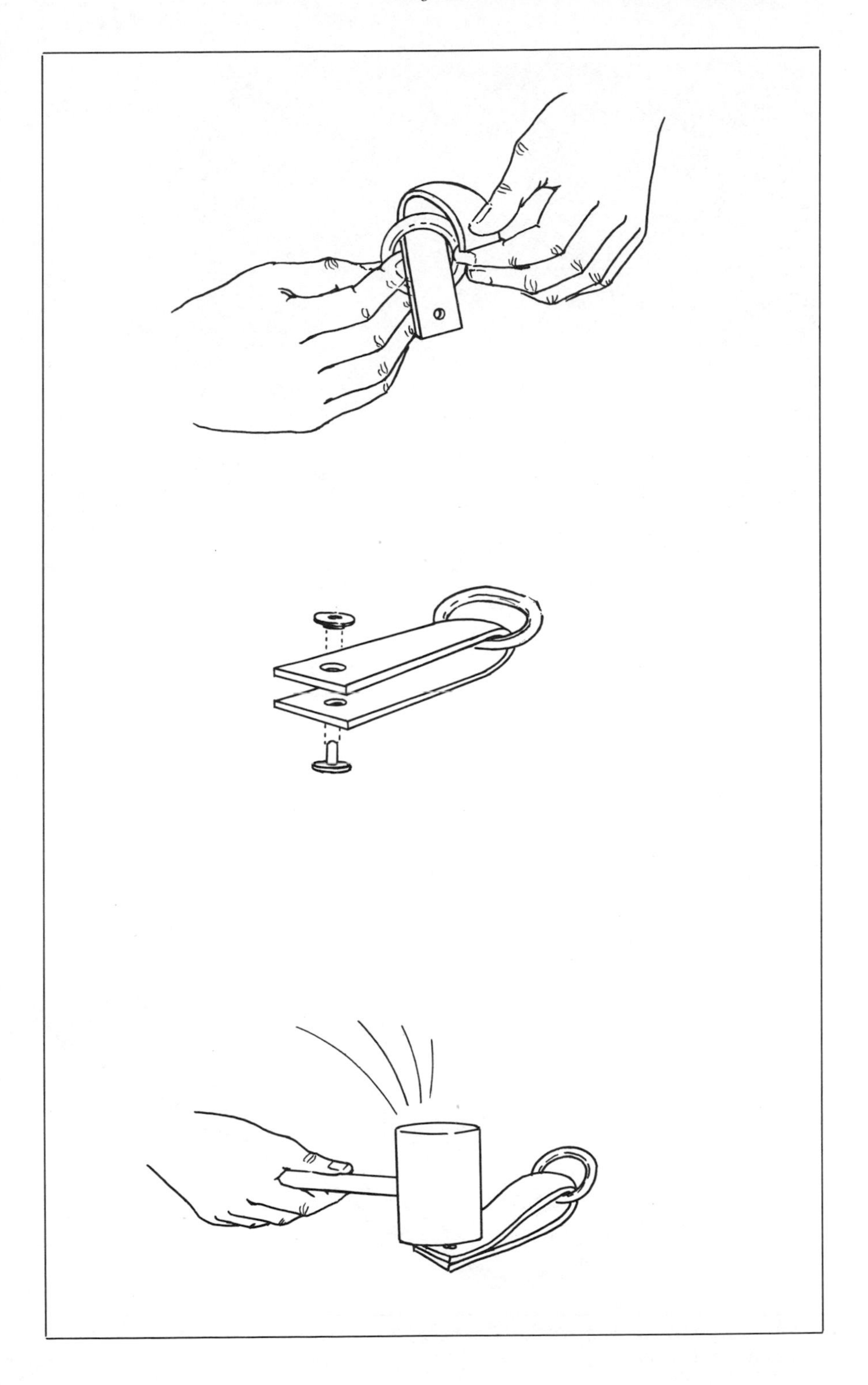

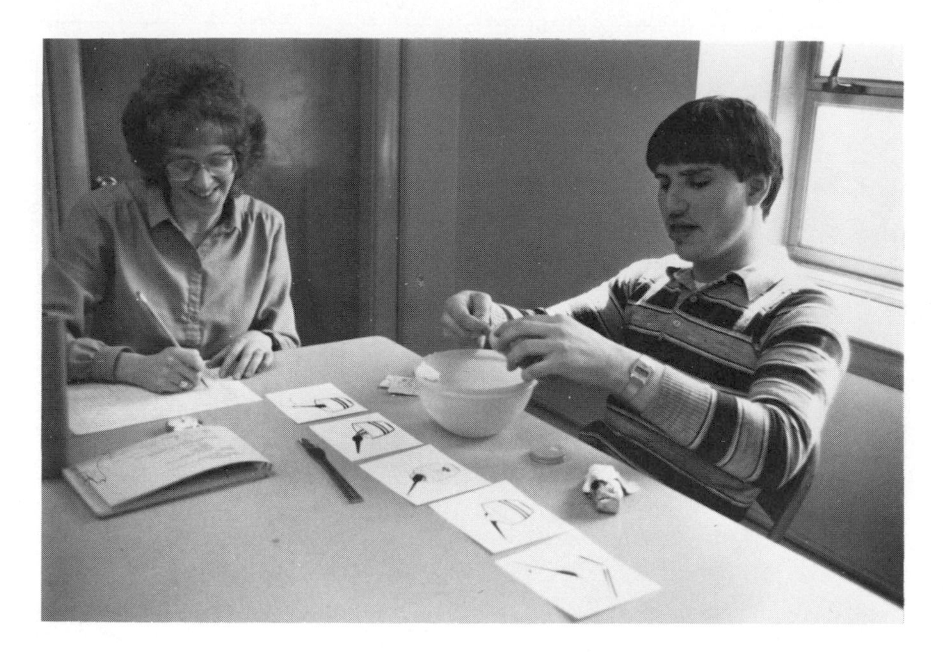

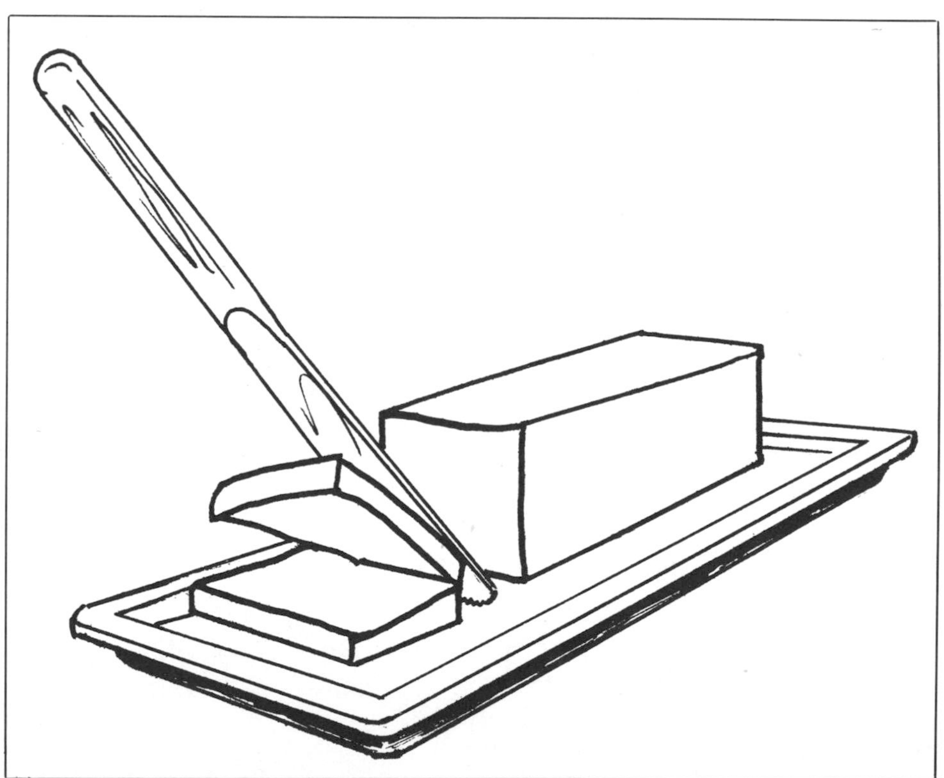

*Fig. 3-24. Task 15, Food Preparation. Following the directions on five cards, student prepares honey butter.*

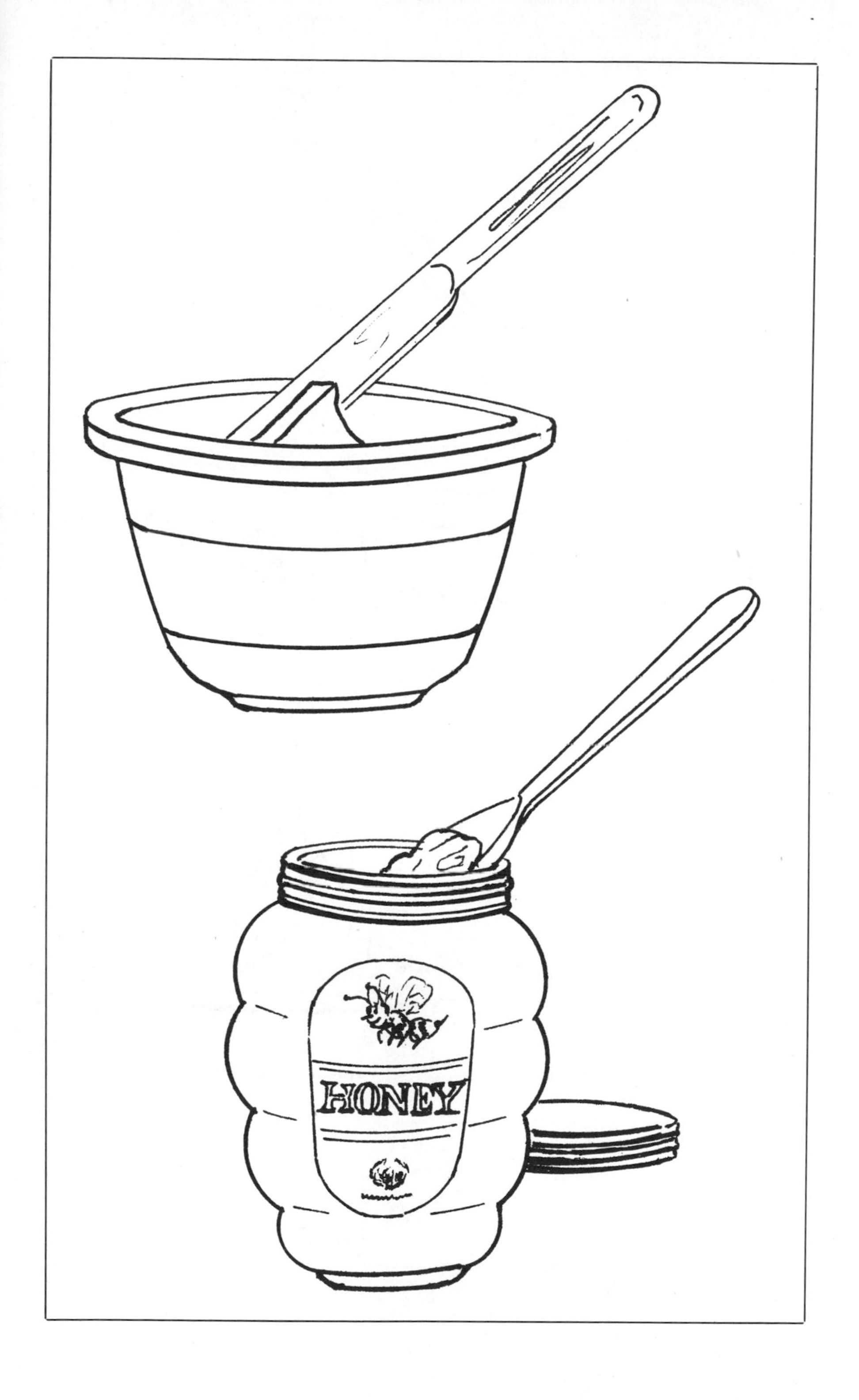
HONEY

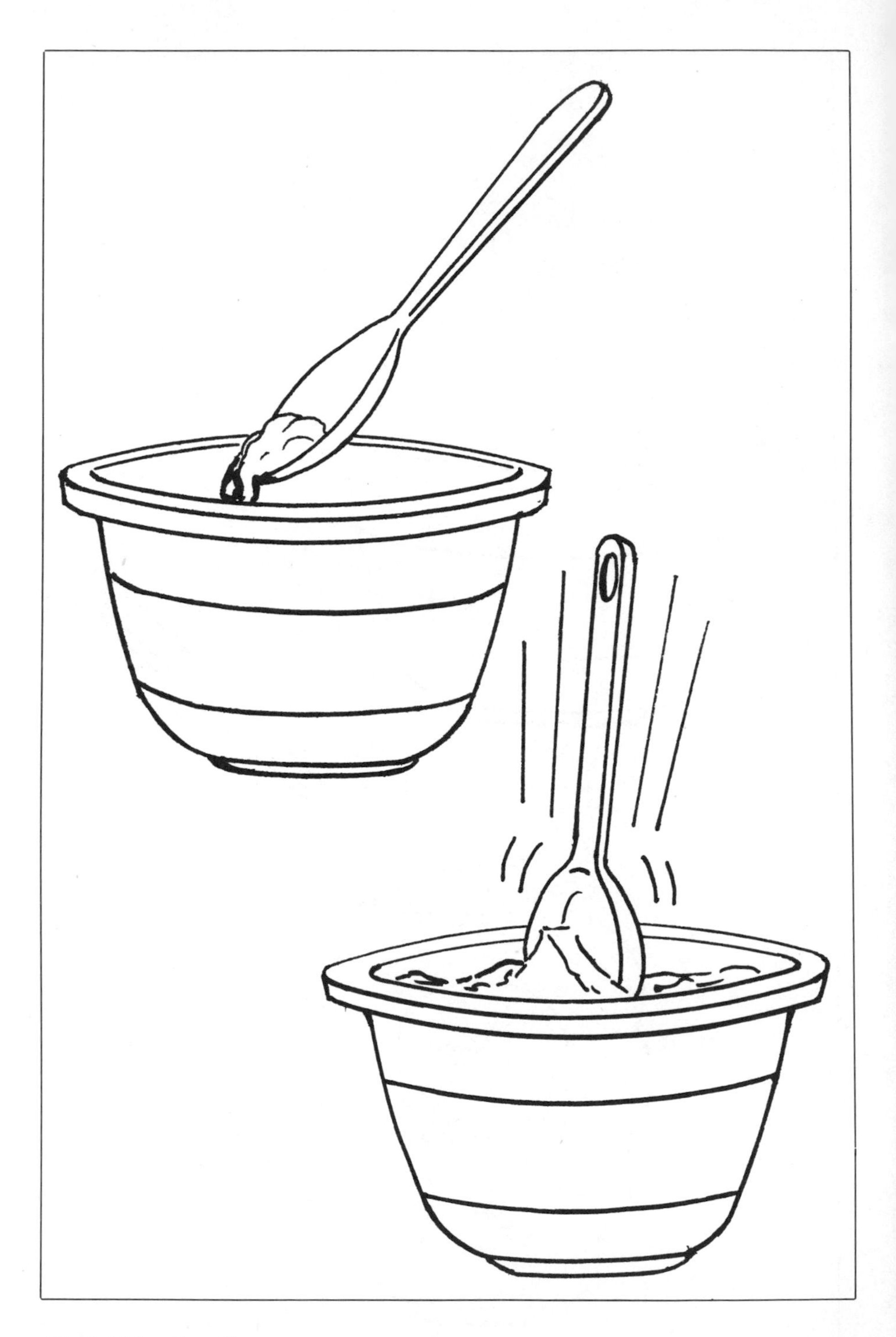

*Fig. 3-24 (continued)*

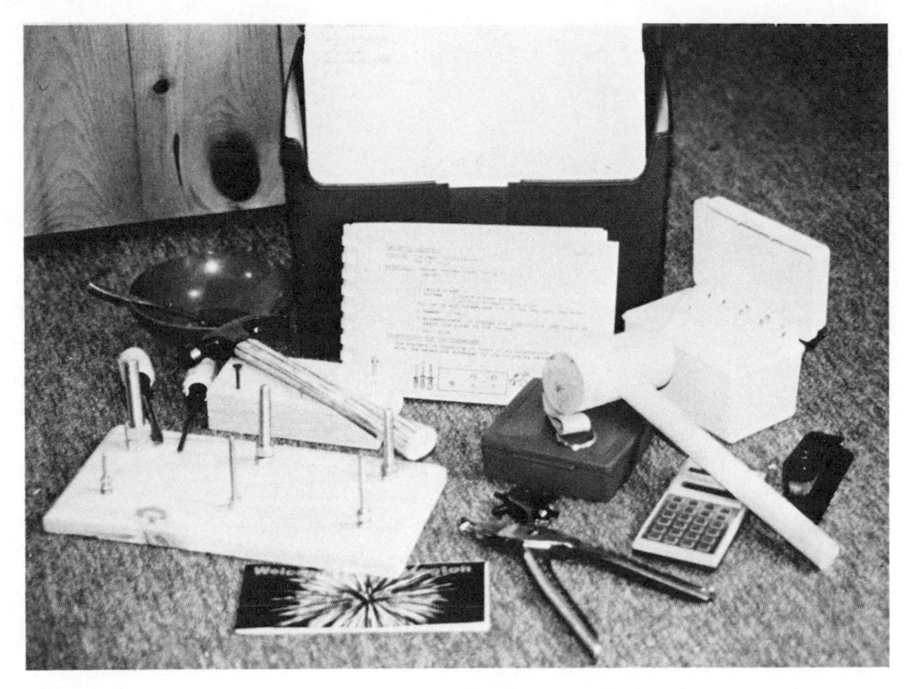

*Fig. 3-25. All the items necessary for the JPSA, shown with the plastic carrying case.*

MATERIALS REQUIRED

All the materials for the assessment are readily available from an occupational therapy department, hardware store, and stationery shop (Fig. 3-25). The total cost of the materials if you were to purchase each item is approximately $50. All illustrations and the profile sheet have been provided in this book, and you may copy them for your use. Please note that illustrations have specific sizes and may need to be enlarged.

A "shopping list" by task for all the materials needed to construct a JPSA follows. All the materials can be carried in a plastic carrying case, with each task neatly housed in a labelled vertical file folder. When assembled the JPSA is easily transportable, weighing only 12 pounds. Some task materials (e.g., hammers, wooden board) that are too large for the file folders can be positioned inside the carrying case.

*General Items*

1 plastic carrying case (10½″ × 9″ × 12″)
17 vertical file folders (9½″ × 11¾″ × 1½″ expansion) (one for each of the 15 tasks and one each for the manual and profile sheets)
17 3½″ × ½″ self-sticking file folder labels
20 profile sheets (see Fig. 3-1).
1 manual (see pp. 70–91) (Suggestion: I keep an extra copy of the instructions for each task in the file folder for the task for easy reference.)
1 stopwatch or clock with a second hand

*Items Needed Only to Construct Assessment*

1 pair of scissors
1 hand or power drill

*Optional Procedures*
Instruction cards and graphics can be laminated very inexpensively at a copy shop to increase their longevity. The manual can be spiral bound inexpensively, again at a copy shop.

*Task 1. Quality Control*
16 2½″ nails
10 odd-size and bent nails

*Task 2. Filing*
26 white cards (3″ × 5″), each bearing one of the following words: age, book, chef, date, employee, form, greater, help, in, janitor, keep, left, mechanic, nurse, off, pencil, quick, read, store, typist, use, visit, work, Xerox, year, zip
1 two-sided instruction card (4¼″ × 5½″) with the following on side 1:

HERE ARE 26 CARDS WITH WORDS ON THEM. THEY ARE MIXED AND MUST BE PUT IN ALPHABETICAL ORDER FROM A TO Z. WHEN YOU HAVE THEM

on side 2:

ARRANGED, PUT THEM IN A PACK AS THEY ARE RIGHT NOW. ANY QUESTIONS? IF NOT, BEGIN.

1 (plastic file box 5¼″ × 3½″ × 3″)
1 set of *A* to *Z* guides for 3″ × 5″ index cards
1 instruction card (4¼″ × 5½″) with the following on one side:

HERE ARE 13 CARDS WITH LAST NAMES. PUT THESE CARDS IN ALPHABETICAL ORDER IN THE FILE BOX.

13 white lined (3″ × 5″) index cards each bearing one of the following names in the left-hand corner:

ADAMS, C.; BANKS, C; DINAN, K.; EVANS, W.; GREEN, G.; GRAY, A.; HALL, J.; JONES, L.; JOHNSON, J; MANN, D.; PETERS, C.; STEVENS, P.; WILLIAMS, E.

6 white (5″ × 3″) cards, each with one of the following words written in capital letters:

MONEY, MATCH, MAIL, MAIN, MISS, MUCH

1 instruction card with the following information printed on one side:

HERE ARE 6 CARDS WITH WORDS. PUT THESE CARDS IN ALPHABETICAL ORDER IN THE FILE BOX.

*Task 3. Carpentry Assembly*
1 pine board (6″ × 4″ × 2″)
1 hammer (4 oz)
1 blade-head screwdriver
1 Phillips-head screwdriver
1 6 × 2″ Phillips Screw
1 6 × 2″ flat-head blade screw
1 6 × 1½″ Phillips Screw
1 1″ 4d nail
1 1½″ 4d nail
1 2″ 4d nail

The wooden board, nails, and screws are typically consumable items; however, it may be possible to recycle the screws and the board.

*Task 4. Classification*
1 9″ × 12″ illustration of a restaurant kitchen (Fig. 3-8)
17 4½″ × 5″ cards: 12 drawings relating to a restaurant kitchen; 5 unrelated drawings

*Task 5. Office Work*
1 standard-size stapler
6 standard-size business cards
5 sheets (8½″ × 11″) white paper
5 business size white envelopes
17 sheets (3½″ × 6″) red construction paper
5 sheets (3½″ × 6″) pink construction paper
5 sheets (3½″ × 6″) green construction paper
11 sheets (3½″ × 6″) orange construction paper
5 sheets (3½″ × 6″) yellow construction paper
6 standard-size paper clips
1 two-sided instruction card (4½″ × 5½″) with the following information printed in bold type

[side 1] YOU ARE TO TAKE 3 RED CARDS, 2 ORANGE CARDS, 1 GREEN CARD, 1 PINK CARD, AND 1 YELLOW CARD AND PLACE THEM IN A PILE. TAKE ONE

[side 2] PAPER CLIP AND CLIP THE PILE TOGETHER. MAKE 4 MORE PILES FOLLOWING THE SAME PROCEDURE. PUT EACH PILE INTO AN ENVELOPE.

The business cards and white paper are consumable. When you are assembling your materials, you may want to gather a stock of these items. To eliminate the cost of purchasing business cards and white paper, I have approached local printers and copy shops asking for donations of these supplies.

You will find that most of these companies are happy to give away these surplus items.

*Task 6. Telephone Directory*
1 9″ × 11″ telephone directory
1 pencil
1 3″ × 5″ index card with the following information:

NAME ______________________________
ADDRESS ______________________________
______________________________
TELEPHONE NUMBER ______________________________

1 white business-size envelope
1 pen
1 stamp

The index card, envelope, and stamp are consumable. Again, to cut down on expenses, approach paper suppliers or stationery shops for donations of envelopes and index cards. Stickers found in ads from record companies or from the Easter Seal Society can be substituted for stamps.

*Task 7. Factory Work*
1 5½″ × 11″ × 1″ wooden board (Fig. 3-13)
1 5⁄16″ × 3″ carriage bolt and 2 matching nuts
1 3⁄8″ × 3″ carriage bolt and 2 matching nuts
1 ½″ × 3″ carriage bolt and 2 matching nuts
1 ¼″ × 3″ machine screw and 2 matching nuts
1 8/32″ × 3″ machine screw and 3 matching nuts
1 6/32″ × 3″ machine screw and 3 matching nuts
1 small plastic bowl (You may substitute a small plastic margarine container.)

*Task 8. Environmental Mobility*
1 map of Washington, D.C., (14″ × 23″) (available free from the following address: National Parks Service, Washington, D.C. Ask for the "Welcome to Washington, D.C." map.)
1 broad-tip black marking pen or black crayon
1 piece of clear plastic cut to the following dimensions: 14″ × 23″
1 instruction card (5″ × 7″) (Develop your own for your own setting. The card might read as follows):

GO OUT THE DOOR.
TURN RIGHT.
WALK THROUGH THE DOOR.
GO DOWN TWO FLIGHTS OF STAIRS.
YOU WILL BE ON THE FIRST FLOOR.
TURN RIGHT.

GO THROUGH THE DOOR.
WALK DOWN THE HALL.
JUST BEFORE THE DOOR IN THE HALL, TAKE A LEFT AND AN IMMEDIATE RIGHT.
WALK DOWN THE HALL UNTIL YOU SEE THE MAILBOXES ON THE LEFT.
LOOK IN THE MAILBOX MARKED
[therapist's last name].
BRING BACK THE WHITE ENVELOPE THAT IS IN THE MAILBOX.

1 business-size white envelope

*Task 9. Money Concepts*

4 pennies
3 nickels
6 dimes
5 quarters
1 dollar bill
1 cash register receipt with a total reading approximately $2.11–2.24
1 inexpensive magazine (priced under a dollar)

*Task 10. Functional Banking*

1 3½″ × 10″ bank check (Fig. 3-18B)
1 #2 pencil
1 8½″ × 11″ sheet of white paper with the following information in bold print:

NAME ______________________________
1. What is the date on the check? ______________________
2. What is the amount of the check? ______________________
3. To whom is the money being paid? ______________________
4. What is the account number? ______________________
5. Whose account will the money come from? ______________________

1 inexpensive calculator

*Task 11. Time Concepts*

1 3″ × 5″ card with a picture of a clock reading 3:00
1 3″ × 5″ card with a picture of a clock reading 3:30
1 3″ × 5″ card with a picture of a clock reading 4:15
1 3″ × 5″ card with a picture of a digital clock reading 12:40 (Fig. 3-20)

*Task 12. Work Attitudes*

5 3½″ × 4½″ cards each depicting a step in a sequence of a student walking into a fast-food shop and purchasing a meal (Fig. 3-21)

*Task 13. Body Scheme*

1 8½″ × 11″ sheet of paper with a drawing of a teenaged boy (Fig. 3-22)
5 identical drawings cut into the following parts: 5 heads, 5 torsos, 10 arms, 5 pairs of legs, 10 feet

*Task 14. Leather Assembly*

1 standard-size rotary leather hole punch
1 wooden leather mallet (1½″ × 4″)
2 key rings
6 sets of small rivets
2 1″ × 3″ 7-oz leather strips
1 plastic box (4″ × 4″ × ½″) to hold rivets, leather, and key rings

The leather, key rings, and rivets are consumable items. The leather strips, however, can be cut from scrap leather. Make sure that you are using a sharp hole punch to facilitate use.

*Task 15. Food Preparation*

1 stick of margarine (Take it out at the beginning of the testing session to soften.)
1 small jar of honey
1 small mixing spoon
1 teaspoon
1 butter knife
1 small plastic bowl
1 box of crackers (Keep these on hand, but leave only a small package in the assessment box.)
5 4¼″ × 5½″ instruction cards (Fig. 3-24)

WRITING THE EVALUATION REPORT

When the test is completed, the therapist has sufficient information to devise a treatment plan. To expedite the write-up procedure and to facilitate clarity in communicating results, I have devised a format that is concrete yet descriptive enough for both educators and laypersons to comprehend. This format is illustrated in the sample evaluation reports that follow this section.

After the therapist has reviewed the profile sheet and calculated the number of circled checks in each column, he or she is able readily to complete the report. This typically takes 15 to 30 minutes, depending on the complexity of results.

The completed version of the evaluation report, including the profile sheet, is placed in the student's chart, with copies sent to pertinent individuals: parents, teachers, academic supervisor, other therapists. In addition, when appropriate the therapist may verbally convey results to these persons.

The following are examples of completed evaluation reports, which may help to clarify the JPSA. The first example describes a student I will call Stacey, who will be further discussed in Chapter 4 in a case study (p. 125). I hope these discussions will assist you in conceptualizing the dynamics of the occupational therapist's role in an educational setting directed at work-related programming.

*Sample Evaluation Report 1**

Name: Stacey
Chronological age: 15 years

*Sample Evaluation Reports 1 and 2 were provided by Nancy Mazonson, M.S., OTR.

Stacey was given the Jacobs Prevocational Skills Assessment on February 15 and 17 and March 1, 1984.

EVALUATION BATTERY
The assessment consists of 15 informal tasks involving functional ability in the following skill areas: fine motor coordination, eye-hand coordination, motor planning, figure-ground discrimination, sorting, classification and sequencing, decision making, problem solving, organizational skills, use of tools, ability to follow directions, conceptual skills, task focus, and work-related behavior (Fig. 3-26).

IMPRESSIONS AND OBSERVATIONS
Stacey was cooperative and has pleasant interaction skills. She appeared motivated to perform well and maintained good task focus throughout the test session. At times when the task was difficult, she appeared anxious and seemed to lack confidence in her abilities. Before the evaluation Stacey was able to take an active, responsible role in scheduling the test sessions.

Stacey was unsystematic in her approach to most tasks, showing difficulty in sequencing and organization. She had difficulty in following two- or three-step written or oral directions, which may be related to problems in reading comprehension and in memory. Stacey seemed to be able to follow best a combination of oral and visual directions. She used visual cues in problem solving to compensate for memory problems. Stacey's manipulation of small objects appeared awkward, and she seemed to have problems with visual scanning.

STRENGTHS
1. Cooperative, motivated
2. Adequate work attitudes
3. Adequate task focus
4. Ability to use visual cues for beginning problem solving
5. Beginning-level concepts of money

WEAKNESSES
1. Poor organizational skills
2. Inconsistent in following multistep directions
3. Poor memory
4. Poor visual scanning
5. Weak in acknowledging difficulties
6. Weak in problem solving and decision making
7. Poor in matching
8. Poor in alphabetizing
9. Poor fine motor coordination
10. Weak in classification and sequencing

RECOMMENDATIONS
It is recommended that Stacey be placed in a highly supervised work setting to improve the following procedures: organization, problem solving, sequencing, and decision making. It is recommended that Stacey be seen in a small group twice per week in occupational therapy to work on functional money skills, direction following, and the ability to assess strengths and weaknesses.

*Sample Evaluation Report 2**
Name: Keith
Chronological age: 17 years

Keith was given the Jacobs Prevocational Skills Assessment on February 24, 1984.

Date(s)____________________

| Tasks: | Fine Motor Coordination | Eye-Hand Coordination | Motor Planning | Figure-Ground | Sorting | Classification / Sequencing | Decision Making | Problem Solving | Organizational Skills | Use of Tools |
|---|---|---|---|---|---|---|---|---|---|---|
| Quality Control: 1 | ✓ | | | ✓ | ✓ | | ✓ | | (✓) | |
| Filing: 2 A. | ✓ | | | | ✓ | (✓) | ✓ | (✓) | (✓) | |
| B. | ✓ | | | ✓ | ✓ | ✓ | ✓ | ✓ | ✓ | |
| C. | ✓ | | | | ✓ | ✓ | (✓) | ✓ | ✓ | |
| Carpentry Assembly: 3 | ✓ | (✓) | (✓) | ✓ | | | ✓ | ✓ | | ✓ |
| Classification: 4 | ✓ | | | | | ✓ | ✓ | ✓ | | |
| Office Work: 5 A. | ✓ | ✓ | ✓ | | | ✓ | (✓) | ✓ | ✓ | ✓ |
| B. | ✓ | ✓ | ✓ | | | (✓) | | ✓ | ✓ | |
| C. | (✓) | ✓ | ✓ | | | ✓ | | ✓ | (✓) | |
| Telephone Directory: 6 A. | ✓ | ✓ | | ✓ | | ✓ | | | ✓ | |
| B. | ✓ | ✓ | | | | | | | ✓ | |
| Factory Work: 7 | (✓) | ✓ | ✓ | ✓ | | | ✓ | ✓ | | |
| Environmental Mobility: 8 A. | ✓ | ✓ | ✓ | ✓ | | | | ✓ | ✓ | |
| B. | | | | | | | | (✓) | (✓) | |
| Money Concepts: 9 A. | | | | | | | | | | |
| B. | | | | | | | | | | |
| C. | (✓) | | | ✓ | | | ✓ | ✓ | | |
| D. | ✓ | | | ✓ | | | ✓ | ✓ | ✓ | |
| Functional Banking: 10 A. | ✓ | ✓ | | ✓ | | | (✓) | | | |
| B. | ✓ | ✓ | | ✓ | | | ✓ | | | ✓ |
| Time Concept: 11 A. | | | | | | | | | | |
| B. | | | | ✓ | | | | | | |
| C. | | | | | | | | | | |
| Work Attitudes: 12 A. | | | | ✓ | | (✓) | ✓ | | ✓ | |
| B. | | | | | | | ✓ | ✓ | | |
| Body Scheme: 13 | ✓ | | | | | | | ✓ | ✓ | |
| Leather Assembly: 14 | (✓) | ✓ | ✓ | ✓ | | ✓ | | | ✓ | ✓ |
| Food Preparation: 15 | ✓ | ✓ | ✓ | | | (✓) | (✓) | | | (✓) |

✓ sitting posture
cooperative, pleasant

*Fig. 3-26. The JPSA form completed for Stacey's evaluation.*

Name: Stacey

| Ability to Follow Directions | | | Conceptual Skills | Task Focus | Behavioral Observations | Time |
|---|---|---|---|---|---|---|
| Visual | Written | Verbal | | | | |
| | | (✓) | | (✓) | ↓ use of model, missed 2 | 1:40 |
| | (✓) | | (✓) | ✓ | ↓ scanning | 2:20 |
| | (✓) | | (✓) | ✓ | | 2:50 |
| | (✓) | | (✓) | ✓ | | :30 |
| | | | | ✓ | awkward manipulation of tools | 4:40 |
| | | ✓ | | ✓ | | :30 |
| | | | | ✓ | | 1:00 |
| ✓ | | ✓ | | ✓ | | 2:20 |
| | ✓ | | (✓) | ✓ | became disorganized easily | 2:50 |
| | | ✓ | | ✓ | | 4:40 |
| | | (✓) | ✓ | ✓ | handwriting ↓ | 2:30 |
| | | (✓) | | ✓ | needed cue to replace bolts | 6:00 |
| | | ✓ | | ✓ | | 2:20 |
| | (✓) | | | ✓ | | 3:00 |
| | | ✓ | (✓) | ✓ | has very basic understanding | :30 |
| | | ✓ | (✓) | ✓ | | :30 |
| | | ✓ | (✓) | ✓ | needed cues | :30 |
| | | ✓ | (✓) | ✓ | ↓ concept making change | :30 |
| | ✓ | ✓ | ✓ | ✓ | | 2:50 |
| | | (✓) | ✓ | ✓ | appears familiar with use of calculator | 1:50 |
| | | ✓ | ✓ | ✓ | | :10 |
| | | ✓ | ✓ | ✓ | | :10 |
| | | ✓ | | ✓ | slow, but was able to answer correctly | :20 |
| | | ✓ | | ✓ | | :40 |
| | | ✓ | | ✓ | disorganized use of table top space | — |
| ✓ | | ✓ | | ✓ | | 5:00 |
| ✓ | | | | ✓ | | 3:00 |
| ✓ | | | | ✓ | awkward use of tools | 5:20 |

↓ self confidence
easily disorganized

Date(s) ____________

| Tasks: | Fine Motor Coordination | Eye-Hand Coordination | Motor Planning | Figure-Ground | Sorting | Classification / Sequencing | Decision Making | Problem Solving | Organizational Skills | Use of Tools |
|---|---|---|---|---|---|---|---|---|---|---|
| Quality Control: 1 | ✓ | | | (✓) | ✓ | | ✓ | | (✓) | |
| Filing: 2 A. | ✓ | | | | ✓ | ✓ | (✓) | ✓ | ✓ | |
| B. | (✓) | | | (✓) | ✓ | ✓ | ✓ | ✓ | ✓ | |
| C. | ✓ | | | | ✓ | ✓ | ✓ | ✓ | ✓ | |
| Carpentry Assembly: 3 | (✓) | (✓) | ✓ | ✓ | | | ✓ | (✓) | | ✓ |
| Classification: 4 | ✓ | | | | | ✓ | (✓) | (✓) | | |
| Office Work: 5 A. | (✓) | ✓ | ✓ | | | ✓ | ✓ | ✓ | ✓ | ✓ |
| B. | (✓) | ✓ | (✓) | | | ✓ | | (✓) | ✓ | |
| C. | (✓) | ✓ | ✓ | | | ✓ | | ✓ | (✓) | |
| Telephone Directory: 6 A. | ✓ | ✓ | | (✓) | | ✓ | | | ✓ | |
| B. | ✓ | ✓ | | | | | | | ✓ | |
| Factory Work: 7 | (✓) | ✓ | (✓) | ✓ | | | ✓ | ✓ | | |
| Environmental Mobility: 8 A. | ✓ | ✓ | ✓ | ✓ | | | | (✓) | ✓ | |
| B. | | | | | | | | (✓) | ✓ | |
| Money Concepts: 9 A. | | | | | | | | | | |
| B. | | | | | | | | | | |
| C. | ✓ | | | ✓ | | | (✓) | ✓ | | |
| D. | ✓ | | | ✓ | | | ✓ | ✓ | ✓ | |
| Functional Banking: 10 A. | ✓ | ✓ | | ✓ | | | ✓ | | | |
| B. | ✓ | ✓ | | ✓ | | | ✓ | | | ✓ |
| Time Concept: 11 A. | | | | | | | | | | |
| B. | | | | ✓ | | | | | | |
| C. | | | | | | | | | | |
| Work Attitudes: 12 A. | | | | ✓ | | ✓ | ✓ | | ✓ | |
| B. | | | | | | | ✓ | ✓ | | |
| Body Scheme: 13 | (✓) | | | | | | | (✓) | ✓ | |
| Leather Assembly: 14 | (✓) | ✓ | (✓) | (✓) | | ✓ | | | ✓ | ✓ |
| Food Preparation: 15 | ✓ | ✓ | ✓ | | | ✓ | (✓) | | | ✓ |

*Fig. 3-27. The JPSA form completed for Keith's evaluation.*

Name: Keith

| Ability to Follow Directions | | | Conceptual Skills | Task Focus | Behavioral Observations | Time |
|---|---|---|---|---|---|---|
| Visual | Written | Verbal | | | | |
| | | (✓) | | ✓ | became disorganized | 2:20 |
| | ✓ | | (✓) | ✓ | poor use of model slow, labored | 6:00 |
| | (✓) | | ✓ | ✓ | | 5:00 |
| | ✓ | | (✓) | ✓ | | 2:00 |
| | | | | ✓ | awkward with tools | 4:00 |
| | | ✓ | | ✓ | | 1:30 |
| | | | | ✓ | | 1:45 |
| (✓) | | ✓ | | ✓ | poor folding | 4:20 |
| | (✓) | | ✓ | ✓ | became disorganized easily | 5:10 |
| | | ✓ | (✓) | ✓ | | 4:10 |
| | | ✓ | ✓ | ✓ | writing slow, but neat | 4:30 |
| | | ✓ | | ✓ | extremely slow movements | 6:00 |
| | | (✓) | | ✓ | required cues (memory) | 3:20 |
| | (✓) | | | ✓ | required assistance | 5:50 |
| | | ✓ | ✓ | ✓ | | :30 |
| | | ✓ | (✓) | ✓ | | :30 |
| | | (✓) | (✓) | ✓ | | 1:30 |
| | | (✓) | (✓) | ✓ | lacks understanding of basic change making skills | 1:00 |
| | ✓ | ✓ | (✓) | ✓ | | 4:00 |
| | | ✓ | (✓) | ✓ | | 1:00 |
| | | ✓ | ✓ | ✓ | | — |
| | | ✓ | ✓ | ✓ | | — |
| | | (✓) | (✓) | ✓ | difficulty c̄ digital | - |
| | | ✓ | | ✓ | O.K. | 1:00 |
| | | ✓ | | ✓ | appropriate responses | - |
| (✓) | | ✓ | | ✓ | unsystematic trial & error attempts | 5:20 |
| (✓) | | | | ✓ | awkward, appeared confused | 4:40 |
| ✓ | | | | ✓ | unsure, needed cues | 4:30 |

conversant, pleasant, nicely groomed

Date(s)______________

| Tasks: | Fine Motor Coordination | Eye-Hand Coordination | Motor Planning | Figure-Ground | Sorting | Classification / Sequencing | Decision Making | Problem Solving | Organizational Skills | Use of Tools |
|---|---|---|---|---|---|---|---|---|---|---|
| Quality Control: 1 | ✓ | | | ✓ | ✓ | | ✓ | | ✓ | |
| Filing: 2 A. | ✓ | | | | ✓ | ✓ | ✓ | ✓ | ✓ | |
| B. | ✓ | | | ✓ | ✓ | ✓ | ✓ | ✓ | ✓ | |
| C. | ✓ | | | | ✓ | ✓ | ✓ | ✓ | ✓ | |
| Carpentry Assembly: 3 | ✓ | ✓ | ✓ | ✓ | | | ✓ | ✓ | | ✓ |
| Classification: 4 | ✓ | | | | | ✓ | ✓ | ✓ | | |
| Office Work: 5 A. | ✓ | ✓ | ✓ | | | ✓ | ✓ | ✓ | ✓ | ✓ |
| B. | ✓ | ✓ | ✓ | | | ✓ | | ✓ | ✓ | |
| C. | ✓ | ✓ | ✓ | | | ✓ | | ✓ | ✓ | |
| Telephone Directory: 6 A. | ✓ | ✓ | | ✓ | | ✓ | | | ✓ | |
| B. | ✓ | ✓ | | | | | | | ✓ | |
| Factory Work: 7 | ✓ | ✓ | ✓ | ✓ | | | ✓ | ✓ | | |
| Environmental Mobility: 8 A. | ✓ | ✓ | ✓ | ✓ | | | | ✓ | ✓ | |
| B. | | | | | | | | ✓ | ✓ | |
| Money Concepts: 9 A. | | | | | | | | | | |
| B. | | | | | | | | | | |
| C. | ✓ | | | ✓ | | | ✓ | ✓ | | |
| D. | ✓ | | | ✓ | | | ✓ | ✓ | ✓ | |
| Functional Banking: 10 A. | ✓ | ✓ | | ✓ | | | ✓ | | | |
| B. | ✓ | ✓ | | ✓ | | | ✓ | | | ✓ |
| Time Concept: 11 A. | | | | | | | | | | |
| B. | | | | ✓ | | | | | | |
| C. | | | | | | | | | | |
| Work Attitudes: 12 A. | | | | ✓ | | ✓ | ✓ | | ✓ | |
| B. | | | | | | | ✓ | ✓ | | |
| Body Scheme: 13 | ✓ | | | | | | | ✓ | ✓ | |
| Leather Assembly: 14 | ✓ | ✓ | ✓ | ✓ | | ✓ | | | ✓ | ✓ |
| Food Preparation: 15 | ✓ | ✓ | ✓ | | | ✓ | ✓ | | | ✓ |

*Fig. 3-28. The JPSA profile sheet, here shown filled out in the column at the far right with the maximum time limit in minutes for each task.*

Name: ____________________

| Ability to Follow Directions | | | Conceptual Skills | Task Focus | Behavioral Observations | Time |
|---|---|---|---|---|---|---|
| Visual | Written | Verbal | | | | minutes |
| | | ✓ | | ✓ | | 2 |
| | ✓ | | ✓ | ✓ | | 10 |
| | ✓ | | ✓ | ✓ | | 5 |
| | ✓ | | ✓ | ✓ | | 3 |
| | | | | ✓ | | 5 |
| | | ✓ | | ✓ | | 2 |
| | | | | ✓ | | 8 |
| ✓ | | ✓ | | ✓ | | 6 |
| | ✓ | | ✓ | ✓ | | 8 |
| | | ✓ | | ✓ | | 6 |
| | | ✓ | ✓ | ✓ | | 10 |
| | | ✓ | | ✓ | | 12 |
| | | ✓ | | ✓ | | 5 |
| | ✓ | | | ✓ | (variable) | 10 |
| | | ✓ | ✓ | ✓ | | 2 |
| | | ✓ | ✓ | ✓ | | 5 |
| | | ✓ | ✓ | ✓ | | 5 |
| | | ✓ | ✓ | ✓ | | 5 |
| | ✓ | ✓ | ✓ | ✓ | | 10 |
| | | ✓ | ✓ | ✓ | | 4 |
| | | ✓ | ✓ | ✓ | | 1 |
| | | ✓ | ✓ | ✓ | | 2 |
| | | ✓ | | ✓ | | 2 |
| | | ✓ | | ✓ | | 5 |
| | | ✓ | | ✓ | | 5 |
| ✓ | | ✓ | | ✓ | | 10 |
| ✓ | | | | ✓ | | 12 |
| ✓ | | | | ✓ | | 8 |

EVALUATION BATTERY

The assessment consists of 15 informal tasks involving functional ability in the following skill areas: fine motor coordination, eye-hand coordination, motor planning, figure-ground discrimination, sorting, classification and sequencing, decision making, problem solving, organizational skills, use of tools, ability to follow directions, conceptual skills, task focus, and work-related behavior (Fig. 3-27).

IMPRESSIONS AND OBSERVATIONS

Keith was cooperative and pleasant throughout the testing session. He presented himself as a charming, mature young gentleman and engaged easily in social conversation.

During the test Keith said that he understood instructions; however, his performance showed otherwise. He did not ask for assistance with tasks or clarification of instructions when it was clear that he was unsure how to continue with the test items. Keith worked close to the table at a very slow, steady pace. His task focus was good.

Keith had difficulty following two- and three-step oral, written, and visual directions. Performance of tasks involving visual and oral directions broke down when an auditory or visual memory component was introduced.

Fine motor coordination is a problem area for Keith. While he was able to complete all tasks, fine motor movements were slow and labored and appeared to require concentration.

Keith's conceptual skills of alphabetizing and money use were limited. Difficulty arose when he was asked to alphabetize words beginning with the same letter. He was also unable to perform simple calculations involving coin values under $1.00. He had difficulty with matching skills but was able to complete concrete tasks involving classifying and sequencing.

Keith's performance broke down when multiple visual stimuli were presented, perhaps because of difficulty with figure-ground discrimination and visual perception.

STRENGTHS

1. Cooperative and friendly
2. Socially pleasant
3. Good task focus
4. Good classification and sequencing skills
5. Adequate sorting of concrete items
6. Functional eye-hand coordination

WEAKNESSES

1. Poor fine motor coordination
2. Weak in problem solving and decision making
3. Inability to recognize or verbalize his needs
4. Difficulty following oral, written, and visual directions
5. Poor memory
6. Weak in alphabetizing
7. Poor in money use
8. Weak in using written directions
9. Poor figure-ground discrimination
10. Poor motor planning

RECOMMENDATIONS

It is recommended that Keith continue with his present occupational therapy schedule of two small group sessions per week and his volunteer job in the school resource room (filing, photocopying, acting as a receptionist) once per week with consultation provided by the occupational therapist. It is also recommended that in all classrooms and workshops material be presented using a combined format of simplified oral, visual, and written directions.

SUGGESTED GOALS AND TREATMENT

1. To improve fine motor coordination; proper use of oral, written, and visual directions; problem solving; and decision making through fabrication of a date book and other age-appropriate craft and leisure activities.
2. To improve fine motor coordination and motor planning skills (incorporating memory) through babysitter's training course and other work-related training, such as cooking and sewing.
3. To improve figure-ground discrimination, alphabetizing, communication, problem-solving, and decision-making skills, Keith will participate in school yearbook activities and continue part-time work in the resource room, where occupational therapy consultation will be provided.
4. To improve Keith's ability to verbalize his needs through proper feedback and reinforcement during the above activities.

## References


1. Anastasi, A. Psychological Testing (3rd ed.). New York: Macmillan, 1968.
2. Bottersbusch, K. F., and Sax, A. B. *A Comparison of Commercial Vocational Evaluation Systems.* Menomonie, Wisconsin: Materials Development Center, Stout Rehabilitation Institute, University of Wisconsin, 1980.
3. Gerber, P. J. "Learning Disabilities and Vocational Education—Realities and Challenges," in K. P. Lynch, W. E. Kiernan, and J. A. Starks (Eds.). *Prevocational and Vocational Education for Special Needs Youth: A Blueprint for the 1980s.* Baltimore: Paul H. Brookes, 1982. Pp. 185–197.
4. Hopkins, H. L., and Smith, H. D. *Willard and Spackman's Occupational Therapy* (6th ed.). Philadelphia: Lippincott, 1983.
5. Institute for the Crippled and Disabled (ICD) Rehabilitation and Research Center. TOWER (Testing, Orientation, and Work Evaluation in Rehabilitation). Write to ICD, 340 East Twenty-fourth St., New York, N.Y. 10010.
6. Kester, D. L. "Prevocational and Vocational Assessment," in H. L. Hopkins and H. D. Smith. *Willard and Spackman's Occupational Therapy* (6th ed.). Philadelphia: Lippincott, 1983.
7. Lynch, K. P., Kiernan, W. E., and Stark, J. A. (Eds.). *Prevocational and Vocational Education for Special Needs Youth: A Blueprint for the 1980s.* Baltimore: Paul H. Brookes, 1982.
8. Trombly, C. A., and Scott, A. D. *Occupational Therapy for Physical Dysfunction.* Baltimore: Williams & Wilkins, 1977.

# Appendix:
# Jacobs Prevocational Skills Assessment Manual

In this section, the manual for the Jacobs Prevocational Skills Assessment is presented. You may photocopy these pages; spiral binding will facilitate use.

INTRODUCTION OF ASSESSMENT TO STUDENT
The therapist should read the following to the student before beginning the assessment:

I am going to be giving you an OT assessment, which consists of 15 different tasks relating to work. Each task is timed, and I will let you know during each task when your time is up. Please try each task and do the best you can. Throughout the assessment I will be writing some notes to help me remember what you have done. After you have completed the whole assessment, we will set up another time to meet. At that meeting I will be able to explain the results to you. Do you have any questions before we begin? [Wait for a response.] Then let's begin.

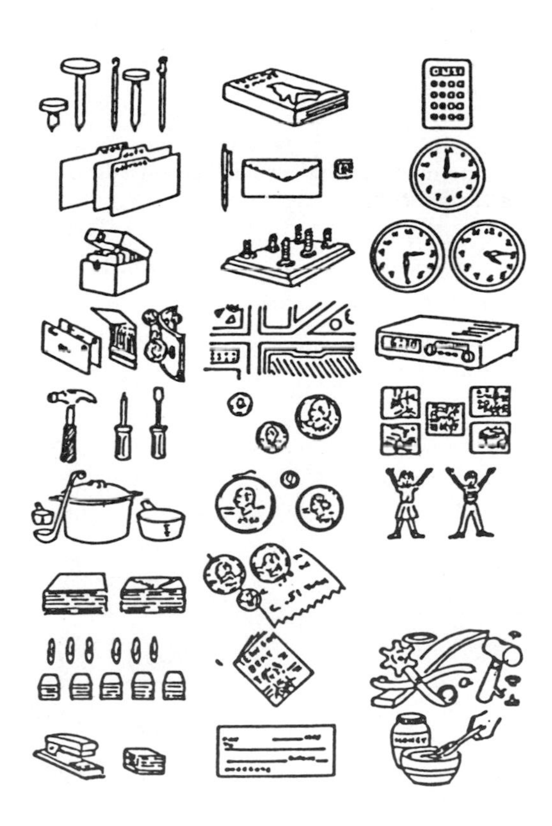

**Task 1**

QUALITY CONTROL

*Purpose*
Sorting
*Materials:*
16 2½-inch nails
10 odd-size and bent nails
*Instructions*
The student is seated to the left of the therapist. The 26 nails are randomly arranged on the table in front of the student, at his or her midline.

After the materials are arranged, the therapist picks up one of the 2½-inch nails in his or her right hand and shows it to the student, saying:

Please find all the nails that look the same as this nail. Put all the same nails here. [Point to the right side of the table.] Put all the different nails here. [Point to the left side of the table.] The different nails are ones that are bent or much thinner or thicker than this nail. [Show the student one of the 2½-inch nails in the pile.] Do you understand? [Wait for a response.] Please begin. [Place model nail below pile of nails.]

*Timing*
Begin timing the moment the student has acknowledged that he or she understands the task instructions.

**Task 2**

FILING

*Purpose*
Sequencing
Conceptual skills

*Part A*
*Materials*
26 white cards (3″ × 5″), each bearing one word beginning with each letter of the alphabet. Most of the words are related to work.
Instruction card (4¼″ × 5½″)
*Instructions*
If the student is unable to read, the therapist should read instructions aloud. For students who have difficulty comprehending verbal instructions, the therapist may demonstrate both parts.

A written instruction card is placed on the table directly in front of the student, 6 inches from the front of the table. The therapist instructs the student to read the card silently. After the student has read it, the card is removed. The therapist places on the table directly in front of the student, 6 inches from the edge of the table, a well-shuffled stack of cards. The therapist asks, "Do you have any questions? [Wait for a response.] Please begin."

*Part B*
Parts B and C are presented to the student only if he or she was able to attempt the preceding part.
*Materials*
1 (5¼″ × 3½″ × 3″) plastic card file
1 set of *A* to *Z* guides for 3″ × 5″ index cards
13 white lined (3″ × 5″) index cards each bearing a different name with a first initial
1 instruction card (4¼″ × 5½″)
*Instructions*
Written instructions are placed in front of the student as in Part A. After the student has read the instructions silently, the card is removed. The therapist arranges the materials as shown below and asks, "Do you understand? [Wait for a response.] Please begin."

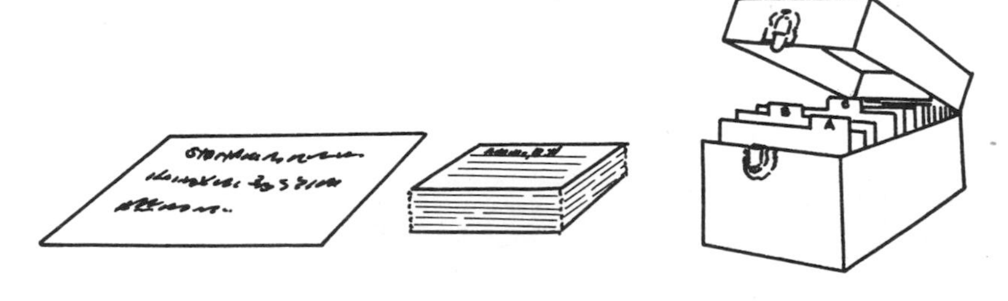

*Part C*

*Materials*

6 white cards (4″ × 3″) each bearing one of the following words written in bold capital letters: MONEY, MATCH, MAIL, MAIN, MISS, MUCH
1 instruction card (4¼″ × 5½″)
1 plastic card file and *A* to *Z* guides from Part B

*Instructions*

Written instructions are placed in front of the student as in Parts A and B. After the student has read the instructions silently, the card is removed. The therapist arranges the materials as in Part B and asks, "Do you understand? [Wait for a response.] Please begin."

*Timing*

Begin timing the moment after you say *begin* in each part.

4

**Task 3**

CARPENTRY ASSEMBLY

*Purpose*
Eye-hand coordination
Use of tools
*Materials*
1 pine board (6″ × 4″ × 2″) with nails and screws as shown below (two nails and three screws are ¾ of the way into the wood):
1 hammer (4-oz.)
1 blade-head screwdriver
1 Phillip's-head screwdriver
1 6 × 2″ Phillips Screw
1 6 × 2″ flat-head blade screw
1 6 × 1½″ Phillips Screw
1 1″ 4d nail
1 1½″ 4d nail
1 2″ 4d nail (single nail placed in board by student)
*Instructions*
The student stands in front of a table of appropriate height, with materials arranged as shown below:

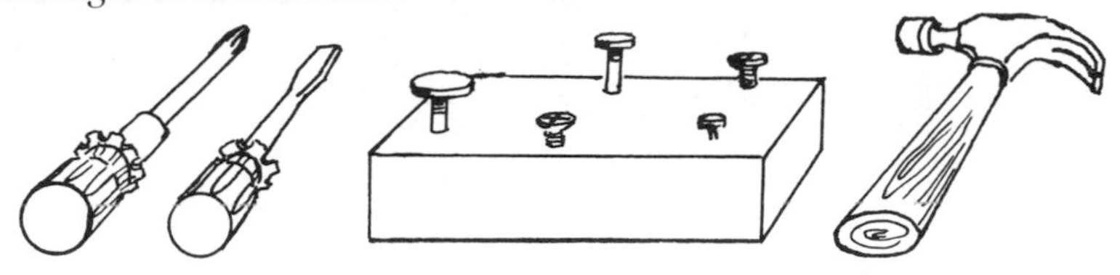

The therapist asks the student the following questions:

What is this? [Point to the blade-head screwdriver.]
What is this? [Point to the Phillip's-head screwdriver.]
What is this? [Point to the hammer.]

If the student is unable to name the tools, the therapist should say

Show me the screwdriver.
Show me the hammer.

The therapist then says

Use the hammer and screwdrivers to make all the nails and screws flat into the wood. Do you understand? [Wait for a response.] Please begin.

After the student has completed this part, the therapist says

Hammer this nail [places a single nail on the table] into the wood. Do you understand? [Wait for a response.] Please begin.

*Timing*
Begin timing the moment after you say *begin.*

**Task 4**

CLASSIFICATION

*Purpose*
Classification
*Materials*
1 illustration (9″ × 12″) of a restaurant kitchen (optional use)
12 cards (4½″ × 5″) each bearing a drawing of an item related to a restaurant kitchen
5 cards (4½″ × 5″) each bearing a drawing of an item unrelated to a kitchen
*Instructions*
The therapist arranges the materials as shown:

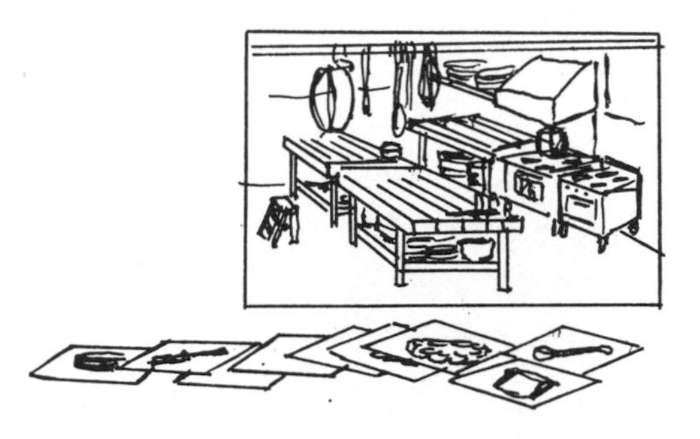

The therapist says:

Find all the cards with items that belong in a restaurant kitchen. Place these cards here. [Point to an area to the right of the materials.] Do you understand? [Wait for a response.] Please begin.

*Timing*
Begin timing the moment after you say *begin.*

**Task 5**

OFFICE WORK

*Purpose*
Organizational skills
Use of tools (Part A)
Ability to follow written directions (Part C)

*Part A*
*Materials*
1 standard-size stapler
6 standard-size business cards
5 sheets white paper (8½" × 11")
*Instructions*
Each part is first demonstrated by the therapist. The therapist demonstrates this part while saying the following:

This is a job that you might do if you worked in an office. Take one business card and staple it at the top of a piece of paper, like this. [The card is also centered at the top of the sheet.] Now you do the same with the other sheets.

Arrange the materials for Part A as shown below:

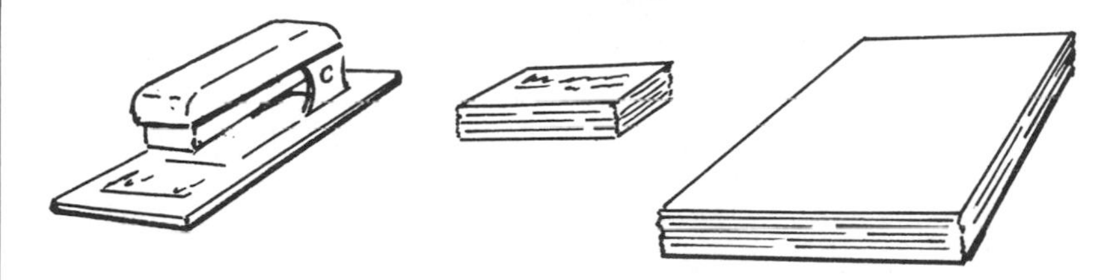

*Part B*
*Materials*
5 white sheets with stapled cards from Part A
5 business-size white envelopes
*Instructions*
Arrange materials as shown below:

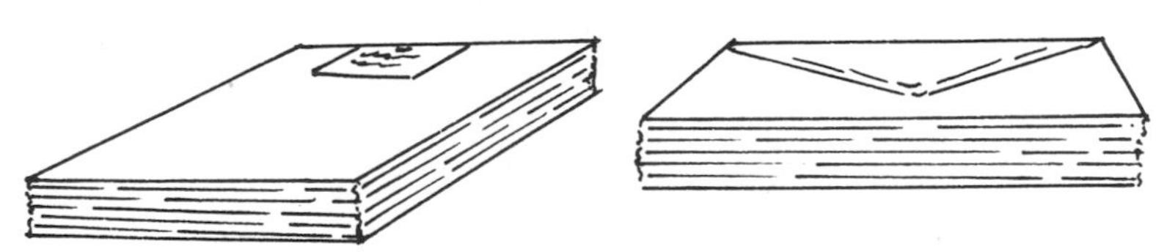

The therapist demonstrates this part while saying the following:

Take one sheet at a time and fold it into thirds. Put this folded sheet into one of the unsealed envelopes. Then put the envelope here. [Point to the right side of the table, 12 inches from the front.] Now you do the same with the other sheets and envelopes.

*Part C*

*Materials*

17 sheets of red construction paper (3½″ × 6″)
 5 sheets of pink construction paper (3½″ × 6″)
 5 sheets of green construction paper (3½″ × 6″)
11 sheets of orange construction paper (3½″ × 6″)
 5 sheets of yellow construction paper (3½″ × 6″)
 1 two-sided instruction card (4¼″ × 5″)
 6 standard-size paper clips
Part B materials (envelopes filled with folded sheets)

*Instructions*

Arrange the materials as shown below:

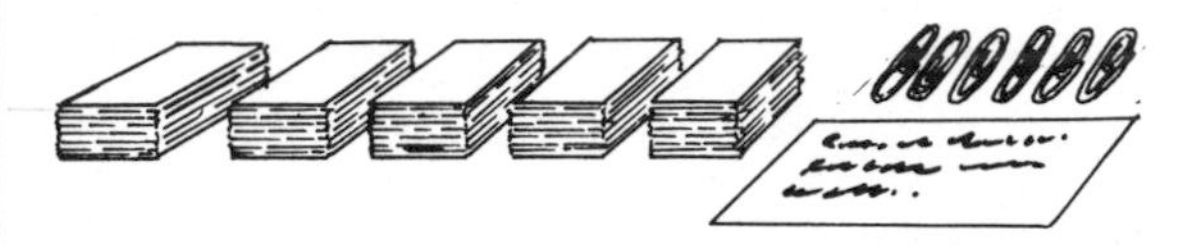

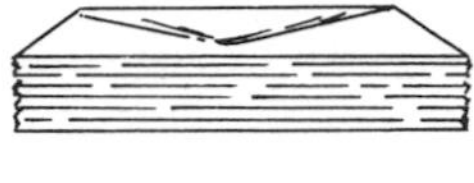

The therapist points to the stacks of paper one at a time from left to right asking the student to name the color of each stack.

Then the therapist places the instruction card on the table and instructs the student to read it silently.

After the student has read the card, the therapist asks, "Do you have any questions? [Wait for a response.] Please begin." The instruction card remains on the table throughout this part.

*Timing*

Begin timing the moment after you complete giving the task instructions.

8

**Task 6**

TELEPHONE DIRECTORY

*Purpose*
Figure-ground discrimination
Organizational skills
Conceptual skills
Fine motor coordination

*Part A*
*Materials*
1 telephone directory (9″ × 11″)
1 #2 pencil
1 index card (3″ × 5″) with the following information in bold print:

NAME ______
ADDRESS ______
______
TELEPHONE NUMBER ______

*Instructions*
Arrange the materials as shown:

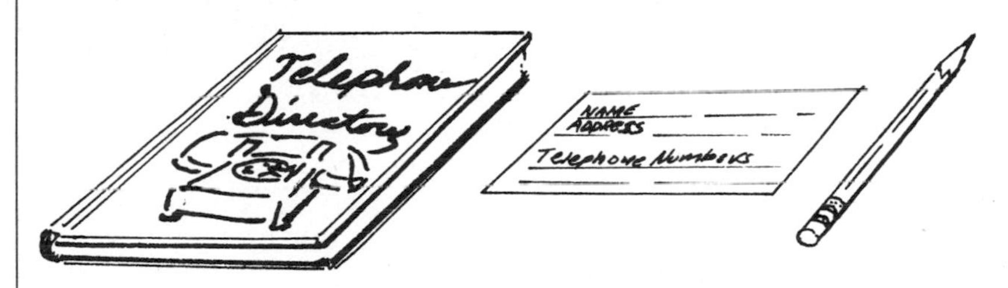


Before performing the assessment, the therapist should look through the telephone directory and select a company name that is written in bold print. This name will be used in both parts of this task.

After the materials are arranged the therapist says:

Here is a telephone directory. Use the telephone directory to look up the address and telephone number of [selected name]. When you have found the address and telephone number, write them on this index card. [Point to the card.] Do you understand? [Wait for a response.] Please begin.

*Part B*
*Materials*
1 white business-size envelope
1 pen
1 postage stamp
1 index card with information from Part A

*Instructions*
Arrange the materials as shown below:

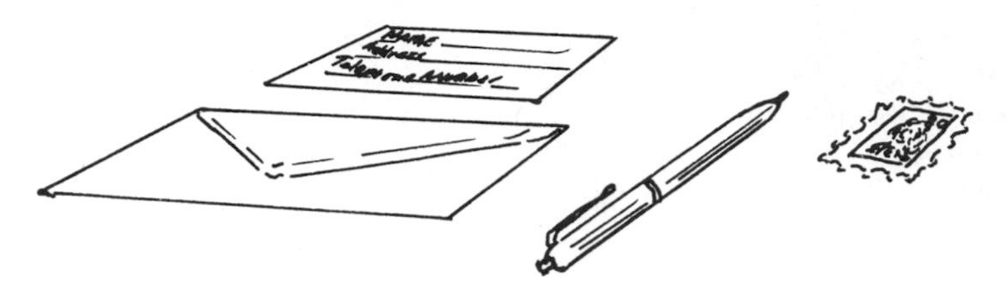

The therapist says the following:

Now we want to send this envelope to [selected name]. Please write the name and address of [name] on the envelope. Write your return address and put this stamp on the envelope, too. Do you understand? [Wait for a response.] Please begin.

*Timing*
Begin timing the moment after you say *begin.*

10

## Task 7

FACTORY WORK

*Purpose*
Fine motor coordination
Matching
Problem solving
*Materials*
1 5½″ × 11″ × 1″ wooden board
1 ⁵⁄₁₆″ × 3″ bolt with 2 matching nuts
1 ⅜″ × 3″ with 2 matching nuts
1 ½″ × 3″ bolt with 2 matching nuts
1 ¼″ × 3″ bolt with 2 matching nuts
1 8/32 × 3″ screw with 3 matching nuts
1 6/32 × 3″ screw with 3 matching nuts
1 small plastic bowl

*Instructions*
The student is seated, and the therapist arranges the materials as shown:

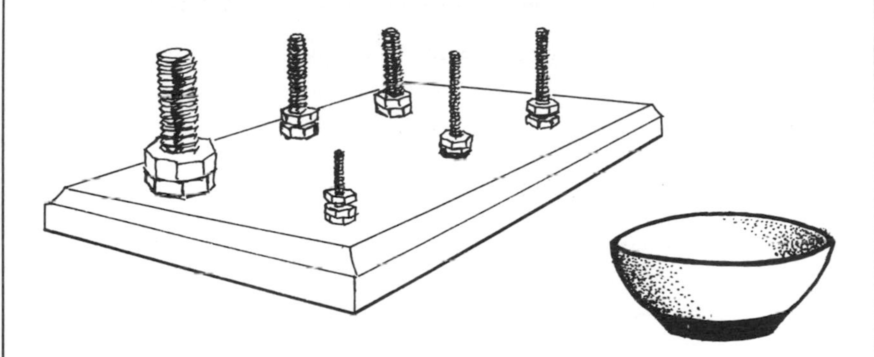

The therapist reads aloud the following directions for the student:

There are six bolts with nuts on them. [Point to the wooden board.] Take *all* the nuts off the bolts and put them into this bowl. [Point to the bowl.] After *all* the nuts are in the bowl, put them all back on the bolts. Do you understand? [Wait for a response.] Please begin.

*Timing*
Begin timing the moment after you say *begin*.

**Task 8**

ENVIRONMENTAL MOBILITY

*Purpose*

Motor planning
Problem solving
Ability to follow written directions

*Part A*

*Materials*

1 map of Washington, D.C. (14″ × 23″)
1 broad-tip black marking pen
1 piece of clear plastic cut to the dimensions of the map (14″ × 23″)

*Instructions*

The materials are arranged as shown below:

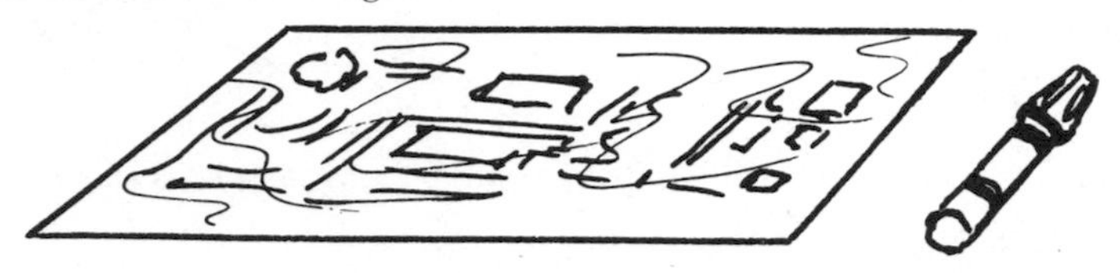

The therapist reads the following instructions aloud:

Please use this marking pen [point to the marking pen] to show the route you would follow when you arrive in Washington, D.C., at the train station [point to the train station on the map] and then want to see the sights first at the White House [point to the White House on the map] and then at the Jefferson Memorial [point to the Jeffereson Memorial on the map]. Please remember to follow the streets and not to cross over the lines. Do you have any questions? [Wait for a response.] Please begin.

*Part B*

*Materials*

1 instruction card (5″ × 7″)
1 envelope

*Instructions*

Before beginning this part, the therapist should have devised an instruction card with a simple step-by-step errand. If the errand is to retrieve an item (the envelope), be sure to place the item in its appropriate place before the task.

The therapist hands the student the instruction card and says:

Please follow the written directions on the card to do an errand for me. Do you understand? [Wait for a response.] Please begin.

If the student is unable to read or comprehend instructions, the therapist should accompany the student on this task while reading instructions aloud for the student to follow.

*Timing*

Begin timing the moment after you say *begin.*

12

## Task 9

MONEY CONCEPTS

*Purpose*
Conceptual skills: number and number quantity, money and money quantity

*Part A*
*Materials*
1 penny
1 nickel
1 dime
1 quarter
1 dollar bill

*Instructions*
When you remove the file for this task, shake it and ask the student, "What does this sound like?"

The therapist removes one penny and places it on the table in front of the student 6 inches from the front of the table and asks, "What is this?"

The therapist removes one nickel from the file and places it on the table to the right of the penny and asks, "What is this?"

The therapist carries out the same procedure with the dime, quarter, and dollar.

*Part B*
*Materials*
4 pennies
2 nickels
3 dimes
2 quarters

*Instructions*
All coins from Part A are removed. The therapist places four pennies on the table 6 inches from the front of the table and centered at the student's midline, and asks, "How much is this?"

The therapist removes three of the pennies and positions two nickels to the right of the penny. The therapist asks, "How much is this?"

The therapist removes all the coins and places one dime and one quarter in a row on the table 6 inches from the front of the table at the student's midline. The therapist asks, "How much is this?"

The therapist leaves these coins on the table and places one quarter, two dimes, two nickels, and four pennies in a row next to them. The therapist asks, "How much is this?"

*Part C*

*Materials*

1 cash register receipt with a total between $2.11 and $2.24
1 dollar bill
5 quarters
6 dimes
3 nickels
4 pennies

*Instructions*

All material from Part B are removed. The therapist arranges the materials as shown:

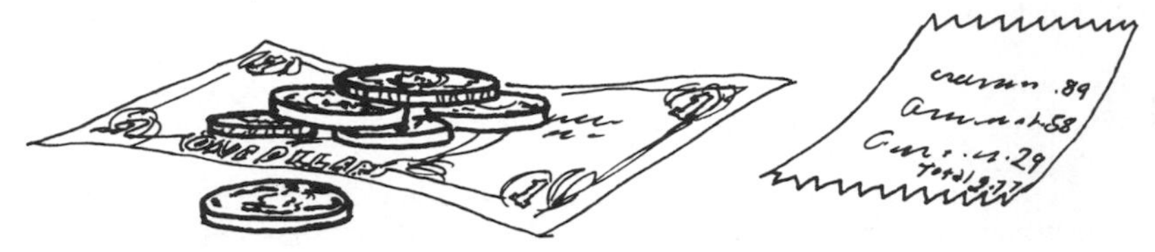

The therapist says, "Please find the total on the cash register receipt and read it out loud."
The therapist continues, "Please find the exact amount of money that you just read on the receipt [Point to the pile of money].

*Part D*

*Materials*

1 inexpensive magazine (priced under a dollar)
All the money from Part C

*Instructions*

The cash register receipt is removed from the table; all the money remains. The therapist holds the magazine in his or her left hand and says:

You are a sales clerk in a store, and I am a customer who would like to buy this magazine. Here is a dollar. [Hand the student the dollar bill from the pile of money on the table.] Please give me the correct change. [Hold out your hand with palm up.]

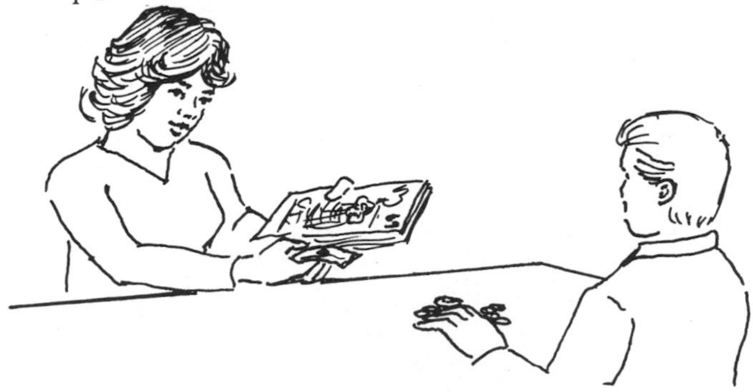

*Timing*

Begin timing after you have completed each question that calls for a response from the student.

**Task 10**

FUNCTIONAL BANKING

*Purpose*
Conceptual skills
Ability to follow written directions
Use of tools

*Part A*
*Materials*
1 bank check (3½″ × 10″)
1 #2 pencil
1 8½″ × 11″ sheet of white paper with the following information in bold print:
NAME ____________
1. What is the date on the check? ____________
2. What is the amount of the check? ____________
3. To whom is the money being paid? ____________
4. What is the account number? ____________
5. Whose account will the money come from? ____________

*Instructions*
The therapist arranges the materials as shown below:

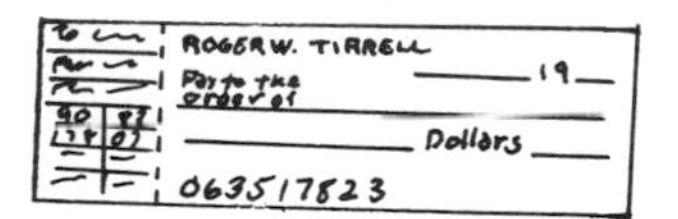


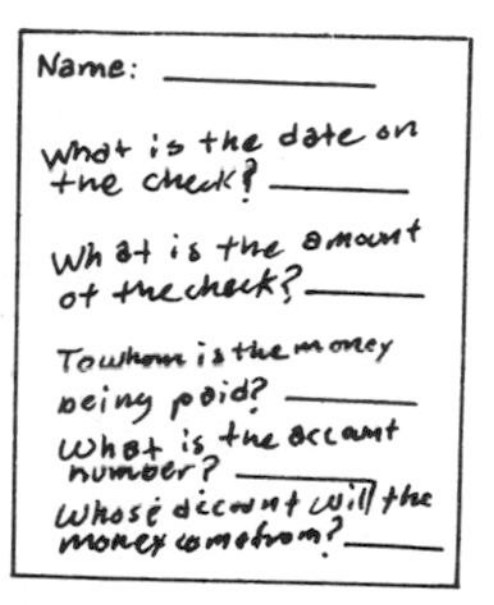


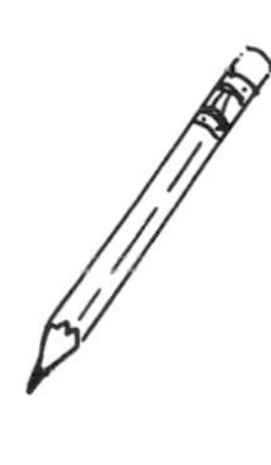

The therapist then says:

Here is a bank check. [Point to the check.] The questions on this paper [point to the paper] are about the bank check. Write the correct answers for each question. Do you have any questions? [Wait for a response.] Please begin.

*Part B*

*Materials*

1 calculator
1 bank check from Part A
1 #2 pencil

*Instructions*

The therapist removes the question sheet from Part A and arranges the materials as shown:

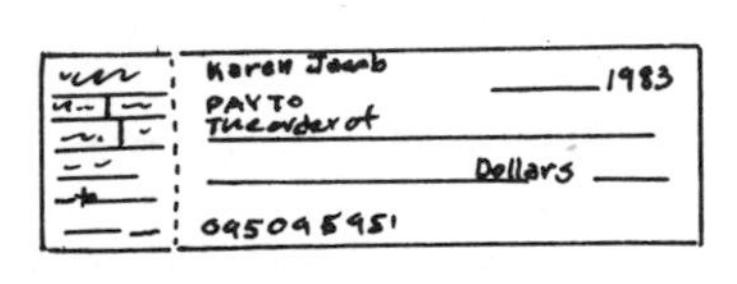


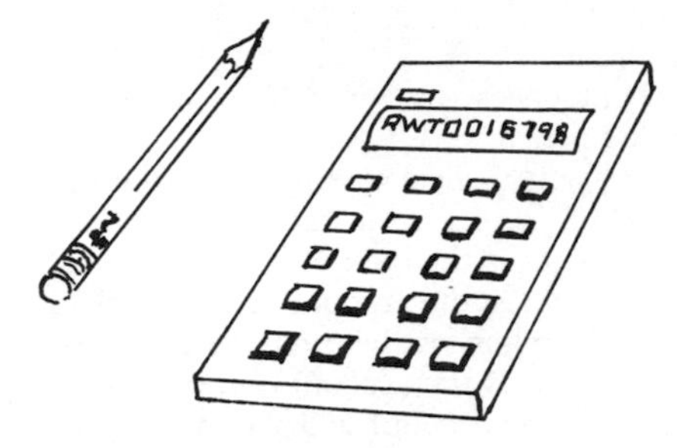

The therapist instructs the student:

Please use this calculator [point to calculator] to find the balance in this account after the check is paid. Please tell me the amount out loud. Do you have any questions? [Wait for a response.] Please begin.

*Timing*

Begin timing the moment after you say *begin.*

**Task 11**

TIME CONCEPTS

*Purpose*
Conceptual skills

*Part A*
*Materials*
1 3″ × 5″ card with a drawing of a clock reading 3:00 (clock #1)
1 3″ × 5″ card with a drawing of a clock reading 3:30 (clock #2)
1 3″ × 5″ card with a drawing of a clock reading 4:15 (clock #3)

*Instructions*
The therapist places clock 1 on the table 6 inches from its edge and centered in front of the student. The therapist asks, "What time is it?" [Point to the clock.]

The therapist follows a similar procedure with clocks 2 and 3.

*Part B*
*Materials*
Clocks 2 and 3
*Instructions*
Clocks 2 and 3 are placed next to each other on the table 6 inches from its edge and centered in front of the student. The therapist says, "It is in the afernoon. Which clock has the later time?"

*Part C*
*Materials*
1 3″ × 5″ card with a drawing of a digital clock reading 12:40
*Instructions*
All items from Part B are removed, and the digital clock card is place on the table 6 inches from the edge and centered in front of the student. The therapist says:

Please look at this clock. If you are taking a break at this time [point to clock], what time would it be after 30 mintues?

*Timing*
Begin timing the moment after you have completed each question.

**Task 12**

WORK ATTITUDES

*Purpose*
Sequencing
Work attitude
Decision making

*Part A*
*Materials*
5 cards (3½″ × 4¼″) each depicting a step in a sequence of a student purchasing food at a fast-food restaurant

*Instructions*
The therapist places the five cards randomly on the table within the student's reach and says:

These picture cards tell a story, but the pictures are all mixed up. Please put them in order from start [point to the left side of the table] to finish [points to the right side of the table]. Do you have any questions? [Wait for a response.] Please begin.

*Part B*
*Materials*
None
*Instructions*
The therapist removes the cards from the table and says:

You are working at McDonald's. Your job is to keep the shop clean. You are going on your lunch break when a customer drops a cup of coffee on the floor. What should you do? [Wait for response and then go on to next question.]

You have 15 minutes left to work. Your friend comes into McDonald's and says, "No one is looking. Why don't you leave work now?" What do you do? [Wait for a response and then go on to next question.]

You are working at the grill at McDonald's when a fire starts. What do you do?

*Timing*
Begin timing after you have completed giving each question.

## Task 13

BODY SCHEME

*Purpose*
Organizational skills
Visual memory
Position in space
Body scheme

*Materials*
1 8½″ × 11″ drawing of a teenage boy
5 drawings of the boy cut into the following parts: 5 heads, 5 torsos, 10 arms, 5 pairs of legs, 10 feet

*Instructions*
The drawing of the boy is placed on the table 6 inches from the edge and centered in front of the student. The therapist says:

Here is a picture of a boy. Look at this picture carefully. [Leave the picture on the table for 15 seconds and then remove it from the student's view.]

Arrange the five cut drawings of the boy on the table randomly and say:

Put these pieces together to make copies of the boy that was on the paper that was shown before. Do you have any questions? [Wait for a response.] Please begin.

*Timing*
Begin timing the moment after you say *begin.*

**Task 14**

LEATHER ASSEMBLY

*Purpose*
Organizational skills
Fine motor coordination
Use of tools
Reward (Student keeps finished product.)

*Materials*
1 standard-size rotary leather hole punch
1 wooden leather mallet (1½″ × 4″)
2 key rings
6 sets of small rivets
2 1″ × 3″ 7-oz leather strips
1 plastic box (4″ × 4″ × ½″) to hold rivets, leather, and rings

*Instructions*
Before giving this task, familiarize yourself with the construction of the key ring (see Fig. 3-23).

All materials are placed randomly on the table. Before beginning the assembly, the therapist says, "Watch what I do so you can do the same after I finish."

The therapist then demonstrates the construction of the key ring without speaking. When it is completed, the therapist says, "Now you make the same key ring." [Point to the model key ring and them remove it.]

*Timing*
Begin timing after you have completed the instructions.

Please note that since one of the purposes of this task is to reward the student, you should assist the student in completing the task if he or she is having difficulty.

20

**Task 15**

FOOD PREPARATION

*Purpose*
Ability to follow visual directions
Use of tools
Reward

*Materials*
1 stick of softened margarine
1 small jar of honey
1 small mixing spoon
1 teaspoon
1 butter knife
1 small plastic bowl
1 box of crackers
5 4¼″ × 5½″ cards showing how to make honey butter

*Instructions*
The illustration cards are placed on the table in a row from card 1 to card 5. All other materials are arranged randomly on the table. The therapist instructs the student

Please follow the cards to make honey butter. When you have finished making the butter, spread it on *two* crackers. You may eat the crackers with the butter when you are finished. Do you understand? Please begin.

*Timing*
Begin timing the moment after you say *begin.*

# 4. Work-Related Programs for Children and Adolescents

As indicated in Chapter 2, work-related programming should be initiated at an early age. This is particularly imperative with the "special needs" child. Throughout the United States, this policy is beginning to take hold, with academic curriculum and therapy being keyed more to work. Occupational therapy is beginning to take a more active role in this type of programming.

However, many occupational therapists face the problem of what to use to assess the child's functioning. Although many standardized and nonstandardized evaluations are available (see Chap. 3), few if any have been established primarily for the child or adolescent. Frequently the therapist must establish his or her own evaluation for use with the pediatric or adolescent population. The Jacobs Prevocational Skills Assessment (JPSA), which was discussed in detail in Chapter 3, is an example of such an assessment. Its versatility (its ability to be adapted to the various needs of learning-disabled children), its limited duration, its high-interest tasks, and its reward characteristics have made it a useful instrument in evaluation and program development.

In this chapter a small sampling of work-related occupational therapy programs being applied with various pediatric and adolescent populations will be presented. Although the programs described do not reflect the entire spectrum of disabilities served by the occupational therapist, taken as a whole they may contain the elements necessary for developing programs for any specified population.

## Little People's School

In 1970 the Little People's School was established as a private, nonprofit day school for students aged 3½ to 15 years with severe learning difficulties and language and hearing problems. The school serves 85 communities in the Boston area. It is certified by the Department of Education of the Commonwealth of Massachusetts for special needs children, conforming with Massachusetts Public Law 766 and U.S. Public Law 94-142.

Since 1979 the Little People's School has provided work-related occupational therapy programming to a preadolescent and adolescent learning-disabled population.* The work-related program was established to meet the changing needs of the occupational therapy population. Because of these students' ages, the need had arisen to begin planning programs that would assist in developing the behaviors and skills important for future vocational tasks and job placement.

The first step in the process of program development was to assess students' level of functioning. As indicated in Chapter 3, no assessments were available that could be utilized with a learning-disabled adolescent population. Therefore an assessment had to be developed. I devised the JPSA to meet this need. This 15-task evaluation assesses the student's ability in a variety of work-related areas (see Chap. 3 for an in-depth look at this instrument).

After the student has completed the JPSA, an interest inventory is sent to his or her home to ascertain leisure skills and interests. Information gathered from the assessment, the interest inventory, classroom observations, and informal discussions with the student and staff was used in developing the occupational therapy programs at the Little People's School. These programs include an arts and crafts fair, assorted crafts (e.g., needlepoint), business skills, food service skills, horticulture, job simulation, leathercraft, leisure and life skills, and woodworking. This is not an all-inclusive list of available activities. For example, the Little People's School has established a work activity center (see p. 113). Many other activities can readily be adapted to a work-related skills focus.

Because of limited funds, in developing each activity I investigated community and school resources. For example, for the business skills activity we needed equipment and supplies to simulate an office environment—typewriters, office furniture. IBM Corporation was contacted for typewriters because it has a special needs program that provides renovated electric typewriters at a reduced cost to persons with physical disabilities. In addition, IBM will provide, at a small cost, a spastic key guard, which is a shield that covers the keyboard and has holes cut out over the keys to prevent misstrikes. The key guards were not only useful for occupational therapy students who have cerebral palsy or motoric problems but were beneficial in some manner for the majority of students, by providing tactile input and making figure-ground distinctions easier. For more information on the IBM special needs program, contact your local office for eligibility criteria.

Stone & Webster Engineering Corporation was contacted for the donation of office furniture. The Corporation gladly gave us its obsolete items—typing tables, secretaries' desks, time clocks, filing racks, metal stamps—which were received as treasures for our program. We have an ongoing relationship with

*There are four common types of learning disabilities: (1) reading disabilities, which usually indicate perceptual difficulties; (2) language and writing problems—difficulty reproducing written symbols or repeating sounds; (3) problems with concepts and abstractions—an inability to find commonalities in beings or objects; and (4) behavior problems—distractibility, short attention span, inability to sit still, unwillingness to cooperate.

Stone & Webster, which generously donates outdated equipment and material for our students.

Local copy shops were contacted for surplus paper items. One such company eagerly kept for us a box of assorted scrap paper, which we carted away weekly.

## THEORETICAL FRAMEWORK

In each occupational therapy program, activities are presented in sequential order based on the hierarchical stages of play specified in the occupational behavior approach (see Chap. 2). These three stages are as follows:

1. *Exploratory play* is the earliest kind of play behavior; the individual is motivated by curiosity and interest in novelty. He or she "plays" with the many aspects of an object. In this process, the individual learns not only about the objects, but about his or her own capabilities and limits.
2. *Competency behavior* is a skill-building stage. In this stage one practices newly acquired skills in an effort to achieve mastery.
3. In the *achievement* stage the individual is engaged in interacting with the environment with an emphasis on performance, using an external standard of excellence and taking risks.

The rationale for using this model is that play is the antecedent to work. Gayle Thompson has devised a clinical model of vocational development that has been most beneficial in formulating the program (Fig. 4-1).

To ensure continuity in the occupational therapy program between the school's divisions (elementary and secondary), all occupational therapy is now based on a work-related skills training model. What this means in fact is that along with the student's academic curriculum, the majority of learning experiences provided have a direct relationship to career or prevocational development. It is hoped that by infusing these basic work skills at an elementary and middle school age, we will have a longer period of time for reinforcement. The difficulty one finds in attempting to provide vocational programming originating at a secondary level will, it is hoped, be alleviated by initiating this early training.

## OCCUPATIONAL THERAPY

### *Arts and Crafts Fair*

The goal of work-related occupational therapy programming is exemplified by our arts and crafts fair. The fair was created as an opportunity for students to make a transition into a work role, with exposure to other students, family, and the local community, within the confines of a safe, structured environment. This was all done within the milieu of the fair and its preparation (Fig. 4-2).

Preparation for the fair, which was originally held every spring, began

**Phase 1**

INITIATION: AWARENESS, INTEREST, MOTIVATION

*Models*
Hershenson's social-amniotic and self-differentiation stages
Reilly's exploration stage
Mosey's individual interaction (pregroup) and parallel group

*Goals*
Client feels safe and supported, discovers interests, becomes motivated, and seeks to become identified with the group of "workers" in the setting

*Climate*
Supportive, relatively free, nonstressful
Planned variety and novelty in surroundings to invite interest and exploration
Opportunity to explore, repeat, imitate successful models
Observable models of involvement; workmanlike, craftsmanlike, sportsmanlike behavior
Group members accept person first as visitor, then new member

*Therapist's Role*
Provides for client dependence and establishment of trust
Assistive, moving to some independence
Encourages, supports efforts
Gives guidance, provides some basic instruction

*Activity Attributes*
Exploration and engagement
Short-term, allowing for experimentation with variety of materials and products
Controllable materials and predictable products
Minimal tool use—either common tools or a few specialized or new tools
Choices available within activity materials and products
Use of different processes or independence in repeated processes
Exploration of what can be done (or will work) with certain materials

*Fig. 4-1. Clinical model of vocational development. (Courtesy Gayle Thompson, M.Ed., OTR.)*

**Phase 2**

MEMBERSHIP: SKILL AND HABIT DEVELOPMENT

*Models*
Hershenson's competence stage
Reilly's competence stage
Mosey's parallel, project, and egocentric cooperative groups

*Goals*
Client learns work skills and develops work habits and interpersonal behaviors, e.g., appropriately seeks feedback, accepts supervision, works cooperatively; acquires identity as a worker; finds areas of abilities and skills

*Climate*
Teaching-learning
Activity viewed as important in adult world
Role models of workers in instructors (staff and volunteers) and in peer groups
Opportunity to compare own performance with that of others
Specific knowledge of results of performance (work, habits, interpersonal)

*Therapist's Role*
Gives systematic instruction in work skills, tool use, and tool care
Gives clear orientation as to expected habits
Structures group interaction, provides model for task and maintenance roles, reinforces client in assumption of group and partner roles
Moves toward supervisor role
Provides feedback on skill and habit development and interpersonal attributes
Assists in problem solving and encourages independent problem solving

*Activity Attributes*
Skill development and problem solving
Products perceived as valued by adults
Longer-term, requiring delay of gratification and problem solving
Projects require planning, calculation, and organization of production
Emphasis on accomplishing whole processes
Creative expression is modified by tools and nature of materials
Problems require detection, correction, and assessment of results

**Phase Three**

TRANSITION: EXPERIMENTATION AND CHOICE

*Models*

Hershenson's independence stage
Reilly's achievement stage
Mosey's cooperative and mature groups

*Goals*

Client seeks to meet standards of quality and production, identifies realistic areas of aspiration and development, and moves toward making choice

*Climate*

In protective setting, client expected to meet standards of workmanship and to demostrate work habits acceptable in true work environment
In trial work placements, client tests work skills and habits with those of other workers
Independence and initiative are reinforced
Client participates in shop maintenance, assists others, or functions as a foreman

*Therapist and Client Roles*

Therapist as work supervisor; client as apprentice, sometimes foreman
Therapist as resource supporting independence in work and community job experimentation

*Activity Attributes*

Recognizing and attempting to meet standards
Advanced performance in areas of interest and skill selected by client
Transference of developed skills to real work tasks
Experimentation in real worker roles
Groups focusing on community and vocational reentry

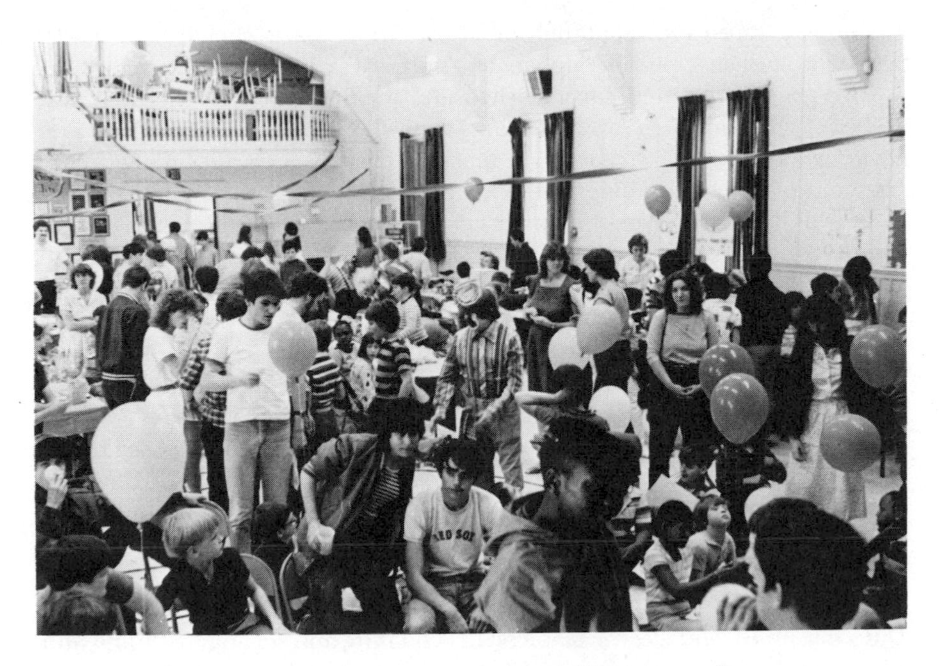

*Fig. 4-2. Little People's School arts and crafts fair, held semiannually.*

after Christmas vacation. Students from this time on prepared items that would be sold, for example, cookbooks, belts, plants, needlepoint projects. As the date of the fair approached, students in the food service program made their baked goods and other products. All aspects of the fair—setting prices, placing price tags on items, establishing student work schedules, advertising, setting up decorations, selling merchandise, and clean-up—were attended to by the students under the supervision of the therapist. In addition, there was an extra incentive for students' participation in the fair, a salary. This money came directly from the fair's proceeds.

The fair was such a success that we now hold it twice a year—before Christmas and during the spring—and it is now a school-wide event. We have encouraged local participation and have sold, on a limited basis, craft projects from other community programs that serve special needs persons, for example, Fernald State School (see Chap. 5).

*Business Skills*

The purpose of the business skills program is to expose students to typing as a means of communication. In addition, the development of typing skills strengthens fine motor and eye-hand coordination, visual discrimination, and memory.

Students are introduced to typing either individually or in groups of up to four. They are first allowed to explore the keyboard and are then instructed to type their own names. For the student who is unable to do this from memory, a typed representation of his or her name is shown as a guide. Next, the student types the alphabet in both capital and small letters.

Two texts were found particularly useful for these groups. The first, Jack Heller's *Typing for the Physically Handicapped: Methods and Keyboard Presentation Charts* is in two parts. The first part contains a discussion of effective methods of teaching typing to the handicapped. The second part contains 19 sets of keyboard presentation charts and drill lines for all possible combinations of missing fingers, for example, three fingers on the left hand and two on the right. Although this text is expensive ($100), the publisher has granted duplication rights to all illustrations [4]. The second text I found helpful was a linguistically oriented typing program called "Type It," developed by Joan Duffy, Learning Disabilities Supervisor for the Arlington Public Schools, Arlington, Massachusetts.*

When the student has gained some competency in typing and is beginning to use visual memory to find appropriate characters, he or she begins to type recipes for the school cookbook. This cookbook is subsequently duplicated and sold at the semiannual arts and crafts fair (Fig. 4-3).

In conjunction with typing, students are introduced to basic secretarial tasks: (1) the use of small office equipment such as photocopy machines, Ditto machines, and electric staplers; (2) collating and sorting; (3) filing and retrieving; (4) dictionary use; and (5) use of the telephone directory.

*Food Service*

Groups of two to three students are introduced to the kitchen by means of a simple step-by-step recipe book developed for these students (Fig. 4-3). The progression in the kitchen includes (1) safety and sanitation; (2) basic food preparation: spreading, pouring, opening, measuring and common abbreviations, and mixing; (3) knife skills; (4) basic kitchen appliance use: electric mixer, electric toaster oven, gas stove; (5) basic cooking: baking, frying and grilling, simmering, broiling; (6) setting a table; (7) serving meals; and (8) taking orders.

After the student has developed competency with the simple recipe book, he or she is introduced to regular step-by-step cookbooks and recipes cut off boxes or out of magazines. Finally he or she brings in a recipe that has been tested at home. Parents are encouraged to reinforce cooking skills at home with their children.

Role playing is an important aspect of these sessions. The roles of waiter or waitress, busboy or busgirl, salad maker, chef, host or hostess, and short-order cook are introduced.

These student groups prepare all the baked goods for our semiannual arts and crafts fair and during the fair cook egg rolls, pizza, and tacos.

*This program can be obtained from the author, c/o Arlington Public Schools, Arlington, Massachusetts 02174.

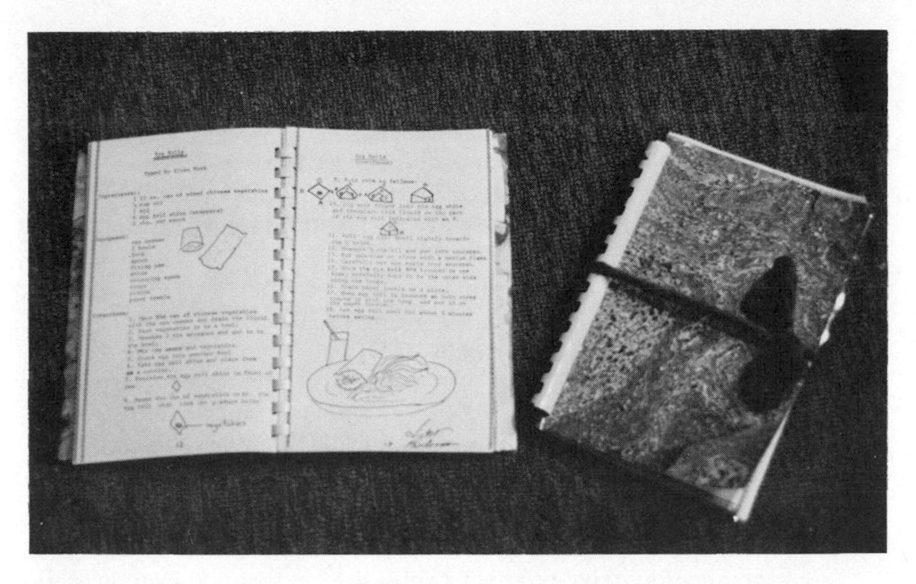

*Fig. 4-3. Simple step-by-step cookbook developed by and for Little People's School students.*

*Horticulture Training*

The horticulture training program has many purposes:

1. To expose the student to the fundamentals of greenhouse operation and processing; plant growth and identification; preparation of soil mixes; and seeding, potting, and planting techniques
2. To develop leisure interests
3. To develop vocational interests
4. To promote social skills such as working cooperatively, solving problems and making decisions in groups, and organizing school tours of the center and field trips to local nurseries

Since space is limited, our horticulture center is composed of three metal wall shelves, each with a 4-foot plant light suspended over it. Despite all odds, we have been able to grow numerous varieties of flowering and foliage plants and vegetables from seeds. In addition, we have grown herbs and bean sprouts, which were used in our food service program. Students in the horticulture training program are also involved in the arts and crafts fair by selling their school-grown plants.

The following sample gradation of simple to complex horticulture activities may be found useful in planning this type of program:

1. Moving plants from one shelf to another
2. Carrying pots to shelves after they have been washed

3. Filling trays with pebbles
4. Arranging flats in stairs
5. Spraying plants with a flower sprayer
6. Filling and carrying watering cans and flower sprayer
7. Determining when pebble tray is dry and filling it with water; determining when individual potted plants are dry and watering them with watering can
8. Fertilizing individual potted plants
9. Washing pots and sorting them according to size
10. Removing dead leaves from plants
11. Weeding flats of seedlings and potted plants
12. Swabbing foliage to eradicate insects
13. Transplanting plants from small pots to larger ones
14. Noting when cuttings have roots and planting them
15. Measuring fertilizer and applying it to plants
16. Taking cuttings from plants
17. Dipping cuttings into root-promoting substance and putting them in sand
18. Staking individual plants
19. Planting bulbs in pebbles
20. Planting seedlings in flats
21. Writing one's own name, the date, and the type of seed for identification
22. Arranging cut flowers in suitable vases
23. Reading a thermometer
24. Measuring the distance from the top of the plant to the plant light
25. Identifying and naming plants with the help of a book
26. Deciding on plant prices for the arts and crafts fair
27. Giving a tour of the horticulture center to other students and staff

*Job Simulation*

Job simulation is another method of reinforcing work skills and behaviors. Many jobs that simulate a work environment are available within the school, for example, office aide, maintenance assistant. The therapist uses these opportunities to have the student perform in a worker role under her supervision. In the case of the office aide, the student may run school errands or use the copy machine.

In addition, we frequently simulate the job of grocery store bagger, which is a realistic and age-appropriate job for some of our students. We have received support for this simulation from local supermarket chains that have given us supermarket supplies (e.g., a shopping cart) and have established programmed instructions on becoming a bagger.

*Leather Craft*

The rationale for using leather craft as a modality included (1) high student interest, (2) free access to equipment (I formerly had a leather business and lent all my equipment to the school), (3) limited cost or donation of supplies, and (4) the therapist's expertise. The occupational behavior model suggested the following sequence of activities:

1. The student is presented with a scrap piece of carving leather (6″ × 8″), a leather mallet, and 12 stamping tools and is allowed to explore this medium.
2. The therapist first demonstrates how to make a ¾-inch-wide name wristband and then instructs the student to make one. This activity entails picking the correct letters for one's name from the alphabet stamping tools, stamping these letters in the correct sequence using a mallet, and returning them to their appropriate position in the alphabet.
3. The student is instructed to make a 1½-inch-wide name belt.
4. The student chooses any appropriate project or one of the following projects: sun visor, wallet, coin purse, comb case.

*Leisure and Life Skills*

The occupational therapy department offered an eight-session leisure and life skills task group to four adolescent girls with the purpose of introducing options for using leisure time. This program evolved from the realization that a vast number of students spend their leisure time watching television or sitting at home with no conception of how to use unstructured time.

In this group the students were given the opportunity to decide on specific topics for each session. Each member, in addition to the therapist, was responsible for teaching topics. Briefly, these included naming the group and brainstorming for topics; a cooking project (Syrian bread); care of clothing—how to iron, fold, and hang clothing properly; making a leather name bracelet; grooming—use of makeup, nail care; babysitting; a needlepoint project; and gardening and flower arranging.

*Woodworking*

Students are exposed to basic woodworking activities by using prefabricated kits to make napkin holders, hot plates, key holders, and other items. The students learn to recognize and use tools and to handle tools safely. They also learn sanding, gluing, staining, varnishing, and sawing.

## Learning Prep School

As the Little People's School administration realized the success of the school's work-related occupational therapy program and the lack of a similar secondary program in the area, the school was expanded in 1980 to include a secondary division. This division, called the Learning Prep School, serves approximately 140 students 15 to 22 years old (Fig. 4-4). It offers a language-based, life-centered curriculum designed to be flexible to meet the needs of the students. The program may lead to a high school equivalency diploma.

In addition to functional academic education, the school offers several work-

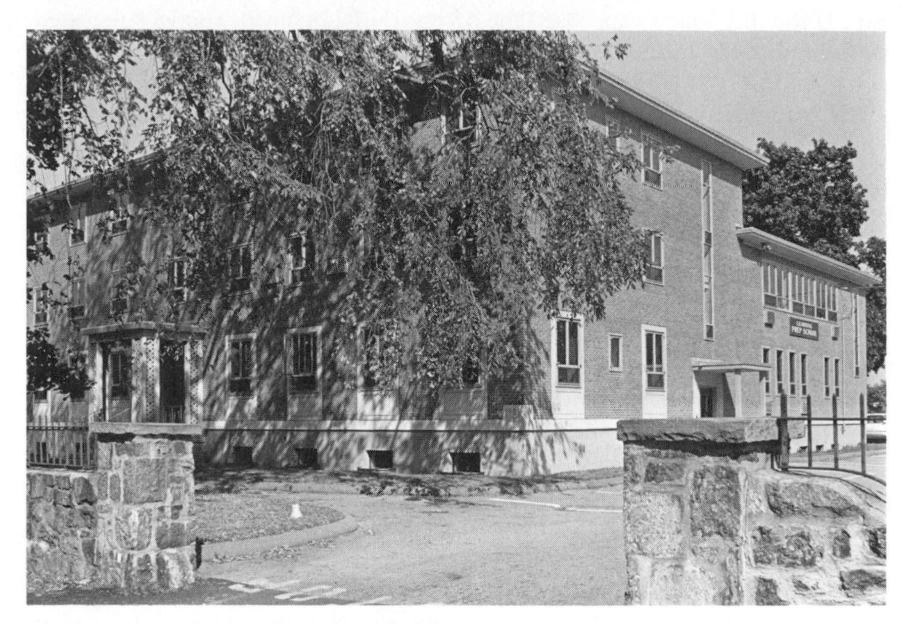

*Fig. 4-4. Learning Prep School, located in West Newton, Massachusetts.*

related programs: a vocational program consisting of ten vocational training workshops; an occupational therapy program that provides both evaluations and treatment in the form of task groups; and a work-study program that provides job placements in the community. These three programs are described in the following sections.

VOCATIONAL PROGRAM

At the time the Learning Prep School was being developed, I was asked to become its vocational coordinator and to develop and implement a vocational program. Because of the success of the occupational therapy program in the lower division, I used it as the basis for the vocational program in the upper division.

The current and projected job market and the types of industry in the local area assisted in determining the choices of vocational areas to be offered in the program. Extensive research was performed by investigating regional vocational and technical schools and exploring the help wanted ads in the local newspapers. Other helpful resources included the Massachusetts Division of Employment Security, the Materials Development Center, Stout Vocational Rehabilitation Institute, University of Wisconsin–Stout (Menomonie, Wisconsin 54751), and the Jewish Vocational Services. After this in-depth search it became apparent that some of the original work-related occupational therapy programs could be expanded into vocational workshops. However, during the development of the programs, positive work behavior as the antecedent to specific skill development was recognized as equivalent in importance to

Student: ____________ Teacher: ____________
Workshop: *Graphic Arts* Signature: ____________
Classes per Week: ____________

FOCUS
(*indicates areas of concentration)

*Illustrating*
____________ Identifying, designing, and illustrating a logo
____________ Identifying and using basic typefaces in advertising
____________ Identifying, designing, laying out, and pasting up an ad
____________ Designing and illustrating an egg-shaped cartoon for advertising
____________ Designing and illustrating a fashion ad, a record album cover, and a magazine cover

*Printing*
____________ Operating the platemaker (installing, checking, and cleaning the electrostatic plates)
____________ Operating the plate processor
____________ Loading, operating, and maintaining the Gestetner Offset Press (switchboard, panel controls, handwheel controls, and feed-out board set-up)

SHOP PERFORMANCE AND BEHAVIOR
____________ Arrives on time
____________ Organizes work area
____________ Uses and cares for equipment properly
____________ Follows directions
____________ Attends to task
____________ Uses time efficiently
____________ Uses skills taught appropriately
____________ Completes a given task
____________ Interacts positively with peers
____________ Interacts positively with instructor

Comments

*Fig. 4-5. Checklist used by graphic arts teacher Roger Tirrell at the Learning Prep School. Note the emphasis on work-related skills and behavior.*

job training. Therefore certain workshops that may not result in job placements were nevertheless included because they facilitate the development of interpersonal skills; responsibility to self, peers, and employers; and self-esteem. All the workshops operate on the premise that the development of work-related skills and behaviors is the basis for future job skills. This is reinforced by the school's system of grading, which reinforces workshop performance and behaviors such as arriving on time, organizing one's work area, attending to the task at hand, interacting positively with peers, and following directions (Fig. 4-5).

The original Learning Prep School workshops were business skills, car-

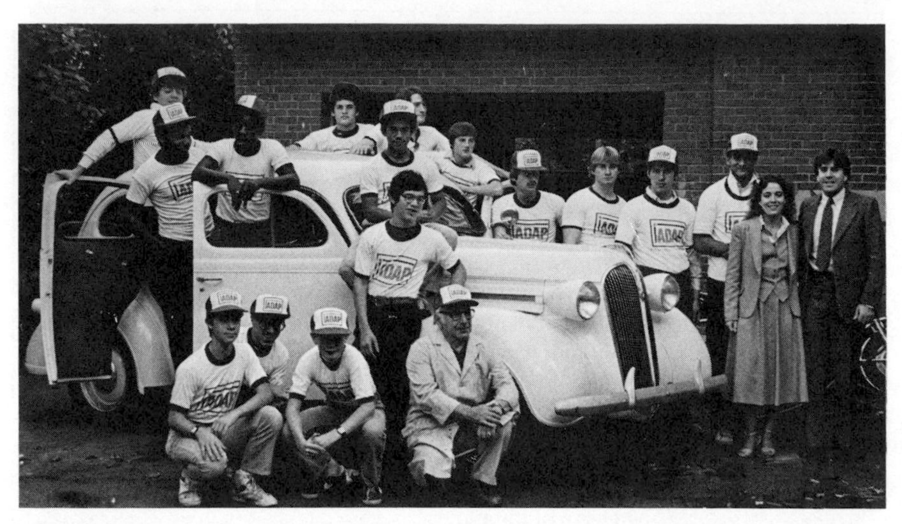


*Fig. 4-6. Learning Prep School students with the 1937 Plymouth donated to the school's automotive workshop.*

pentry, food service, graphic arts, horticulture, masonry, photography, and sewing. However, yearly research performed by the school to keep pace with the current and predicted job market revealed the need to expand or eliminate existing workshops and to develop new ones. Presently the school provides vocational training in the following fields: (1) automotive maintenance, (2) bicycle maintenance, (3) business skills, (4) carpentry, (5) child care, (6) food service, (7) graphic arts, (8) horticulture, (9) building maintenance, and (10) photography.

As with the work-related program for the lower division, the upper division vocational program was faced with limited funding. Once again I turned to the local community for support. For example, ADAP Discount Auto Parts stores donated supplies to begin the automotive maintenance program. Their interest in our school has continued, and in 1983 they donated a 1937 Plymouth, which was refurbished by the students and shortly afterward was sold as a school fund raiser (Fig. 4-6).

The vocational workshops are described below.

*Automotive Maintenance*

Training covers a variety of areas of automobile service, ranging from car washing and simple service-station-attendant functions to small-engine maintenance (Fig. 4-7).

*Bicycle Maintenance*

Students are trained in repairing and servicing bicycles and accessories. The assembly and inspection of parts is an integral part of the program. This

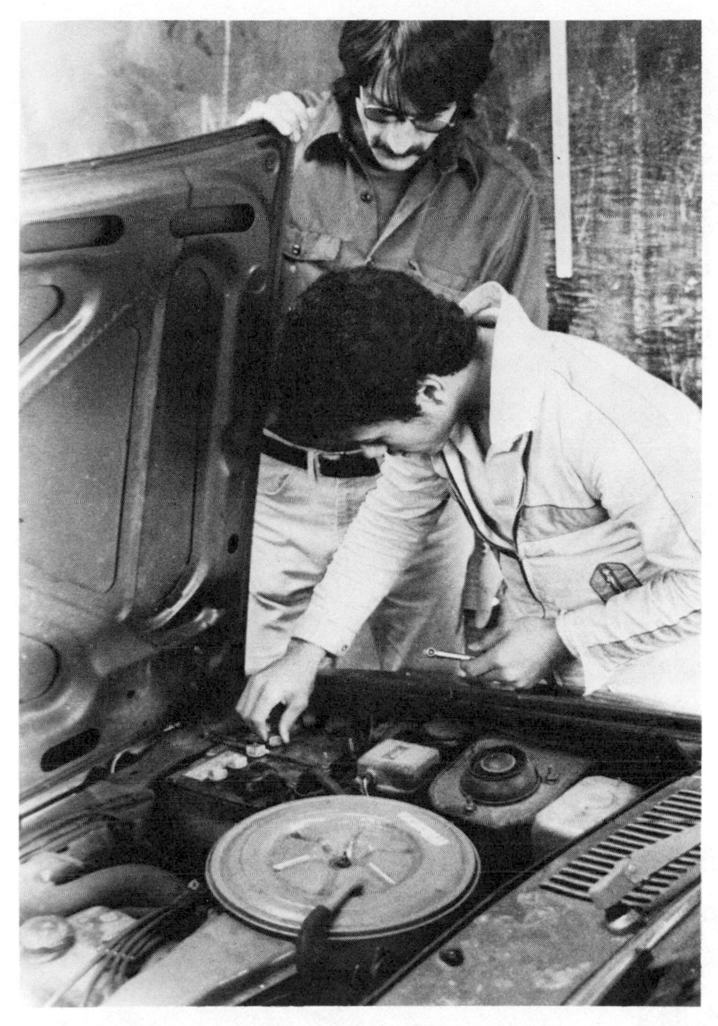

*Fig. 4-7. A class in automotive maintenance at the Learning Prep School.*

workshop offers bicycle "tune-ups" to the staff at prices well below those in the community. With the proceeds the students are able to take periodic bicycle excursions (Fig. 4-8).

*Business Skills*

Activities in the business skills workshop primarily involve clerical tasks and distribution of information or messages by mail, by telephone, or in person. Students who enter this area may receive specialized training in typing, telephone use, and the operation of office machinery (Fig. 4-9). Integrated into

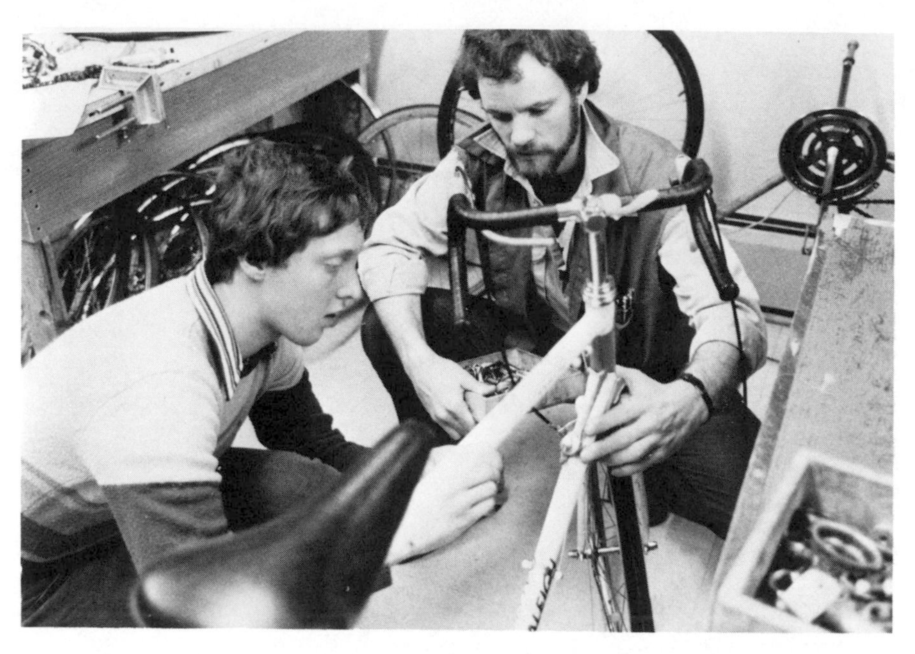

*Fig. 4-8. Student learning bicycle maintenance and repair.*

*Fig. 4-9. Learning Prep School students practicing typing in their business skills workshop.*

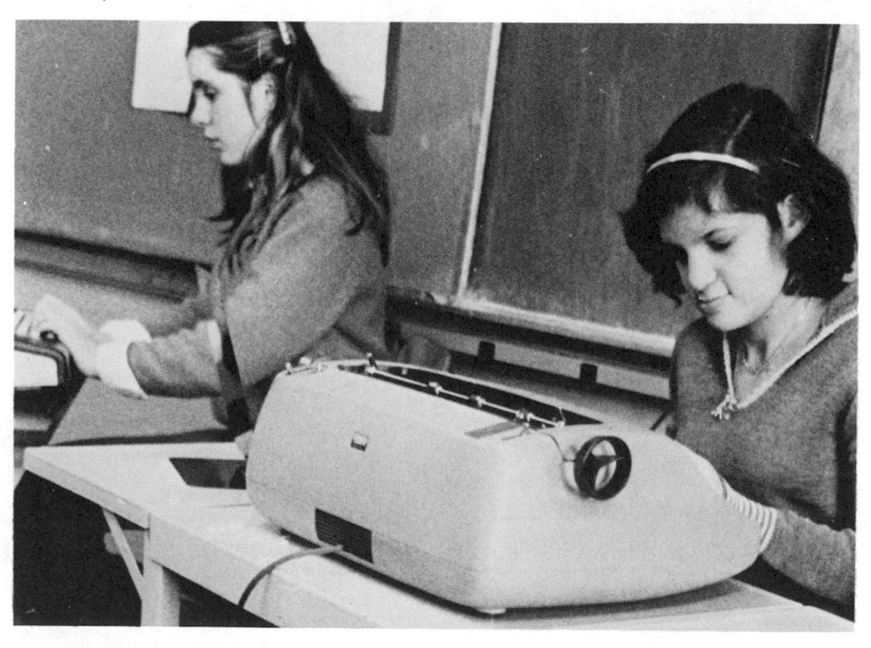

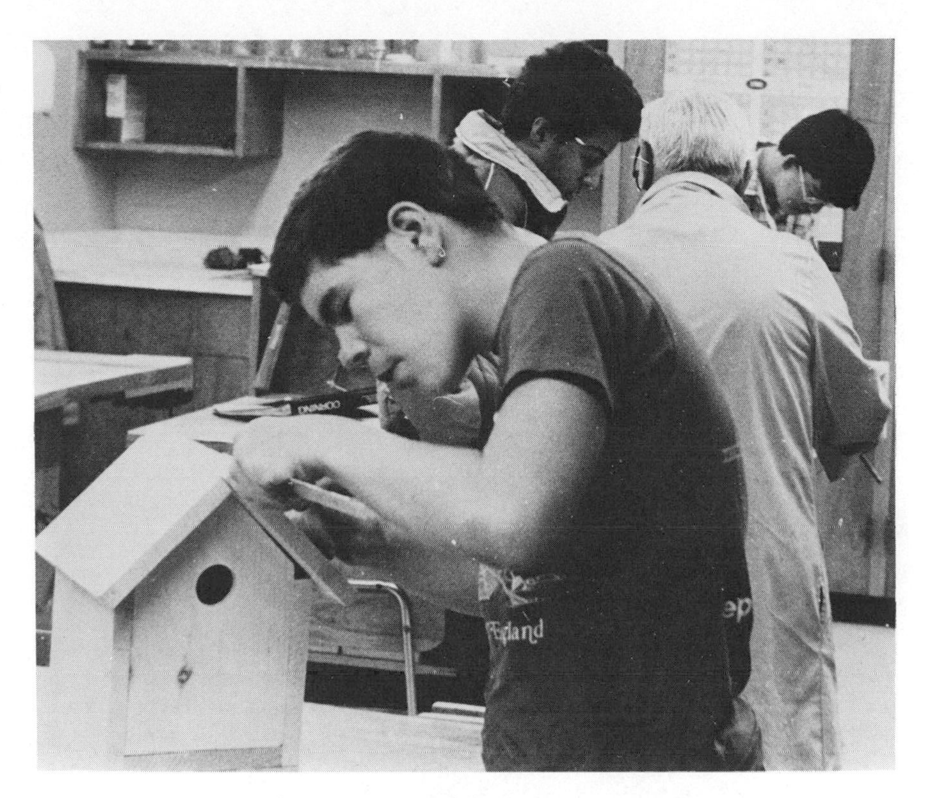

*Fig. 4-10. A project in the carpentry workshop.*

the program is an emphasis on consumerism—checking and savings accounts, budgeting, credit application, charge accounts, and installment contracts.

*Carpentry*

The carpentry program has two levels: a basic course and more advanced apprentice training. Students are first trained in basic drafting, hand and machine skills, and measurements, which enables them to produce a variety of finished wooden projects (Fig. 4-10). The more advanced students have built a free-standing greenhouse and woodshed. The workshop has established a small business that sells its finished products to the public (Fig. 4-11).

*Child Care*

Students are trained to work as child care aides through on-site training at the school's child care center. These students are developing skills such as planning and implementing academic and nonacademic lessons and supervising children during play (Fig. 4-12).

*Food Service*

Students enrolled in the food service workshop are developing the basic skills of food preparation, safety and sanitation, equipment operation, nutritional

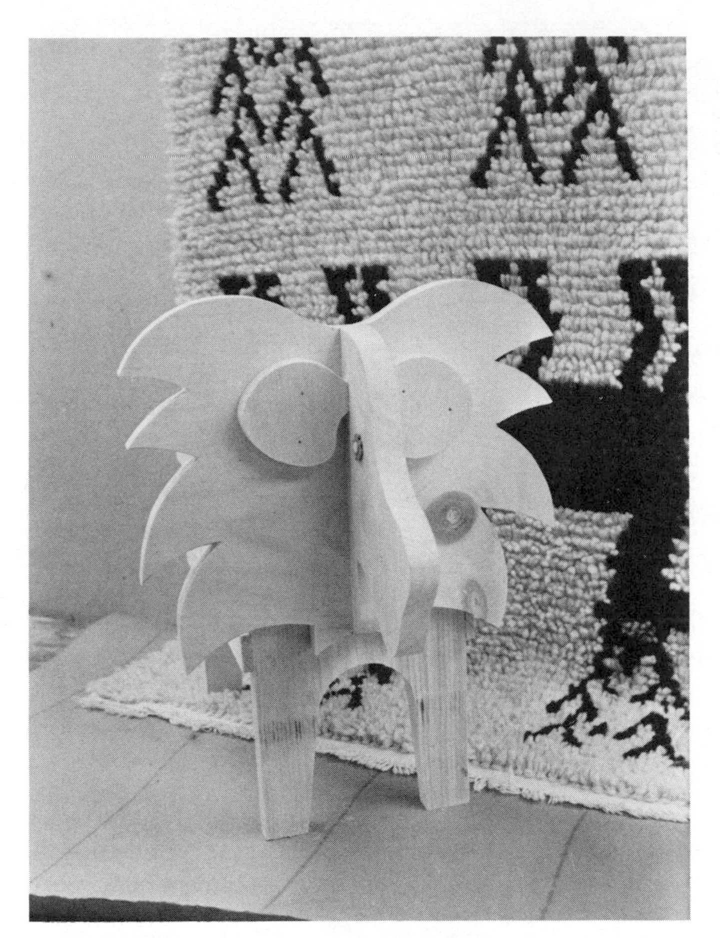

*Fig. 4-11. Wood project constructed and for sale in the carpentry workshop.*

standards, portion control, and customer service. These basic skills have enabled the students, under the instructors' auspices, to operate successfully a medium-scale Federally certified lunch program and salad bar (Fig. 4-13).

*Graphic Arts*

The graphic arts program is designed to teach the fundamentals of printing and design. Students learn to operate a small offset press, an on-line typesetter, and a copy machine. The emphasis is on layout, paste-up, logo designing, and commercial illustration (Fig. 4-14).

*Horticulture*

The horticulture workshop is designed to train students in landscaping and greenhouse skills. Students learn the rudiments of lawn and tree care, land-

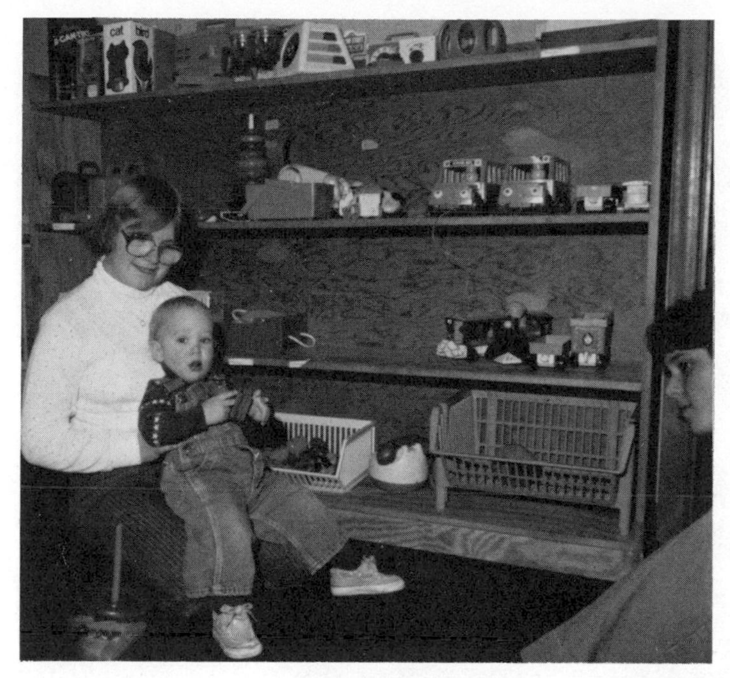

*Fig. 4-12. Student learning child care in the Learning Prep School child care center.*

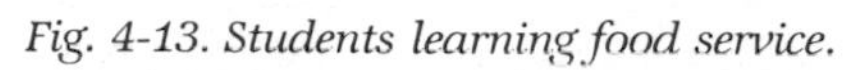

*Fig. 4-13. Students learning food service.*

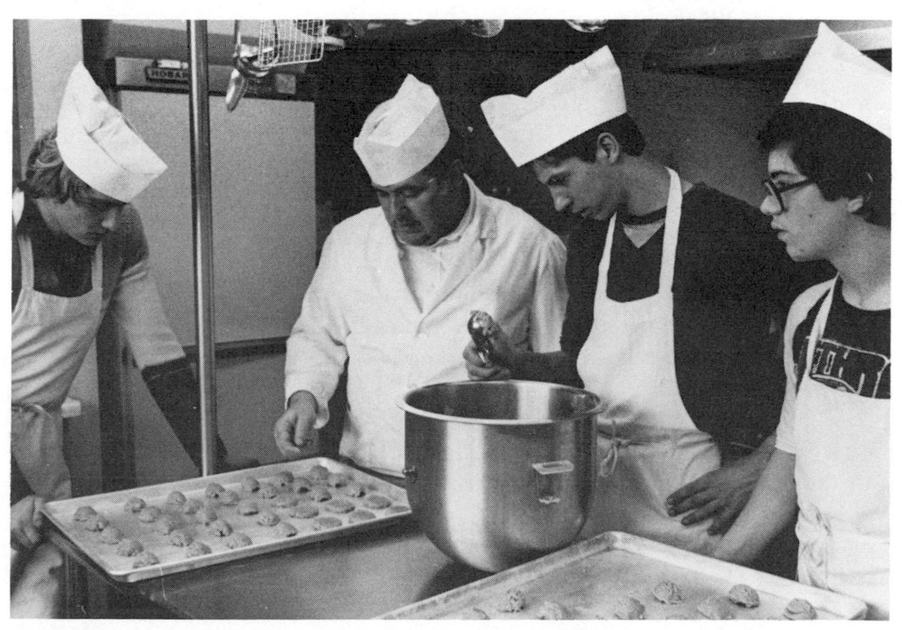

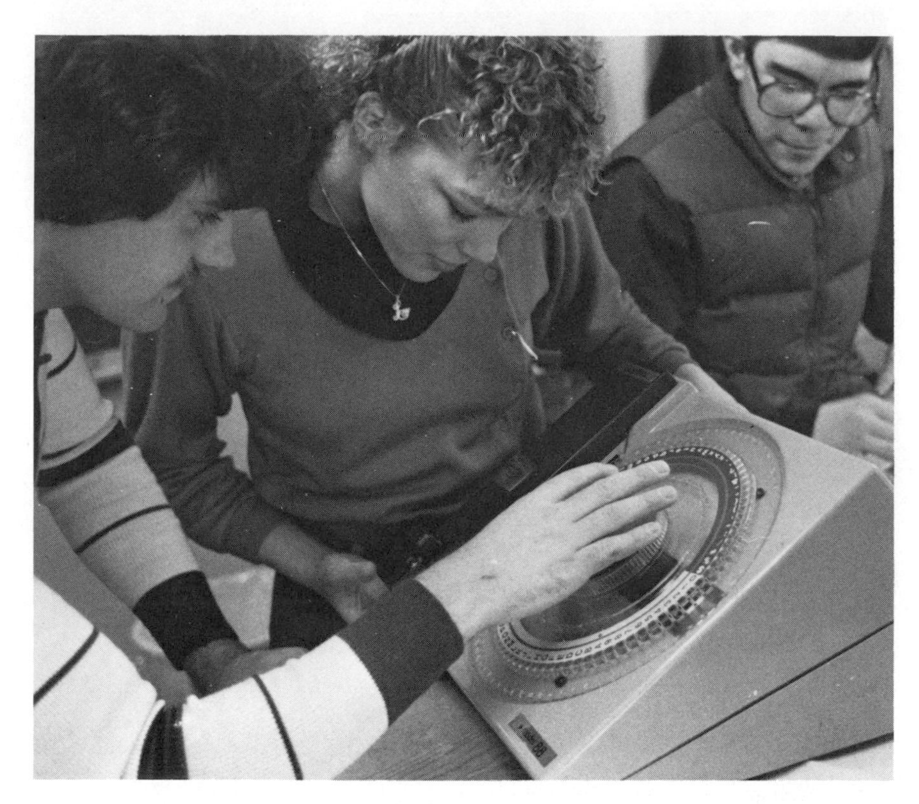

*Fig. 4-14. A class in graphic arts.*

scape design, and proper use and care of mechanical equipment. The school's 14′ × 22′ free-standing greenhouse also affords students the opportunity to develop skills in plant propagation and care (Fig. 4-15).

*Building Maintenance*

Students are trained in many aspects of building maintenance through on-site work. Dusting, sweeping, vacuuming, mopping, waxing floors, and washing windows are some of the activities in the curriculum. The student may also be trained to make minor repairs and become acquainted with cleaning equipment and cleaning agents.

*Photography*

In the photography workshop, students become familiar with basic photographic equipment, techniques, and vocabulary (Fig. 4-16). The development of good picture-taking and darkroom skills is an initial goal that serves as a foundation for a program encouraging creative self-expression and conceptual

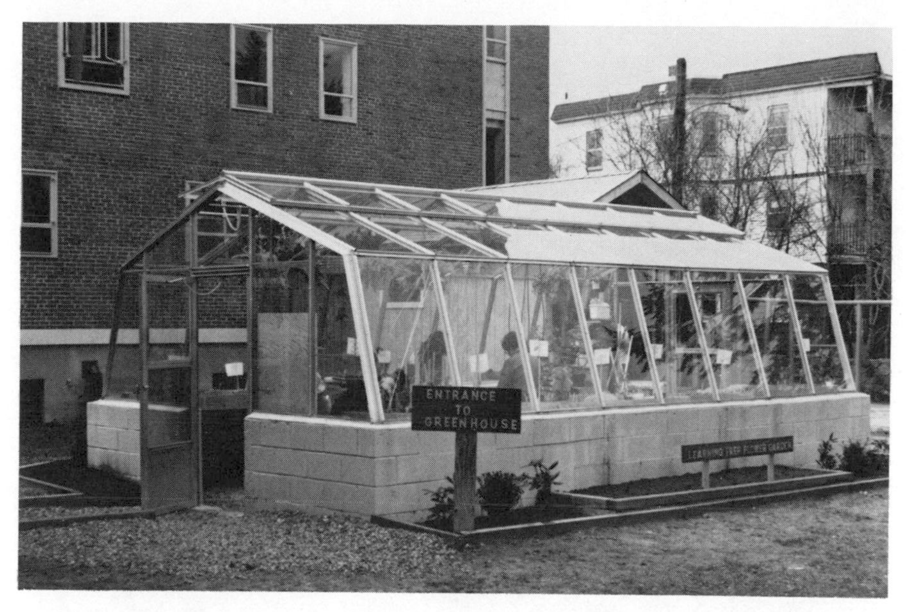


*Fig. 4-15. Greenhouse constructed by students and staff at Learning Prep School and used in developing horticulture skills.*

thinking. Projects include conventional documentary and studio photography in addition to exercises in multimedia work and special effects. In-house projects such as the yearbook and school-related publications are also an extension of the program. The students' work has been successfully displayed at the Carpenter Center for the Visual Arts at Harvard University.

WORK ACTIVITY CENTER

According to a 1977 U.S. Department of Labor study, nearly half of all existing sheltered workshop programs are work activity centers [8]. Historically, such centers serve those who are not prepared to enter a sheltered workshop but who could benefit from exposure to work-oriented activities. Their purpose is to

> provide appropriate and individualized developmental services to the whole person in order to build coping skills and abilities, enhance decision-making processes, foster independent or semi-independent living and develop vocational skills and related behaviors. The uniqueness of the individual will prevail in the program by recognition of strengths, weaknesses and individual personality traits. [1]

At the Little People's School we established a work activity center for the older students (10–16 years) to prepare them for the transition to secondary school; to stress work-related behaviors, skills, and habits such as problem solving, decision making, responsibility, perseverance, cooperative behavior,

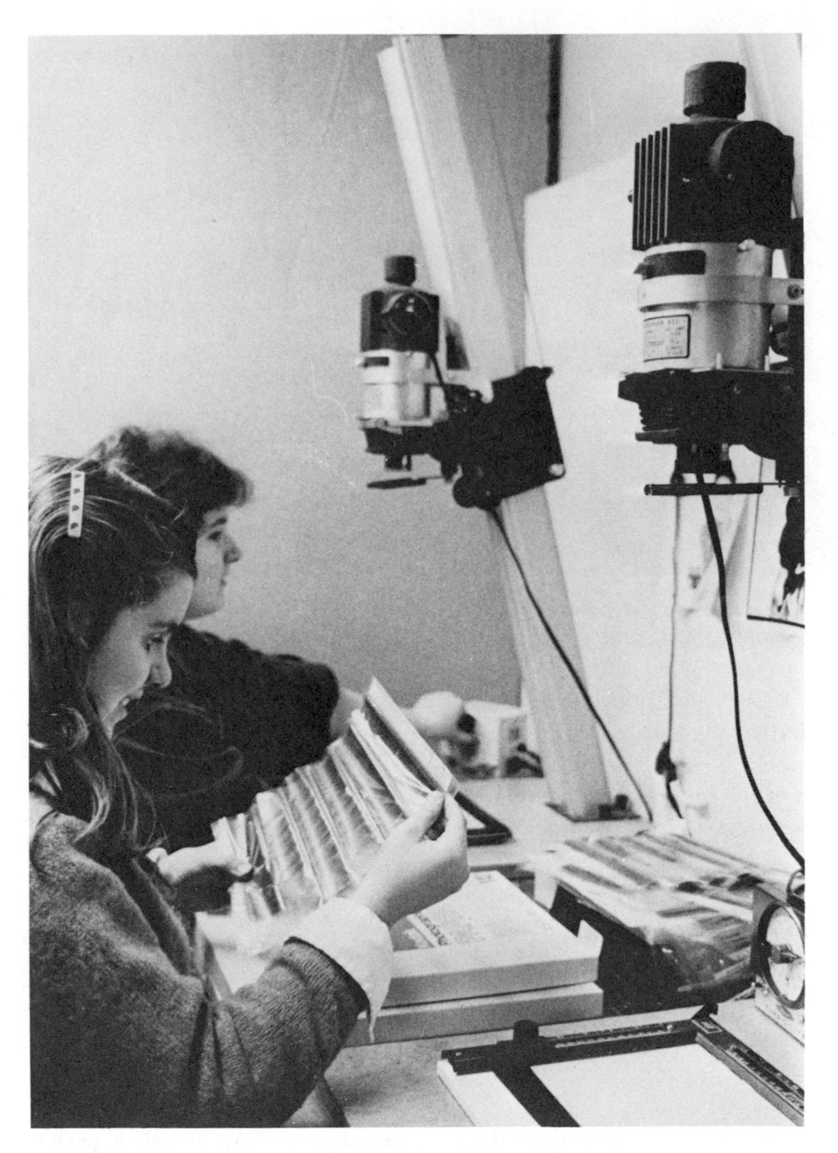

*Fig. 4-16. The darkroom in the photography workshop.*

and quality control; and to provide training in the direction of sheltered work. Because of the success of this program, we have expanded the center to include secondary school students who can benefit from this experience.

During the developmental stages of our center, we approached many local sheltered workshops and work activity centers for tours and assistance. Through one of these contacts, we established a mutually helpful arrangement whereby our center became a satellite program of a large and active local workshop. For us, this arrangement was ideal: It not only eliminated the need for us to establish a certified program, but also provided us with as much subcontract work as we can handle. During periods of contract overload, this local workshop provides us with subcontract work and the students receive remuneration for their production (Fig. 4-17). For periods when subcontract work is not available, the therapists have devised activities that simulate subcontract work, for example, collating, assembling, and packaging.

OCCUPATIONAL THERAPY PROGRAM

Work-related occupational therapy is an integral link in Learning Prep School programming. The occupational therapist functions as the liaison between instructors and vocational and academic administrators. In this capacity the therapist acts as a consultant to personnel who may not have expertise in task and job analysis, adaptive and assistive equipment, techniques of work simplification and activities of daily living. In addition, the therapist uses information from the JPSA to assist staff in developing teaching strategies based on the student's learning style. The therapist also functions as a role model, working side by side with several students or individually with one who may need extra attention. Various staff members including the psychologist, the nursing staff, the counseling staff, and physical and speech therapists collaborate with the occupational therapist to teach social skills through group discussion and modeling in such settings as sex education

*Fig. 4-17. Students doing piecework (rolling and packaging posters) at work activity center.*

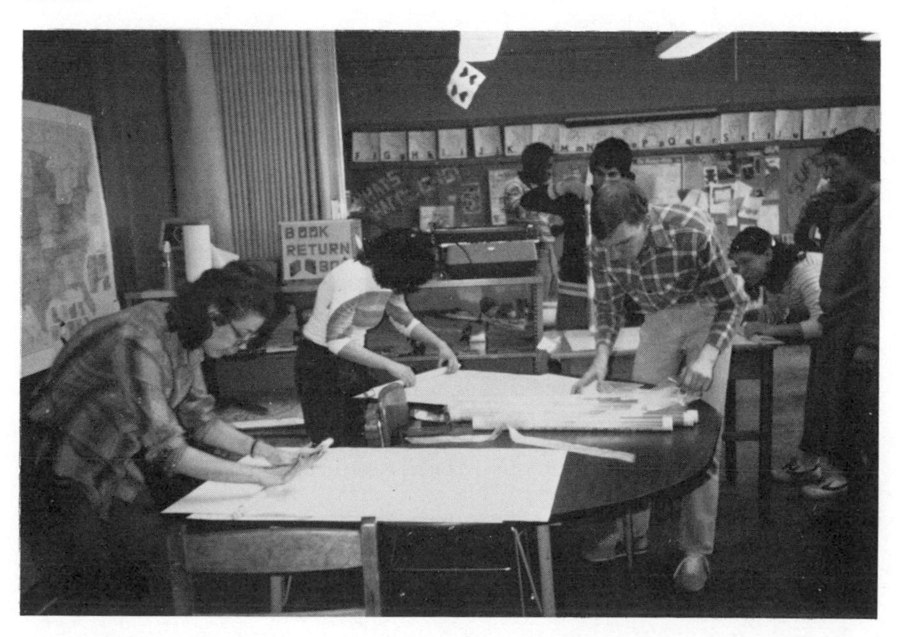

class, the lunchtime feeding program, and cardiopulmonary resuscitation (CPR) classes.

The occupational therapy department also provides evaluations and direct services to students who need remediation in specific work-related skill areas. A list of work-related behavioral objectives (Table 4-1) has been formulated for use as a guide in developing treatment plans and progress notes. Progress notes are written three times yearly with specific objectives selected and rated on a five-point scale. Fig. 4-18 shows a typical progress note.

The treatment offered by the occupational therapy department is in the form of occupational therapy task groups. Students are typically seen in task groups of two to five or six persons in two 45-minute sessions weekly. These group sessions provide a series of learning experiences that will enable the student to make appropriate vocational decisions and develop work habits necessary for eventual employment. Several of the task groups are described in the following paragraphs.

*Babysitter Training*

Social trends such as the trend toward more single-parent families, the increased number of families with both parents working outside the home, and the increased number of older siblings tending to younger family members have expanded the need for well-trained babysitters. For many adolescents, babysitting is one of the first opportunities to earn money and learn job responsibilities. Through the assistance of Laura Hollander, an occupational therapist from Faulkner Hospital in Jamaica Plain, Massachusetts, and

*Table 4-1. Work-Related Behavioral Objectives of Occupational Therapy*

I. Behavioral and Social
   The student
   A. Demonstrates oral and motor awareness
   B. Demonstrates oral and motor control
   C. Displays independence in performance of activities of daily living
   D. Displays awareness of appropriate repertoire of leisure activities
   E. Increases the frequency of appropriate informal social contacts
   F. Increases the frequency of appropriate social contacts with peers in a simulated work environment
   G. Controls disruptive behavior during therapy
   H. Controls frustration

II. Learning
   The student
   A. Performs matching and sorting tasks
   B. Performs classification tasks
   C. Performs alphabetizing tasks
   D. Demonstrates the ability to perform functional linear, liquid, and solid measurement
   E. Demonstrates the ability to perform functional money tasks
   F. Demonstrates the ability to perform one-to-one correspondence and number quantity tasks

III. Motor.
The student uses compensatory strategies to
A. Demonstrate fine motor coordination
B. Demonstrate eye-hand coordination
C. Demonstrate ocular motor control
D. Demonstrate appropriate sitting posture
E. Demonstrate the ability to use common tools, e.g., hammer, stapler

IV. Communication
The student
A. Demonstrates the ability to communicate basic needs appropriately
B. Demonstrates the ability to follow
1. two- to three-step visual directions
2. two- to three-step verbal directions
3. two- to three-step written directions
4. two- to three-step visual and verbal directions
5. two- to three-step visual and written directions
6. two- to three-step verbal and written directions
7. visual directions of three or more steps
8. verbal directions of three or more steps
9. written directions of three or more steps
10. visual and verbal directions of three or more steps
11. visual and written directions of three or more steps
12. verbal and written directions of three or more steps

V. Production
The student
A. Maintains task focus
B. Carries out two- to three-step tasks in the proper sequence
C. Carries out tasks of three or more steps in the proper sequence
D. Adjusts work pace with supervision
E. Adjusts work pace independently
F. Accurately and consistently completes a specific task after having demonstrated the ability to perform the task
G. Demonstrates flexibility in adapting to changes in the therapeutic program
H. Independently maintains continuous work during a therapy session
I. Monitors the quality of work produced in a therapy session

VI. Independence
The student
A. Demonstrates the ability to use a model or sample to complete a task
B. Displays organizational skills
C. Develops and applies compensatory strategies to adapt activities for functional ability
D. Starts work independently
E. Begins work promptly upon receiving instructions
F. Solves problems in a simulated work setting
G. Makes decisions in a simulated work setting

VII. Visual and perceptual
The student uses compensatory strategies to perform activities involving
A. Figure-ground skills
B. Spatial relations
C. Directionality

*Fig. 4-18. Occupational therapy progress note.*

**Prevocational Occupational Therapy Progress Reports**
**April to June 1984**

Name: Keith Date of Birth: 2/5/65
I.D. #: 3340
Frequency of Treatment Sessions: Two per week
Modalities Used in Treatment: Craft and leisure activities, school yearbook, lunchroom cashiering
Tests Administered: Jacobs Prevocational Skills Assessment

Key
1 = Rarely (Student displayed this behavior 0–20% of the time in therapy.)
2 = Occasionally (Student displayed this behavior 21–40% of the time in therapy.)
3 = Approximately half the time (Student displayed this behavior 41–60% of the time in therapy.)
4 = Frequently (Student displayed this behavior 61–80% of the time in therapy.)
5 = Consistently (Student displayed this behavior 81–100% of the time in therapy.)

| Therapy Goals Addressed This Term | 1 | 2 | 3 | 4 | 5 |
|---|---|---|---|---|---|
| *Learning* | | | | | |
| The student | | | | | |
| 1. Performs alphabetizing tasks | | x | | | |
| 2. Demonstrates the ability to perform functional money tasks | | | x | | |
| *Motor* | | | | | |
| The student uses compensatory strategies to | | | | | |
| 1. Demonstrate fine motor coordination | | x | | | |
| *Communication* | | | | | |
| The student | | | | | |
| 1. Demonstrates the ability to communicate basic needs appropriately | | | x | | |
| 2. Demonstrates the ability to follow: | | | x | | |
| a. two- to three-step verbal directions | | | x | | |
| b. two- to three-step visual and written directions | | | x | | |

| | | | | | |
|---|---|---|---|---|---|
| *Independence* | | | | | |
| The student | | | | | |
| 1. Solves problems in a simulated work setting | | x | | | |
| 2. Makes decisions in a simulated work setting | | x | | | |
| *Visual and Perceptual* | | | | | |
| The student uses compensatory strategies to perform activities involving | | | | | |
| 1. Figure-ground skills | | | x | | |

COMMENTS

Improvement has been noted in Keith's ability to assess accurately his personal strengths and weaknesses. Keith more frequently asks for assistance from both peers and supervisors in a simulated work setting and has responded to suggestions that he choose work tasks that emphasize his areas of strengths.

RECOMMENDATIONS

It is recommended that Keith's performance continue to be monitored by the occupational therapy department. A home program has been devised by the therapist and given to Keith's parents to be used by him over the summer vacation.

the local chapter of the American Red Cross, we have developed a week-long intensive babysitter training program. This is open not only to the occupational therapy population, but to any Learning Prep School student, up to a maximum enrollment of 15.

In this training program, the students are guided through a sequence of hands-on exercises on topics such as telephone protocol, ethics and contracts, child development, accident prevention, diapering, mealtime, bedtime, discipline, mouth-to-mouth resuscitation and clearing of obstructed airways, fire safety (a local fire captain discusses what to do in case of fire), and safety (a local police sergeant discusses safety precautions, e.g., never leaving a child alone).

For those students able to and interested in learning CPR, we schedule a certification course in the following weeks. Thus far 12 students have been CPR certified (Fig. 4-19).

*Library Group*

The library group has set up and maintains the student library. Occupational therapy students perform tasks such as sorting books according to subject, labelling them (based on the Dewey Decimal System), and placing pockets containing cards inside the books. We hope this group will eventually become a functional pool of librarians.

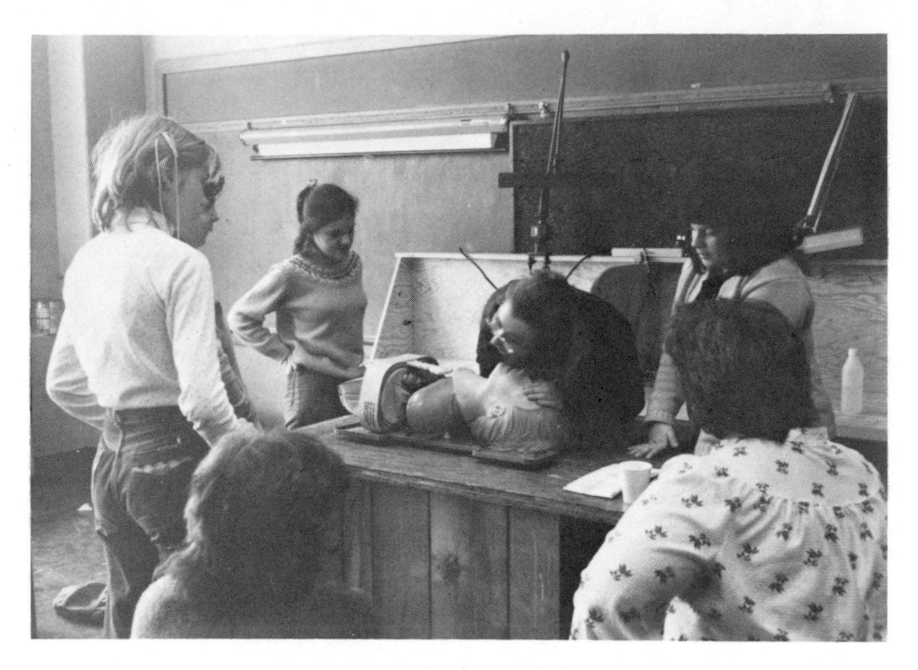

*Fig. 4-19. Students practicing cardiopulmonary resuscitation during babysitter training class.*

*School Store*

Twice a week during class break, which lasts 20 minutes, two occupational therapy students operate a school store (Fig. 4-20). These students sell school supplies such as pencils and notebooks and refreshments such as fruit juice and cookies. Job responsibilities, which have been delineated by the students, include recording sales, checking inventory, tallying money, packaging items, and dealing with customers. A simulated banking system has been developed to monitor the store's profit, which I am happy to say is steady.

*Yearbook*

Occupational therapy produced the first school yearbook in 1982. Students serve as the production staff, determine the book's content, and schedule and monitor deadlines for various contributors such as the photography workshop and the printer. By selling advertising space in the yearbook, the students have been able to reduce the cost of the books and make this a financially independent venture.

*Lunchroom Cashier*

Before working in the lunchroom, students have the opportunity to practice in occupational therapy the job responsibilities of a lunchroom cashier—social interaction, money skills. Once the student feels ready, he or she enters the lunchroom setting to perform this job under the therapist's supervision.

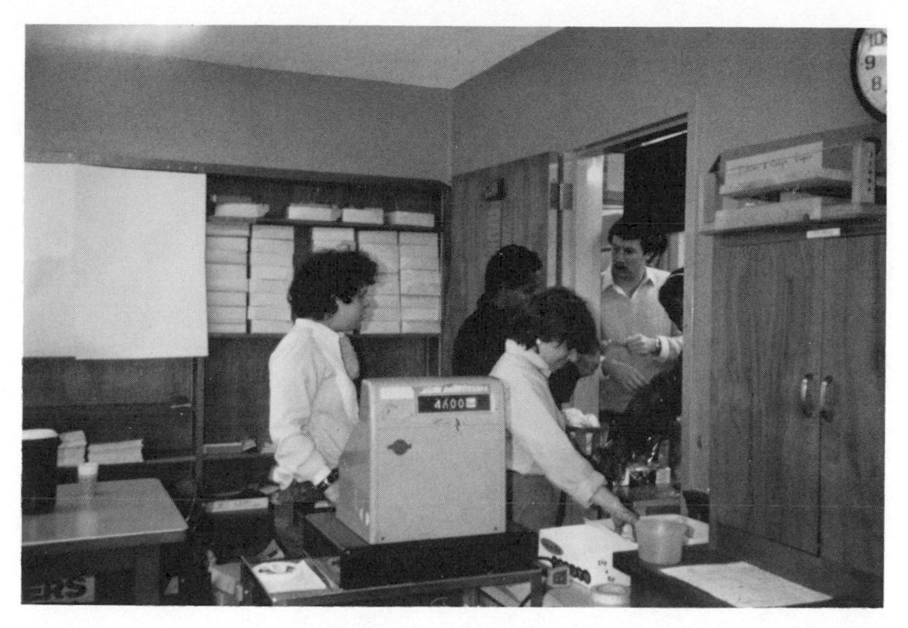

*Fig. 4-20. Students working in the Learning Prep School store.*

This group has devised a system for keeping a record of those who owe lunch money, and it is the group's responsibility to dispense collection notices!

*Cookie Group*

Students were given the task of setting up a functional business enterprise. After many brainstorming sessions, they elected to establish a "cookie-gram" company, which bakes large (and delicious) chocolate-chip cookies and customizes them with frosting messages (Fig. 4-21).

Students are responsible for all aspects of this business and learn to cope with working under pressure occasionally, for example, during a large-volume holiday season. This has been a very successful group; after only one year in business it is in the black.

*Volunteer Program*

Basing this program on the transitional employment program model, discussed in greater detail in Chapter 5 (see pp. 146–147), the occupational therapist selects volunteer jobs (e.g., cafeteria aide) for appropriate occupational therapy students (Fig. 4-22). Once the job has been obtained, the following procedure is followed:

1. The therapist performs the job for a day or two to gain an understanding of what is required and what will be expected from the student.
2. The therapist performs the job side by side with the student.

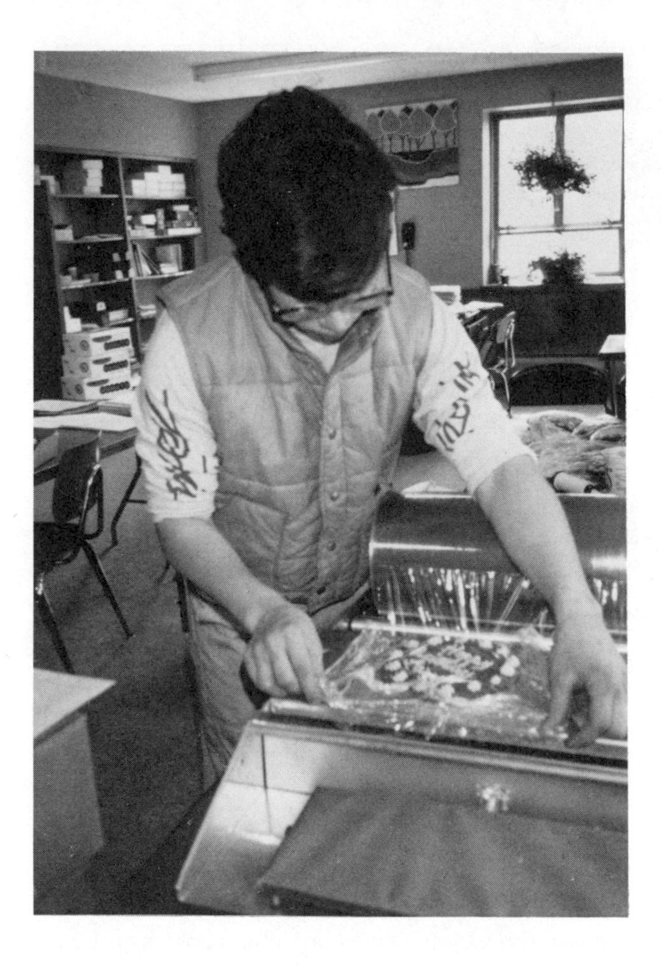

*Fig. 4-21. Student shrink-wrapping a "cookie-gram."*

3. The therapist watches the student perform the job.
4. The student performs the job without the therapist and eventually commutes to the job site independently.

*Craft Group*

The craft group is the lowest-level occupational therapy group. Group members engage in repetitive and structured craft and art activities, for example, leather craft, weaving, model assembly, sewing, and the traditional yearly construction of a colorful school banner, which is hung in the students' cafeteria. Typically the other items produced are sold at the semiannual arts and crafts fair.

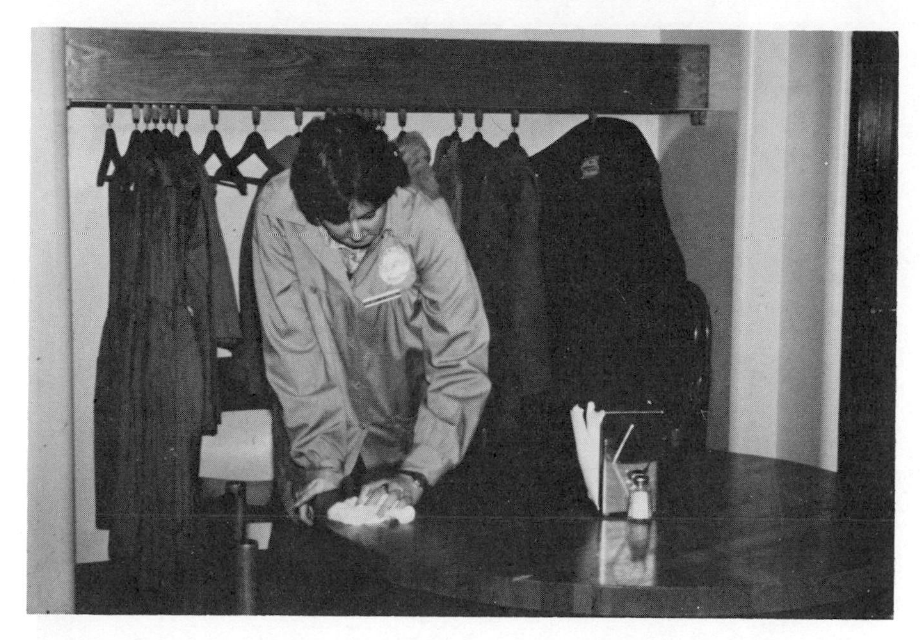

*Fig. 4-22. Student working as a volunteer cafeteria aide at Newton-Wellesley Hospital, Newton, Massachusetts.*

## WORK-STUDY PROGRAM

In an additional administrative capacity as Job Placement and Development Coordinator, I have had the opportunity to apply my occupational therapy skills across the occupational choice process. The ultimate goal of our programs is to realize the greatest potential of all the students. When a student has learned the necessary prerequisite vocational skills and behaviors, he or she is eligible for the work-study program. This program has three components and may be viewed as a transition in the occupational choice process from career exploration to realistic career choice.

### *Volunteer Training*

Volunteer training in the work-study program is an expanded version of the occupational therapy volunteer program (i.e., it involves more students and more time on the job). Volunteer positions are provided one or two days per week to expose students to various worker roles. Placement has been provided at local facilities such as hospitals and nursing homes and at the National Spinal Injury Foundation.

### *In-house Work-Study*

In-house training in positions such as child care aide, office and maintenance assistant, and lunchroom cashier is provided on an alternate-week basis. The

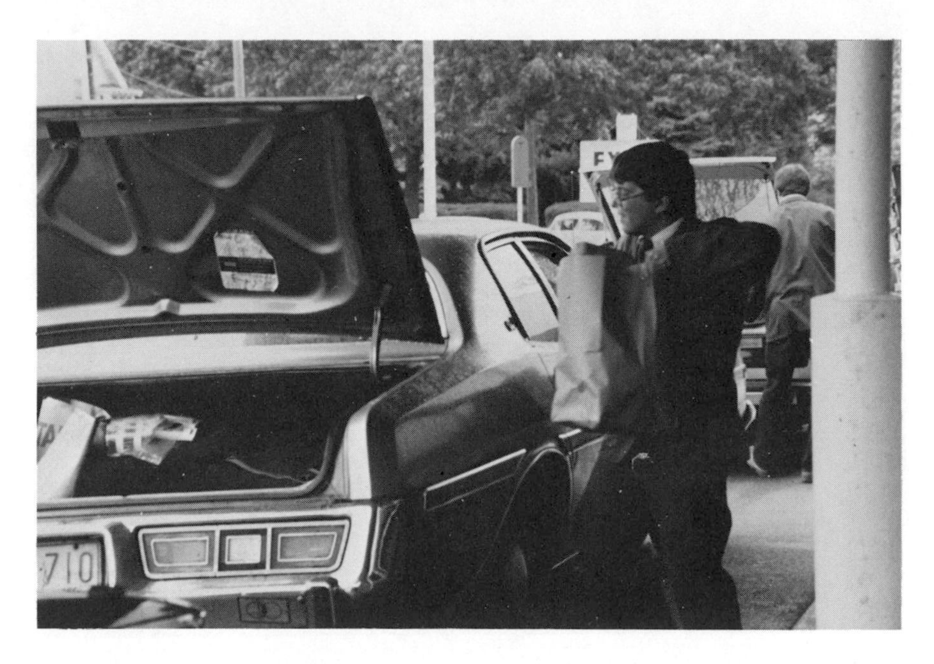

*Fig. 4-23. Under the work-study program a student is a bundler-bagger at a local supermarket.*

therapist consults with the staff at these job sites to assist them in developing programming that will facilitate the student's success in the "real" work world.

*Work-Study*

Students are placed in jobs appropriate to their skill levels and interests in their local communities on an alternate-week basis. Once placed in a job the student may progress through the normal advancements of that position. To date, community response to hiring students has been excellent; many students are gainfully employed in the greater Boston area (Fig. 4-23).

FUND RAISING

Common in education, particularly the private sector, is limited funding. I have been able to use small school fund raisers both to finance programs and equipment and to reinforce students' work-related behaviors and skills outside the school setting.

The Learning Prep School has fund-raising drives periodically to support, for example, the purchase of computers or recreational equipment. On these occasions we may raise funds by selling products such as cloth calendars, pot holders, beach towels, community theater tickets, and ads in our yearbook in the students' local communities. Participating students have the opportunity to practice social skills, by contacting persons in their communities; communication skills, by explaining what they are selling and why; and money skills. A prize program has been devised as a motivator so that students who sell the most receive a direct benefit from their efforts.

The Learning Prep School program has been nicely conceptualized by Nancy Mazonson in a model that also shows the parallel development of interests outside school and the occupational choice process (Fig. 4-24). The following case study will also assist in illustrating the occupational therapy program. The student, Stacey, was discussed in Chapter 3; her results on the JPSA were presented on page 62 and 63. You may find it beneficial to refer to that section.

*Case Study**
Name: Stacey
Chronological age: 17

CLINICAL PICTURE
Pregnancy was unremarkable. Stacey was born after a 12-hour labor, an Rh baby with jaundice. Postnatal developmental milestones were within normal limits: sitting up at 6 to 7 months, walking at 14 months, toileting at 3 years. Language development initially was within normal limits; however, vocabulary, phrasing, and sentence development was delayed.

MEDICAL HISTORY
No illnesses or hospitalizations. Stacey began to receive speech therapy at age 3. Therapy continued until age 5½, when she entered kindergarten, at which time language and academic delays were noted and special school placement began. At age 13, Stacey entered the Little People's School.

SOCIAL
Stacey lives with her mother and two sisters.

EMOTIONAL DEVELOPMENT
Stacey presently receives group and individual counseling at school to address feelings of low self-esteem. Stacey has used denial as a defense mechanism and has fabricated stories about her social life to appear normal to her peers. Stacey exhibits unrealistic expectations and denial of the limitations of her disability.

SCHOOL PROGRAM
At present Individualized Educational Plan goals for Stacey are as follows:

*Language.*
To improve receptive and expressive language, emphasizing vocabulary, understanding of concepts, grammar, and functional language.

*Reading.*
To improve comprehension, vocabulary, and recognition of parts of speech.

*This case study was provided by Nancy Mazonson, M.S., OTR, Learning Prep School, West Newton, Massachusetts.

| | | | | |
|---|---|---|---|---|
| Occupational Choice Process | Fantasy and exploration stage | Tentative choice stage | | Final stage |
| Learning Prep School Activities | Vocational workshops<br>OT groups<br>Cookie-gram group<br>School store<br>Library group<br>Yearbook<br>Craft group<br>Cashier group<br>Arts and crafts fair<br>School fund raisers | → Vocational Workshops<br>In-house jobs<br>Cashier<br>Child care (volunteer)<br>Office assistant<br>Maintenance assistant<br>Volunteer work<br>Babysitter training | → Narrower range of vocational workshops<br>Child care ($)<br>Maintenance ($)<br>After-school job placement<br>Summer job placement | → Work/Study Job<br>Apprentice training program |
| Parallel Development Outside School | | Volunteer Work<br>Babysitting<br>Yard work<br>Paper Route | After-school job<br>Summer job | |

*Fig. 4-24. Learning Prep School activities in relation to the process of occupational choice and nonschool activities. (Courtesy Nancy Mazonson, M.S., OTR.)*

*Math.*
To improve money, banking, and budgeting skills.

*Study Skills.*
To improve dictionary skills, use of contextual clues to deduce word meanings, use of encyclopedia and reference pages, and letter-writing skills.

*Career Awareness.*
To improve awareness of career options.

*Vocational.*
Participation in three workshops: photography, food service, and child care.

GOALS OF THERAPY

*Speech Therapy.*

1. To discriminate between grammatical and nongrammatical sentences with 90 percent accuracy within a structured setting
2. To construct grammatical sentences in present and past tenses in conversation with 80 percent accuracy
3. To use self-monitoring skills to improve discrimination, identification, and correction of errors
4. To use turn-taking and listening skills in group conversation through the use of written and spoken sentences and paragraphs, role play, group discussion, and peer feedback

*Counseling*

1. Individual—To improve expression of feelings and self-esteem
2. Group—To improve expression of feelings concerning the social stresses of adolescence and understanding and implementation of appropriate behavior in a variety of social settings

*Occupational Therapy*

1. To improve ability to assess strengths and weaknesses
2. To improve problem-solving and decision-making skills
3. To improve ability to use visual cues in following directions, sequencing, and memory
4. To improve ability to follow three-step directions
5. To improve fine motor skills
6. To improve functional money skills

OCCUPATIONAL THERAPY PROGRAM

Stacey's occupational therapy activities are performed in a small group setting that simulates a work environment. Tasks involve measuring, manipulation of small objects, following written and oral directions, planning, decision making, and functional use of money.

Stacey's programming in occupational therapy has followed a progression of increasing difficulty. At ages 15 and 16 she participated in a variety of small task groups: cashiering group, production and craft work, girls club. By age 16 Stacey has developed the work skills and behaviors necessary for successful functioning in a highly supervised work environment. She has shown a particular interest in the child care vocational workshop and has expressed her desire to work in the area of human services in the future. As a result it has been recommended that Stacey become an assistant (apprentice) in the child care center, with expanded work hours. This placement is monitored by the occupational therapist, who provides consultation to the child care su-

**Work Behavior Checklist**

Name: ______________________________
Date: ______________________________

| | | |
|---|---|---|
| ___ | 1. Attendance | Coming to work on the days you are supposed to |
| ___ | 2. Punctuality | Coming to work on time<br>Coming back from break on time |
| ___ | 3. Starting work independently | Starting work by yourself without needing help |
| ___ | 4. Independent work skills (initiative, follow-through) | Working on your own<br>Finishing jobs you start |
| ___ | 5. Attention span | Keeping your mind on your work |
| ___ | 6. Use and care of tools and equipment | Taking care of tools and equipment and using them correctly |
| ___ | 7. Organizational work area | Keeping your work area neat and organized |
| ___ | 8. Problem solving, judgment | Making good decisions if there is a problem |
| ___ | 9. Quality of work | Always doing a good job<br>Taking care of everything that needs to be done<br>Being thorough |
| ___ | 10. Work pace, work endurance | Working at a good speed—not too fast, not too slow<br>Being energetic and staying with the job |
| ___ | 11. Flexibility | Being able to make changes in the way you do the job<br>Being able to do things in a new or different way |
| ___ | 12. Meeting deadlines | Being able to have something finished or ready by a certain time |
| ___ | 13. Safety rules | Remembering safety rules |
| ___ | 14. General appearance | Dressing nicely for work<br>Looking clean and neat for work<br>Following the rules if there is a dress code |
| | Other: | |

*Fig. 4-25. Work behavior checklist. (Courtesy Nancy Mazonson, OTR.)*

pervisors, so that programming and work responsibilities can be designed to foster growth in the areas of need assessed by the Jacobs Prevocational Skills Assessment.

In the child care setting Stacey can learn diapering, toileting, meal preparation, and clean-up procedures and how to maintain a time sheet. Supervision feedback on performance and self-assessment can be done on a weekly basis through the use of a work behavior checklist designed by the therapist (Fig. 4-25).

As implied by the variety of programs discussed in this book, the occupational therapist may assume many different roles in the context of prevocational programming. In the following example, therapists have determined the need for additional evaluations and training of students to make an ongoing program more comprehensive.

TREATMENT SETTING

Located throughout the state of Colorado are Community Center Board programs, which provide services to low-functioning, developmentally disabled persons. The Margaret Walters School is one such program, addressing the needs of persons aged to 21 years with IQs of 50 or below who have various diagnoses: Down's syndrome, developmental delays, mental retardation (etiology unknown), cerebral palsy, high-risk infant. The school is actually just one arm of a larger organization called Jefferson County Community Center, a birth-to-death program consisting of several residential facilities, three workshops, two schools, and an intensive-care facility for those who would otherwise be in a nursing home.

The prevocational occupational therapy program, which was developed at the school by Sherry Olin and Mary Haldy, evolved from an ongoing Work Experience and Study (WES) program. The WES program, developed for students aged 18 to 21 years, involves a continuum of classroom study through in-house job placement to community job placement.

Therapists observing the WES program realized there was a need for an additional, more comprehensive evaluation to facilitate a better match between a student's strengths and an in-house or community job. Such an assessment was developed and became one of the major components of the current prevocational occupational therapy program. Other components include job task analysis, consultation, a decision-making group, and program planning.

OCCUPATIONAL THERAPY EVALUATION

Students' physical capacities, behavioral skills, interests, and tool use are evaluated to determine the students' strengths and weaknesses and to aid in making recommendations for job placement.

*Physical Capacities*

The department uses an adapted version of the Physical Capacities Evaluation developed by the Delaware Curative Workshop, Wilmington, Delaware, to determine ability and functional tolerances in standing, sitting, lifting, and repetitive work [5]. In addition the Purdue Pegboard, the Minnesota Rate of Manipulation Test, and the Bruininks-Oseretsky Test of Motor Proficiency are given. Finally, range of motion testing and sensory testing are done.

*Behavioral Skills*

The Comprehensive Occupational Therapy Evaluation Scale (COTE scale) is used to assess behavior in various situations [2]. The scale defines 25 observable behaviors that "are particularly relevant to the practice of occupational therapy" [2]. These behaviors are divided into three categories: general behavior, interpersonal behavior, and task behavior. For example, under task behavior, decision making is evaluated in the following manner [2]:

Decision Making:
0 —Makes own decisions
1 —Makes decisions but occasionally seeks therapist approval
2 —Makes decisions but often seeks therapist approval
3 —Makes decision when given only two choices
4 —Cannot make any decisions or refuses to make a decision

Each of the behaviors on the scale is rated from 0 to 4, with 0 representing normal function or an absence of problem behavior and 4 indicating a severe problem. Scores are totaled, and ratings can range from 0 to 100; higher scores indicate more severe problems. The COTE scale can be used to measure the student's progress in treatment programs.

*Interests and Tool Use*
An interest checklist is completed by each student individually. The student is also asked to perform workshop tasks, for example, hammering, bolting, stapling, punching holes, to determine his or her functional level of tool use.

JOB ANALYSIS
Before making a job placement, the therapist may arrange a visit to the proposed job site to analyze potential jobs, focusing on the following skill areas: (1) fine motor coordination, (2) gross motor coordination, (3) perceptual skills, (4) academic or cognitive skills, (5) social interactions, (6) tactile skills, and (7) tool use. For example, a day care aide job would be analyzed in the following manner:

| *Skill* | *Job-Requirement* |
| --- | --- |
| S | Friendly and playful interaction skills |
| S | Giving direction, and keeping children involved in activity, finding new activities |
| S | Self-control and patience |
| S | Handling fights |
| S | Independence and decision making |
| Tac | Touching children |
| P | Finding toys and supplies on shelves and putting them away |
| P | Tolerating noise and confusion |
| P | Putting servings on plates and placing plates on table |
| A | Memory for names |
| A | Counting |
| FM | Fine motor (picking up small items, eg., puzzles) |

Key: S = social, Tac = tactile, P = perceptual, A = academic, FM = fine motor.

Through this process of job analysis, students have been appropriately placed in jobs such as cafeteria server, hotel and nursing home laundry helper, dishwasher, groundskeeper, day care aide, and maintenance assistant.

CONSULTATION

The therapist may assume the role of consultant to the teaching staff to discuss such issues as appropriate job placement of students.

DECISION-MAKING GROUP

Under the direction of a therapist, groups composed of several students who hold in-house or community jobs develop cooperative work habits, independence, and initiative. Students decide on an activity and then share the responsibility for its organization and implementation. In time the group becomes increasingly independent of the therapist. Eventually the therapist is able to determine which students will be successful candidates for different community or sheltered workshop jobs.

PROGRAM PLANNING

Therapists at the Margaret Walters School are involved in program planning to meet the long-term goal of extending the occupational therapy program to students aged 13 to 17, with the explicit purpose of developing or improving prevocational skills at an earlier age. It is hoped that earlier exposure will facilitate an easier transition into the WES program.

*Case Study**

Name: David

Chronological age: 20 years

REASON FOR REFERRAL

David was referred to occupational therapy for an assessment of strengths and weaknesses in fine and gross motor areas for current and future job placement.

BACKGROUND INFORMATION

David is a 20-year-old with a diagnosis of mental retardation, etiology unknown. He also had a ventricular heart defect and has undergone two heart catheterizations. He has a mild sensory hearing loss bilaterally and usually wears a hearing aid in the left ear.

David was in special education programs from 1970 to 1975 before entering the Community Center Program.

OBSERVATIONS

David has participated in a weekly group meeting of several vocational students to increase independent decision-making skills. In this group David has demonstrated mature behaviors; he socializes appropriately with peers and staff, takes responsibility for his own actions, and is very cooperative. He is interested in most tasks and carries them to completion with few or no reminders. He is able to check his work and usually corrects his errors independently. David needs approval and guidance at times when making decisions or solving problems.

David's main interests are hiking and checkers. He usually listens to music and watches television after school. He has said that he would like to have more to do in his spare time.

*This case study was provided by Sherry Olin, OTR, and Mary Haldy, OTR, Margaret Walters School, Arvada, Colorado.

TESTING RESULTS

*Physical Capacities.*

The physical capacities test measures strength, endurance, balance, and ability to perform gross motor tasks. David demonstrated fairly good balance and endurance during the squatting and stooping activities, although he did say his legs became a little tired. He climbed a stepladder easily and safely while carrying a paint can and maneuvered a fully loaded wheelbarrow with control.

David handled 35 pounds easily, both lifting and carrying. He lifted using good body mechanics. Grasp strength as measured by a dynamometer was 50 pounds with the right (125 lb is the norm) and 35 pounds with the left (117 lb norm). Pinch grasp was measured as 10 pounds with the right (22.5 lb norm) and 6 pounds with the left (21 lb norm). David has more strength in the larger muscles proximally (shoulders) than in the fine muscles distally (fingers). Also noted was a slight tremor in David's hands when he was placing and displacing small items on shelves.

*Range of Motion.*

David has no joint limitations that would hinder his ability to perform gross motor tasks. He is not able to evert and invert his feet fully, but this is probably due to lack of body awareness of the ankle.

*Sensory Testing.*

The sensory test measures stereognosis (tactile discrimination with eyes closed) and pain, temperature, and position sense. David completed all the tasks satisfactorily.

*Right-Left Discrimination.*

David correctly identified the right and left sides of his body and of objects in his environment. He was not able correctly to determine right and left on another person, identifying them as opposite of what they were.

*Hand and Office Tool Test.*

David used a stapler, scissors, hole punch, and paper clip satisfactorily. He had difficulty tearing tape from a tape dispenser at first but learned quickly after a demonstration. David knew how to use a screwdriver but demonstrated poor coordination when attempting to keep the tool in the screw slot. He knew how to use the pliers but it took him some time to make them do what he wanted. He also had trouble using two tools at once (e.g., screwdriver and wrench). He used a hammer satisfactorily.

*Bruininks-Oseretsky Test of Motor Proficiency.*

The Bruininks-Oseretsky test measures speed, dexterity, and strength of limbs together with visual motor abilities. David scored at a 10 years 5 months level in upper limb coordination (target throwing and kinesthetic awareness of arms). Visual motor control fell at 7 years 11 months, upper limb speed and dexterity at 7 years 2 months, and speed of response at 5 years 8 months. These results indicate that David can plan how to use his arms but performs tasks at a slow rate. The visual motor tests indicate the presence of perceptual problems (especially shape reproduction) and some difficulty with fine motor control of a pencil.

*Minnesota Rate of Manipulation Test, Purdue Pegboard and Grooved Pegboard.*

Tests of fine motor dexterity and manipulation indicate that David has average ability in this area. He was able to manipulate the test items satisfactorily at an average rate of speed.

*Academic Skills.*
David demonstrated some difficulty discriminating between typewritten letters and numbers. His ability to match names and addresses is fair. During this task he looked over his work upon completion, found his own errors, and corrected them. David counted 20 items easily. He has learned safety words by rote but is unable to do any other reading.

SUMMARY
David's areas of strength include gross motor endurance and functional strength, balance, and overall body awareness. Cooperation, ability to relate to others, and ability to learn from demonstrated tasks or his own mistakes are also positive traits. David's fine motor abilities are fair: His speed is average, and he has some tremoring.

RECOMMENDATIONS
David would be successful in a job requiring gross motor skills such as janitor, groundskeeper, or kennel worker. He could also learn jobs using fine motor skills such as packaging or other workshop tasks, but his slow working pace would affect his success. Because of his high social skills and ability to accept responsibility, it is felt that David could succeed at a community job.

## James Whitcomb Riley Hospital

Many new programs are being established to provide work-related programming and assessment for the physically disabled teenager and young adult. One example is a program developed by the occupational therapy department at James Whitcomb Riley Hospital for Children in Indianapolis, Indiana [5]. Briefly, this program consists of three segments: (1) prevocational and vocational consultation—discussions that allow for the formulation of realistic work-related planning; (2) prevocational evaluation—assessment of physical functioning, work behaviors, and skills; and (3) an individually developed prevocational program. Although each program is individually tailored, two basic worker behavior segments—personal communication and coping with criticism—are included in all programs [5].

## Handicapped Employment Training Assistance Unit

Another example of a program developed for physically disabled teenagers and young adults has a group emphasis. It is the Handicapped Employment Training Assistance (HETA) Unit, established in 1978 by the Crippled Children's Association of South Australia. HETA trainees "are carefully monitored through a group work/work assessment programme until they have the skills to make realistic job choices, gain employment and maintain themselves in the work force" [6].

The program consists of three units that have been devised in a developmental progression; successful completion of one unit allows for entry into the next [3]. The first unit involves *group sessions* that assist trainees in setting goals that can be achieved within a group discussion framework. For example, the trainee might set the goal of presenting himself or herself in a positive manner during a job interview. In the second unit, on *job assessment placements*, trainees have the opportunity to test out in actual work situations the work skills and behaviors they have gained through the group sessions. HETA has 325 employers to draw on for placement, and each trainee receives several two-week placements (an average of three placements per trainee). Finally, for trainees who have completed at least three successful job assessment placements but remain unemployed, the *future employment unit* offers a job-finding club. "Members are encouraged to actively seek work, develop meaningful recreation activities and maintain and develop new skills" [6].

In the HETA units, the occupational therapist plays a key role in the comprehensive evaluation of trainees, as a resource person, and in counseling. Modapts* (Modular Arrangement of Pre-determined Time Standards) are commonly used to evaluate work ability. In addition, general physical functioning is assessed.

As a resource person, the occupational therapist interprets medical information for the staff member team in terms of the limits it sets on work options and assists the vocational coordinator in the choice of appropriate job assessment placements. In some instances the therapist makes simple adaptations to a job placement, for example, ramps, telephone head set, volume control phone. These occasions are at a minimum because the program's philosophy is to find positions that are appropriate to the trainee's remaining abilities.

The therapist has a small case load for counseling, which takes place in group sessions. "As an extension of this involvement in groups the occupational therapist is responsible for the development and cataloguing of the programme kits. Activities and games that have been developed to demonstrate concepts such as risk taking, consensus, confidence etc. are documented in kit form in order that the ideas and materials can be used more than once" [6].

HETA has had a high success rate with trainees. Approximately 65 percent of its trainees have been successfully placed in open employment [6].

## References

1. Bergman, A. *A Guide to Establishing an Activity Center for Mentally Retarded Persons.* Washington, D.C.: President's Committee on Employment of the Handicapped, 1977.
2. Brayman, S. J., Kirby, T. F., and Misenheimer, A. M. Comprehensive occupational therapy evaluation scale. *Am. J. Occup. Ther.* 30:94, 1976.
3. Crippled Children's Association of South Australia, Handicapped Employment Training Assistance Unit brochure. Andrew T. Kyprianou, Programme Director, HETA, The Regency Park Rehabilitation Centre for the Disabled, Days Road, Regency Park, South Australia 5010.

*Information on Modapts can be obtained by writing to Australian Association of Pre-determined Time Standards and Research, 525 Elizabeth Street, Sydney, N.S.W., Australia 2006.

4. Heller, J. *Typing for the Physically Handicapped: Methods and Keyboard Presentation Charts*. New York: Gregg Division/McGraw-Hill, 1978.
5. Hopkins, H. L., and Smith, H. D. *Willard and Sparkman's Occupational Therapy* (6th ed.). Philadelphia: Lippincott, 1983.
6. Lyons, T. HETA—A Groupwork Approach to Work Preparation for the Young Physically Handicapped. Presented at the Australian Association of Occupational Therapists Twelfth Federal Conference, August 1982.
7. Occupational Therapy Department, James Whitcomb Riley Hospital for Children. *Planning for the Future—Prevocational Programs for Disabled Youth*. Indianapolis: Indiana University Hospital, 1982.
8. Wright, G. N. *Total Rehabilitation*. Boston: Little, Brown, 1980.

# 5. Programs for Adults

*. . . In our society, the twenties are a time of work preparation, job exploration, and settling in, while the thirties are years of work advancement.*

*H. L. Hopkins and H. D. Smith*

## Programming for Adults with Psychosocial Problems

Many variables must be considered in planning and implementing a work-related program for adults with psychosocial dysfunctioning. Because of their fear of failure, these clients often have difficulty making transitions and adapting to change. Often a therapist will notice that a client decompensates when a change in routine occurs, for example, entry into a "work" program. Other types of problems that are encountered by these clients with regard to work may involve their inability to organize, manage time requirements, get along with others (especially authority figures), and solve problems [10].

The therapist must continually be aware of inconsistencies in behavior and work performance evidenced by the client because of the psychotic process or medication given to treat it. Changes in medication or inconsistent use or even disuse may have a profound effect on the client.

Work-related assessments used with those with psychosocial dysfunctions should provide the opportunity for the client to work with other people. Unfortunately this ability is not always evaluated in these assessments and must be ascertained during therapy. At the New York Veterans Administration Medical Center, a portion of the Jacobs Prevocational Skills Assessment (see Chap. 3) has been adapted and found a useful instrument with a population of veterans with physical or psychiatric disabilities or both.

The programs presented in this chapter illustrate the diversity in treatment facilities and program implementation. Not only are the traditional hospital and community mental health center discussed, but forensic psychiatry and correctional institutions are also included. Once again, it is hoped that you will gain insights from these program descriptions that will be useful in your own practice.

### Veterans Administration Medical Center

NEW YORK VA MEDICAL CENTER*

A prevocational program for veterans with psychiatric or physical disabilities (or both) has been developed at the New York Veterans Administration Med-

*Most of the information presented on the New York Veterans Administration Medical Center was prepared by Lauren Kirson, OTR.

ical Center. The program, which is open to both inpatients and outpatients, includes a daily workshop, a work incentive program, and community work alternatives.

The occupational therapy prevocational program involves four levels of care: screening, evaluation, treatment, and disposition. The program has helped veterans to explore vocational goals and to adapt to work (work adjustment).

Occupational therapy, physical therapy, corrective therapy, and educational therapy are all sections of the rehabilitation medicine service (RMS) and are responsible to the chief of RMS, who is a physiatrist.

The occupational therapy department, headed by the chief occupational therapist, comprises an assistant chief occupational therapist; three psychosocial occupational therapists, each assigned to a separate psychiatric inpatient ward; four physical dysfunction occupational therapists, three of whom are involved with general physical disabilities rehabilitation, the fourth being a hand therapist; and a prevocational occupational therapist. A case manager, who is responsible to the chief of RMS, assists patients with outside vocational and educational referrals and works closely with the prevocational occupational therapist.

*Referrals to Prevocational Occupational Therapy*

Referrals are made from the RMS through the physical dysfunction therapists and from the psychiatry service through the psychosocial therapists. Outside the RMS, referrals are made on a consultation basis and are usually a part of the medical team's treatment plan for the patient.

At the time of referral, the prevocational therapist requests medical background information about the patient from the occupational therapist making the referral or the staff member requesting the consultation. The patient's medical record is also used for initial data gathering. At the time of the referral the treatment team discusses the purpose and possible goals for the patient in prevocational treatment and the treatment team's probable discharge plans for the patient.

Before the initial prevocational evaluation, screening information is provided by the occupational therapist to the prevocational therapist. For physical disabilities patients, this information includes the initial occupational therapy evaluation, a functional summary, and, when available, a self-report. These items provide information about the following areas: (1) independent living and daily living skills and performance, (2) sensorimotor skills and performance, (3) cognitive skills and performance, (4) therapeutic adaptations, (5) leisure skills, and (6) any specialized evaluation results available. For psychosocial dysfunction patients the screening information includes the patient's history and course of hospitalization, present psychiatric status, and results of the following assessments: the Barth Time Construction [2], Comprehensive Occupational Therapy Evaluation (COTE) scale scores [5], and a self-report.

The areas assessed in screening are:

1. Self-care
2. Homemaking and maintenance
3. Work or school
4. Leisure time and work-play balance
5. Social interpersonal skills (group)
6. Social relations
7. Psychological intrapersonal skills (individual)
8. Sensory motor and psychomotor functions

*Prevocational Evaluation*

As part of the prevocational evaluation, the patient is *interviewed* by using the screening sheet shown in Fig. 5–1 to obtain specific information about his or her educational, vocational, and leisure history and to aid in determining treatment goals. It is also important to find out if the patient is service connected, as service-connected veterans are eligible for more benefits. The veteran is also asked about his or her plans with regard to living situation, work, training, school, or volunteering.

In addition to the interview, a set of *structured tasks* is used to assess (1) sensorimotor skills including gross and fine coordination, strength, endurance, sensory integrative skills including figure-ground discrimination, visual motor integration, and praxis; and (2) cognitive skills including concentration, attention span, memory, and problem solving. The following tasks are administered:

The patient is presented with *a small box of screws* of various sizes. The therapist chooses one screw and asks the patient to pick a certain number of screws of the same size.

The patient is shown *pieces of colored paper* and is asked to identify one color at a time. Next the patient is given simple written directions to arrange the colored paper in a certain order.

The patient is first given *12 cards*, each bearing a word starting with a different letter of the alphabet, and is asked to put the cards in alphabetical order. Then the patient is given another set of cards, this time with words all starting with the same letter, and again is asked to alphabetize them.

The assessment tasks that have just been described are similar to those from the Jacobs Prevocational Skills Assessment. Lauren Kirson, who attended my session at the annual American Occupational Therapy Association in Philadelphia in 1982, felt that the assessment could be used with a mixed population with both psychosocial and physical dysfunctions.

Tiled Trivet Assessment.

The following materials are required for the tiled trivet assessment [21]:

8″ × 8″ piece of cardboard
Box of tiles of assorted colors, sizes, and shades
Glue
Sample of a tiled trivet with light-against-dark pattern of any hue

**Prevocational Program Screening Sheet**

PERSONAL DATA

Date __________

1. Name __________
2. Address __________
3. Social Security No. __________
4. Date of birth __________
5. Service connection __________ (percentage)
6. Diagnosis __________
7. Ward (referring source) __________
8. Primary therapist __________
9. Precautions __________
10. Source of income __________

EDUCATIONAL DATA

11. What level of education did you reach? __________
12. Did you ever attend any special schools? __________
13. Have you ever received vocational training? (State where and when.) __________
14. Do you have any degrees, licenses, or certificates? (Specify type, date, and where received.) __________
15. What subjects did you like when you were in school? __________
16. What subjects did you dislike when you were in school? __________

VOCATIONAL DATA

17. What is the last job that you held? __________
18. When did you work there and for how long? __________
19. State your title and briefly describe your duties. __________
20. What was your reason for leaving this job? __________
21. What other jobs have you held and how long? (Include service duties.) __________
22. What was your favorite job, and why? __________
23. What was your least favorite job, and why? __________
24. How do you learn best on the job? __________
25. In your work experience, did you have any conflicts with your supervisor or other employees? (Please explain.) __________
26. How do you spend your leisure time? (Special interests or hobbies?) __________
27. What would you like to be doing a year from now? __________

YOUR JOB INTERESTS, IN ORDER OF RANK

28. __________
29. __________
30. __________
31. __________

DOCUMENTATION RECEIVED

Consult
Doctor's order
Self-report
Functional summary (Phys. Dys.)

RECOMMENDATION

Placement area:
Starting time and date:

Approved By:

*Fig. 5-1. Screening sheet used in interview for prevocational program at New York Veterans Administration Medical Center, Rehabilitation Medicine Service. (Courtesy Lauren Kirson, OTR.)*

*Fig. 5-2. Prevocational assessment form. (Courtesy New York Veterans Administration Medical Center.)*

**Prevocational Assessment**

Name:
SS#:

Date:
Ward, Area:
Supervisor:

Rating Scale: 5 = excellent or high; 1 = poor or low

| I. WORK SKILLS AND HABITS | *Excellent* | *Very Good* | *Good* | *Fair* | *Poor* |
|---|---|---|---|---|---|
| 1. Attendance | 5 | 4 | 3 | 2 | 1 |
| 2. Punctuality | 5 | 4 | 3 | 2 | 1 |
| 3. Responsibility | 5 | 4 | 3 | 2 | 1 |
| 4. Neatness | 5 | 4 | 3 | 2 | 1 |
| 5. Endurance | 5 | 4 | 3 | 2 | 1 |
| 6. Organization | 5 | 4 | 3 | 2 | 1 |
| 7. Initiative | 5 | 4 | 3 | 2 | 1 |
| 8. Productivity | 5 | 4 | 3 | 2 | 1 |
| 9. Works independently | 5 | 4 | 3 | 2 | 1 |
| 10. Concentration | 5 | 4 | 3 | 2 | 1 |
| 11. Manual dexterity | 5 | 4 | 3 | 2 | 1 |
| 12. Work quality | 5 | 4 | 3 | 2 | 1 |
| II. LEARNING ABILITIES | | | | | |
| 13. Verbal instructions | 5 | 4 | 3 | 2 | 1 |
| 14. Written instructions | 5 | 4 | 3 | 2 | 1 |
| 15. Demonstrative instructions | 5 | 4 | 3 | 2 | 1 |
| 16. Memory, retention | 5 | 4 | 3 | 2 | 1 |
| 17. Recognizes errors | 5 | 4 | 3 | 2 | 1 |

(Continued)

| | | | | | |
|---|---|---|---|---|---|
| III. INTERPERSONAL RELATIONSHIPS | | | | | |
| 18. Accepts supervision | 5 | 4 | 3 | 2 | 1 |
| 19. Works with others | 5 | 4 | 3 | 2 | 1 |
| IV. SOCIAL AND PSYCHOLOGICAL ADJUSTMENT | | | | | |
| 20. Hygiene | 5 | 4 | 3 | 2 | 1 |
| 21. Motivation | 5 | 4 | 3 | 2 | 1 |
| 22. Confidence | 5 | 4 | 3 | 2 | 1 |
| 23. Anxiety tolerance | 5 | 4 | 3 | 2 | 1 |
| 24. Frustration tolerance | 5 | 4 | 3 | 2 | 1 |
| 25. Independence | 5 | 4 | 3 | 2 | 1 |
| 26. Attitude toward work | 5 | 4 | 3 | 2 | 1 |
| 27. Self-esteem | 5 | 4 | 3 | 2 | 1 |

DISPOSITION:

PLAN:

Fig. 5-2 (continued)

The therapist sits on the patient's dominant side, about two feet away, and places the box of tiles in a position to encourage midline crossing. The therapist presents the sample trivet and asks the patient to "make a trivet with the same design and then glue the tiles in place."

A *prevocational assessment form* has been developed to rate the patient's work skills and habits, learning abilities, interpersonal relationships, and social and psychological adjustment after the interview and evaluation tasks (Fig. 5-2).

*Treatment Planning*

After the initial prevocational evaluation is completed a *treatment plan* is made, based on the patient's physical and functional status; work, educational, and leisure history; performance on the evaluation; attitude, motivation, interests, and goals; psychological and social characteristics; and, for inpatients, discharge data and probable discharge plans.

Patients *may be excluded* from the prevocational program if when they are evaluated they display two or more major deficits in the following performance components: motor, sensory integrative, cognitive, psychological, or social functioning. Patients may also be excluded if they are unable to complete satisfactorily a two-week comprehensive assessment in the prevocational workshop.

*Prevocational Treatment*

The *prevocational workshop*, which is supervised by the prevocational occupational therapist, provides patients with work samples in a variety of areas such as clerical work, piecework, mechanical and electrical work, and crafts. These work samples are used to assess a patient's interest and potential in different vocational areas and to improve work skills, work habits, learning abilities, interpersonal relationships, and social and psychological adjustment.

The workshop is open two hours daily, five days a week. Individual schedules are arranged based on the patient's availability (taking into account other scheduled treatment), need for daily structure, treatment plan, and endurance. Each patient's progress is updated once a month, and individual meetings are held with patients as needed to discuss their progress, treatment plans, and possible disposition. The prevocational assessment form (see Fig. 5-2) is used to evaluate the patient's workshop progress.

There are two levels in the workshop. The *ongoing assessment level* is for patients who need longer-term or ongoing comprehensive assessment and exploration of work-related goals. This level can be used to assess a patient's readiness for the Monetary Incentive Program (MIP, discussed below) and to provide work training with ongoing supervision. This level is limited to approximately two weeks. The *skill practice level,* is for patients who, after the initial prevocational evaluation and the two-week workshop assessment, need further treatment in the areas of work skill and habits and require a structured supportive setting with regular supervision. This level can be used to prepare patients for (1) further inpatient services, (2) outpatient referrals through the case manager, (3) the MIP, or (4) community alternatives. This level is limited to approximately six months.

The Monetary Incentive Program, a program of jobs in various services throughout the hospital, gives patients first-hand job experience. The patient is given a choice of assignments and ranks them in order of preference. The prevocational occupational therapist secures the desired position by a visit or phone call to the area and then meets with the MIP area supervisor to brief him or her about the patient. Next, the therapist and patient meet to discuss the work assignment and possible hours of duty, which are finalized in a meeting of the patient, therapist, and MIP area supervisor in the MIP work area. A time card on which the patient records his or her work hours is kept in the MIP work area. The patient and therapist meet weekly to discuss the patient's progress. The therapist also contacts the MIP area supervisor to keep informed of the patient's progress. This program is limited to approximately three months.

Counseling about *work alternatives* such as volunteer or leisure activities in the community, stroke clubs, and senior citizen centers is provided for patients who have been in occupational therapy treatment. In most cases the patient is seen by the prevocational occupational therapist for an initial prevocational assessment. For these patients the stress is on their work history, the skills they still possess, their leisure interests, their community, the availability of transportation, and their ability to use it. In some cases phone calls may be made to obtain openings in community centers or to give patients information about specific community resources. Patients are advised to learn more about resources independently or with family members. Follow-up is provided through meetings with or phone calls to patients to see if they are able to make use of the referrals and to see if further intervention is needed.

*Discharge and Disposition*

When a patient has shown improvement in work skills and habits or has reached a baseline level in work functioning, he or she should be ready for discharge from the program. The patient should also have a better understanding of his or her assets and some acceptance of the limitations as imposed by his or her disability. It is hoped that the patient will have more realistic and specific goals. These goals may take the form of referrals to various community resources. At this point the prevocational therapist works closely with the case manager to make appropriate referrals. Patients are most often referred to the following resources:

1. The Office of Vocational Rehabilitation of New York City, which has offices in the five boroughs, and provides counseling, referral to training centers, and placement
2. The Veterans' Upgrade Center, which provides counseling, testing, and job referrals
3. The VA regional office, which provides outpatient vocational counseling and rehabilitation and houses the Curative Workshop, a sheltered workshop open to service-connected veterans
4. The Job Service of the New York State Department of Labor, which provides testing, counseling, training, and placement
5. Federation, Employment and Guidance Service, which provides counseling, testing, and referral for training or placement
6. The Private Industry Council, which provides training and placement
7. The Employment Program for Recovering Alcoholics, which provides counseling, testing, and referral for training or placement
8. The Division of Substance Abuse Services of New York State, which provides vocational and educational training, testing, and counseling
9. The International Center for the Disabled, which provides counseling, evaluation, testing (TOWER System), prevocational and vocational training, and sheltered workshop training
10. The New York City Board of Education, which provides adult education programs and a directory of educational and leisure programs

*Case Study**

R. D. is a 50-year-old man who was separated from his wife before his admission to the inpatient psychiatric unit of the New York VA Medical Center in May 1982. He has a son aged 12 and a daughter aged 11. R. D. had been living with his family in

*This case study was prepared by Lauren Kirson, OTR, New York Veterans Administration Medical Center, New York, New York.

an unfurnished apartment. The family slept on the floor in blankets. There were no cooking facilities in the apartment.

R. D. has had many psychiatric admissions as a result of marital difficulties and alcoholism. His provisional diagnosis on this admission was depressive reaction secondary to marital discord and alcoholism in a dependent personality.

After two months of treatment on the admissions unit, the patient was transferred to the intermediate unit for further treatment. He was referred for prevocational evaluation on July 19, 1982, by the occupational therapist on that unit. R. D. was seen initially in prevocational occupational therapy on July 23, 1982, when his educational and leisure history were obtained. His education was limited to the sixth grade. The patient's father apparently withdrew him from school after the patient had had to repeat a year because of failing grades.

Before his military service R. D. worked as a short-order cook for about two years. In 1950 he enlisted in the army and was stationed in Alaska, where he worked in communications and saw no military action. He received a rank of private E-2 and was honorably discharged in 1952.

After his discharge he worked as a furniture sprayer. He left this position after six years because he felt that the paint fumes were causing him health problems. For the next two to three years R. D. was either unemployed or worked at odd jobs.

From 1961 to 1965 he worked as an operations engineer at the Hess Refinery, checking temperature readings. During his time of employment at Hess, he became more involved with alcohol abuse and eventually was fired from his position.

After 1965 R. D. worked at numerous odd jobs for short periods of time and spent a great deal of time unemployed. Most recently he worked as a food preparer for four months in early 1982, before his admission to the medical center.

The patient's leisure time is spent watching television and occasionally fishing.

The patient was next given the prevocational structured tasks battery. The results were as follows:

1. Work skills and habits: Score 4—very good with mild impairments noted in organization
2. Learning abilities: Score 3—good with mild deficits noted in ability to comprehend written directions
3. Interpersonal relationships: Score 4—very good
4. Social and psychological adjustment: Score 3—Good with impairments noted in patient's confidence, self-esteem, and anxiety tolerance.

R. D. expressed an interest in future work in the food service area. On the basis of the results of the prevocational assessment, he appeared ready and motivated for an MIP assignment in the food service area.

To assess further the patient's ability to work with foods and to determine whether his skills were commensurate with an MIP assignment, R. D. was given a cooking evaluation, which was to make a simple salad and dressing. (The MIP assignment available to occupational therapy is in the ingredients control unit, which involves working with fruits and vegetables.) The cooking evaluation revealed that R. D. was able to work with foods independently, plan the preparation of food, and use utensils safely and effectively to produce a successful outcome.

The MIP assignment was used to improve the patient's deficit areas (low self-esteem, decreased confidence, poor anxiety tolerance, and weak organizational skills) and to prepare him for possible future employment, perhaps in the food service area.

On August 3, 1982, R. D. began his assignment in dietetics, which was to work in the hospital kitchen three hours daily in the morning. R. D. worked in the ingredients control unit chopping vegetables and making salad plates and had some stock duties. After a month, R. D. increased his assignment time to four hours daily and was willing to work during early morning hours. The patient's MIP area supervisor reported that his attendance and punctuality were excellent and that he was able to complete all assigned tasks well.

R. D. was also a member of the MIP discussion group, in which he participated actively, discussing work-related issues and plans for future employment. He also attended groups on the alcohol rehabilitation unit and was able to control his drinking.

During September the patient came to the prevocational occupational therapist asking for assistance in filling out an application for employment in dietetics at the medical center. The application was completed, and the patient submitted it to personnel. His MIP area supervisor had given the patient a letter of reference recommending him for the position. In October R. D. was notified that he had been accepted for part-time employment in dietetics. He began his part-time job in early November, while still hospitalized, and was then discharged from prevocational occupational therapy. Shortly thereafter, the patient found a furnished room to rent and was discharged from the medical center. The patient has been seen informally in the hospital and has remarked that his job is going well and that he plans to seek another part-time job.

## Psychiatric Rehabilitation Programs

### FOUNTAIN HOUSE

Fountain House is the first psychiatric rehabilitation program established in the United States for the purpose of facilitating the social and vocational adjustment of individuals into the community after psychiatric hospitalization [3]. At Fountain House, which is located in a homelike clubhouse in New York City, over 1,000 persons attend monthly as members of a club, not as "patients." The clubhouse is open seven days a week and provides a prevocational day program that includes six units: (1) thrift shop, (2) snack bar, (3) clerical office, (4) kitchen and dining room, (5) administration, and (6) education. The program is structured to include those activities essential to clubhouse function. Members select activities that are of interest to them and that will provide them with maximum success.

> Fountain House has arranged a world that cannot function unless its members are present and active. Members work on the switchboard and reception desk, and they do maintenance, research, member reachout, and clerical jobs (which include putting out a daily newspaper for members). They run the kitchen and large dining room; they shop for food, prepare and serve more than 250 midday meals, and clean up [32].

Approximately six staff workers are responsible for supervising each unit and providing rehabilitation to its members. In essence, each unit is a smaller Fountain House, having its own responsibilities for each of the services provided by the agency. These services include (1) the Transitional Employment Program (TEP); (2) a reachout program for dropouts and rehospitalized members; (3) an apartment program for members unable to obtain adequate housing; (4) High Point, a farm project located in New Jersey that enables members to learn to garden and care for farm animals; and (5) an evening and weekend social and recreational program.

It is the TEP that is of interest to us and that will provide an example to occupational therapy programs in other facilities.

*Transitional Employment Program*

Each weekday approximately 150 members work, on a half-time basis, in over 40 businesses in New York and New Jersey. Placement has been secured by staff workers who have approached commerce and industry for entry-level positions requiring little training or few skills. These jobs are usually subject to high turnover or absenteeism. Arrangements are made with the employer to fill jobs on a permanent basis rotating employees every three to six months. Two members are assigned the placement, one in the morning, the other in the afternoon; each receives the prevailing wage. The staff worker performs the job for a few hours or days before member placement to understand its requirements thoroughly and then works alongside the member during his or her first days.

TEP has a well-established success record, and agencies now contact Fountain House for employees. Eventually, some members progress from TEP to full-time employment. As Beard [3] has noted, "Transitional employment . . . is an example of a social device which circumvents a series of barriers which all too often prevent employment of many psychiatric patients who have the capacity to perform gainful employment."

Fountain House serves as a model program providing the impetus for the establishment of clubhouses and TEPs both nationally and internationally. In 1977 Fountain House initiated a National Staff Training Program, which provides training opportunities "to stimulate the development of essential community services for the severely disabled psychiatric patient, and to significantly assist in the expansion of rehabilitation opportunities for this underserviced and most needful mentally disabled population" [32].

## McLEAN HOSPITAL OPEN DOOR THRIFT SHOP

McLean Hospital's Open Door Thrift Shop, a community-based retail program, is a derivation of the Fountain House model (Fig. 5–3). McLean is a private, nonprofit inpatient and outpatient facility for psychiatrically disabled clients. Within its rehabilitation services department, a variety of vocational rehabilitation programs, including a hospital-based clerical training program, food service training, and the Open Door Thrift Shop, are provided.

The shop was established in 1973 by an activity therapist as an integral part of the Clinical Vocational Assessment Program. It is an optional component in the training of McLean Hospital occupational therapy students. Donna Gatti, the program's current coordinator, describes the shop this way [13]: "The basic objectives of the program are twofold: to permit formal and informal evaluation of client's social, emotional and basic vocational functioning and to provide a transitional community setting for the habilitation or rehabilitation of work adjustment skills." In most cases the shop represents the first opportunity for clients to practice these skills outside the hospital.

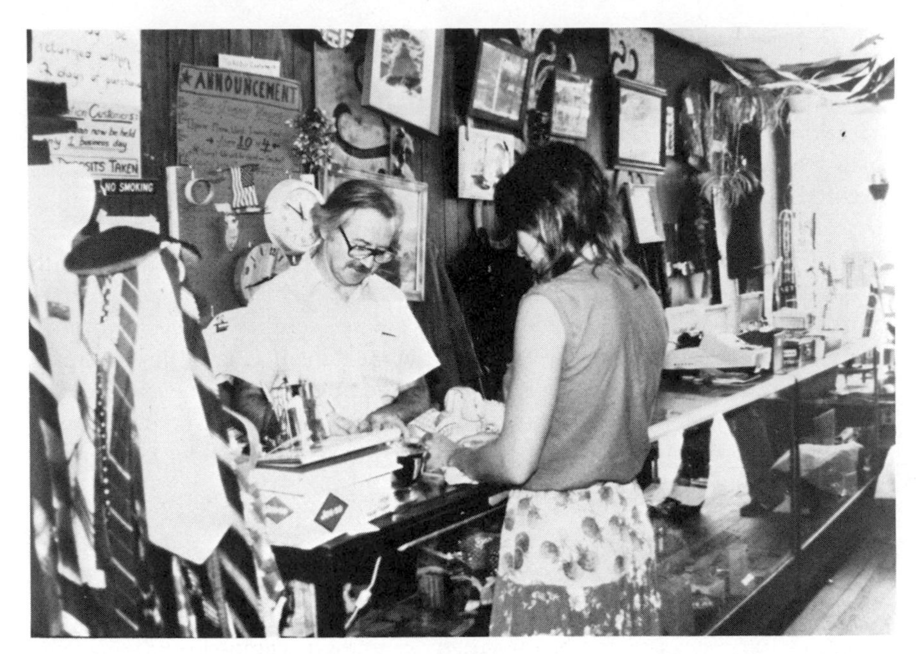


*Fig. 5-3. McLean Hospital's Open Door Thrift Shop, Belmont, Massachusetts. (Photo courtesy of Matthew Gold.)*

It has been effective in helping clients make the transition to more functional community roles.

The shop is located approximately one-half mile from the hospital, with a shuttle provided for the physically disabled. Over 60 patients participate in the program per year for an average three-month period. This amount of time is in keeping with the 1975 Supreme Court decision on Patient Worker Wage and Hour legislation, which specifies a limit of 90 program hours for vocational evaluation and training of patients [27].

Shop tasks are analyzed, and clients are appropriately placed in jobs ranging from simple to complex. Clients work together on the truck that picks up donated merchandise, sort and price items, and, in the shop itself, sell directly to the public. Envelope stuffing, sorting, housekeeping, and activities of daily living such as vacuuming, dusting, and folding clothes are examples of highly structured, simple, one- or two-step repetitive tasks. Cashiering and preparing window and case displays are multistep, less structured tasks that require initiative and judgment.

*Referral Process*

Typically, after an inpatient has had various performance-related assessments, he or she can become eligible for referral to the shop by the rehabilitation counselor. Most clients referred are between the ages of 18 and 30 and have poor or nonexistent work histories; a large number have been hospitalized for more than 90 days.

Name ______________________________ Date __________

1. What is your reason for wanting to work in the Thrift Shop?

______________________________

______________________________

______________________________

2. Do you think you could work on an "outside" job if one were available?

______________________________

3. Please rate yourself in comparison to people you have worked with before.

| | *Above Average* | *Average* | *Below Average* |
|---|---|---|---|
| Attendance | ____ | ____ | ____ |
| Quality of work | ____ | ____ | ____ |
| Quantity of work | ____ | ____ | ____ |
| Ability to deal with co-workers | ____ | ____ | ____ |
| Ability to deal with supervisor | ____ | ____ | ____ |

4. Please list, to the best of your recollection, all previous jobs held, and approximate length of time at each.

*Fig. 5-4. Questionnaire for McLean Hospital clients applying for work in the Open Door Thrift Shop.*

Once referred, the client meets with the program coordinator for an interview, tours the shop, and is introduced to shop tasks. In the interview the client is asked to share both verbally and in written form his or her expectations and goals from participation in the shop and to discuss previous work history. At this time the coordinator discusses general program expectations such as dressing appropriately (in line with community standards), maintaining control over behavior disturbing to other workers and customers, recognizing impending loss of control and returning to hospital, being responsible for arranging appointments that are not in conflict with established work schedule and for making travel arrangements between the hospital and shop, following directions, maintaining a minimum level of verbal communication, and participating in weekly "employee" meetings. At the conclusion of the interview, clients who decide to begin placement complete a brief preemployment questionnaire and receive copies of the mutually arranged work schedule (Fig. 5–4).

Formal work evaluations are conducted monthly, with informal individual meetings held as necessary (Fig. 5–5). There is frequent communication among the program coordinator, the rehabilitation counselor, and hall (i.e., ward) treatment teams. On completion of the program the client is asked to fill out a program evaluation, which not only assists in synthesizing his or her work experience but also provides the coordinator with ongoing feedback on the entire program (Fig. 5–6).

**Evaluation Form**

| PRODUCTION AND WORK SKILLS | *Needs improvement* | *Acceptable* |
|---|---|---|
| Concentrates on tasks | ______ | ______ |
| Follows verbal directions | ______ | ______ |
| Follows written directions | ______ | ______ |
| Retains directions over time | ______ | ______ |
| Accurate in written tasks | ______ | ______ |
| Accurate in use of numbers | ______ | ______ |
| Completes tasks in assigned time | ______ | ______ |
| Paces own time | ______ | ______ |
| Consistent in task performance | ______ | ______ |
| Plans ahead in task assignments | ______ | ______ |
| Establishes task priority | ______ | ______ |
| Organizes two or more tasks | ______ | ______ |
| Able to shift from task to task | ______ | ______ |
| Able to learn new tasks | ______ | ______ |
| Physically coordinated for task | ______ | ______ |
| Physical tolerance (standing/ sitting) | ______ | ______ |
| Can work in a noisy area | ______ | ______ |
| Aware of consumer needs | ______ | ______ |
| Uses tools/equipment properly | ______ | ______ |
| Handles the unexpected | ______ | ______ |
| COOPERATION | | |
| Discusses work problems with supervisor | ______ | ______ |
| Works with fellow workers | ______ | ______ |
| Willing to redo tasks | ______ | ______ |

| MOTIVATION | *Needs improvement* | *Acceptable* |
|---|---|---|
| When in doubt, asks questions | ______ | ______ |
| Checks own work | ______ | ______ |
| Attempts tasks until correct | ______ | ______ |
| Avails self of suggestion to improve | ______ | ______ |
| Uses independent judgment | ______ | ______ |
| Sets own work goals | ______ | ______ |
| Eager to learn | ______ | ______ |
| Shares improvement ideas | ______ | ______ |
| RESPONSIBILITY | | |
| Attends regularly | ______ | ______ |
| Arrives punctually | ______ | ______ |
| Notifies work area when absent | ______ | ______ |
| Takes breaks as scheduled | ______ | ______ |
| Maintains organized work area | ______ | ______ |
| Directs others in tasks | ______ | ______ |
| Follows safety procedures | ______ | ______ |
| Familiar with environment of area | ______ | ______ |
| Accepts work standards | ______ | ______ |
| WORK TRAITS | | |
| Separates personal and work issues | ______ | ______ |
| Appropriate dress/hygiene | ______ | ______ |
| Use of verbal communication | ______ | ______ |
| At ease in work setting | ______ | ______ |
| Uses a sense of humor | ______ | ______ |
| Pride in work completed | ______ | ______ |
| Accepts praise | ______ | ______ |

Patient's Name ____________________ Hall __________ Date ______

Rehabilitation goal ____________________

Placement ____________ Task ____________ Rating ______

Current overall work strengths: ____________________

Areas needing improvement: ____________________

Specific work goals: ____________________

Patient's comment: ____________________

Patient's signature ____________________

Accrued weeks ____________ Hours per week ____________

Staff signature ____________ Counselor's signature ____________

*Fig. 5-5. McLean Hospital Work Evaluation sheet, filled out monthly in conference between client and therapist.*

Name ______________________ Date ____________

1. Please recall as clearly as you can your initial reason for coming to work in the Thrift Shop.

   ______________________

2. Has that goal been met? ______________________

   Why do you think this is so? ______________________

3. Please rate yourself in comparison with your co-workers.

| | *Above Average* | *Average* | *Below Average* |
|---|---|---|---|
| Quantity of work | ____ | ____ | ____ |
| Ability to deal with customers | ____ | ____ | ____ |
| Attendance | ____ | ____ | ____ |
| Ability to deal with co-workers | ____ | ____ | ____ |
| Quality of work | ____ | ____ | ____ |
| Ability to deal with supervision | ____ | ____ | ____ |

Do you think working in the Thrift Shop is: ____ similar to outside jobs
____ not at all like outside jobs

I feel ____ more able
____ less able
to hold an "outside" job than before working at the Thrift Shop.

5. How do you account for this? ______________________

   ______________________

6. Please rate the Thrift Shop as you see it.

| | *High* | *Medium* | *Low* |
|---|---|---|---|
| Amount of pressure on workers from customers | ____ | ____ | ____ |
| Amount of pressure on workers from supervisor | ____ | ____ | ____ |
| Amount of responsibility given to workers | ____ | ____ | ____ |
| Amount of criticism from supervisor | ____ | ____ | ____ |
| Amount of praise or support from supervisor | ____ | ____ | ____ |
| Amount of criticism from co-workers | ____ | ____ | ____ |
| General job satisfaction | ____ | ____ | ____ |
| Value of weekly meetings | ____ | ____ | ____ |

7. What did you find most frustrating? ______________________

   Most fun? ______________________

   Most challenging? ______________________

8. What changes would you like to see in the Thrift Shop?

OTHER COMMENTS

*Fig. 5-6. A program evaluation form, which McLean Hospital clients are requested to complete at the conclusion of their work experience program.*

## Community Mental Health Center

DR. SOLOMON CARTER FULLER CENTER

The Dr. Solomon Carter Fuller Mental Health Center is an example of a comprehensive community center established to meet the mental health and mental retardation needs of residents within a specific catchment area of Boston on either an inpatient or an outpatient basis.

One of the Fuller Center programs of interest to us is the Structured Client

WORK AREA: LAUNDRY

*Job cluster: laundry cleaner*
1. Dust
2. Empty waste baskets
3. Sweep floor
4. Wash floor
5. Wash and wipe walls
6. Wash windows
7. Other related duties

*Job cluster: mangle worker*
1. Load sheets onto rack
2. Stretch sheets flat on rack
3. Feed sheets onto spreader
4. Transfer racks to mangle
5. Feed sheets into mangle
6. Fold sheets coming from mangle
7. Stack folded sheets
8. Other related duties

*Job cluster: pants presser*
1. Operate leg presser
2. Operate trunk presser
3. Operate cuff presser
4. Fold and/or hang pants
5. Transfer completed work
6. Other related duties

*Job cluster: machine operator*
1. Load and unload machines
2. Add detergent
3. Start and stop machines
4. Tend and repair machines
5. Transfer laundry
6. Prepare special washes
7. Sort clean wash by article
8. Other related duties

*Job cluster: material handler*
1. Sort according to article
2. Sort according to building
3. Bundle laundry
4. Package laundry
5. Weigh laundry
6. Load and unload laundry
7. Fold and stack laundry
8. Receive and deliver laundry
9. Classify and mark incoming laundry
10. Other related duties

*Job cluster: shirt presser*
1. Operate sleeve presser
2. Operate collar and cuff presser
3. Operate body presser
4. Operate yoke presser
5. Fold and/or hang shirts
6. Transfer completed work
7. Other related duties

*Fig. 5-7. Duties of a typical hospital job.*

Work Program. Its objective is to provide individualized work-related skills and vocational training to the client to foster a more productive and independent life in the community. The program is coordinated jointly by the director of occupational therapy and the director of inpatient social work.

Three types of work placement are available to clients, depending on their need for supervision:

*Ward jobs.* Closely supervised clients, who are confined to their ward and who may be homicidal or suicidal, may be eligible for one of the two maintenance positions on their own ward. These jobs are supervised directly by the mental health worker.

*Occupational therapy department jobs.* Supervised clients not confined to the ward may be eligible for placement in jobs in occupational therapy equipment inventory and general maintenance in the occupational therapy department. Here, the client is always directly supervised by the occupational therapist.

*Hospital jobs.* Throughout the center graded jobs have been created relying heavily on nonclinicians to supervise clients. The work areas include laundry, clerical, food service, grounds and landscaping, housekeeping, painting, retail and gift shop, and storeroom. Fig. 5–7 shows examples of specific jobs and job responsibilities.

Before placement, clients go through a simulated job application process. They must complete application forms similar to those used by the center for its employees (Fig. 5–8). This is followed by an application interview with the work site supervisor. Typically a postinterview is held with one of the coordinators of the program to agree on the terms of the work assignment

*Fig. 5-8. Application form used in Structured Client Work Program, Dr. Solomon Carter Fuller Mental Health Center, Commonwealth of Massachusetts Department of Mental Health.*

Name: ______________________ Date: ________
Present Address: ______________________
Social Security Number: ______________________

| *Educational Record* | *Dates attended* | *Did you graduate?* |
|---|---|---|
| High school | ________ | Yes ___ No ___ |
| Vocational school | ________ | Yes ___ No ___ |
| Additional training or skills (languages, secretarial, etc.) | ________ | Yes ___ No ___ |

*Employment (list most recent position first)*
Name of company: ______________ Address: ______________
Date of Employment: ______________
Describe your duties: ______________

Reason for leaving: ______________
Name of company: ______________ Address: ______________
Date of employment: ______________
Describe your duties: ______________

Reason for leaving: ______________
What kind of jobs do you like? ______________

Do you have any disabilities that are limiting to you? ______________

Are you receiving or have you ever received workers' compensation or any type of disability payment? Yes ______ No______
Have you ever been a client of Massachusetts Rehabilitation? Yes _____ No_____

1. Client will be at work at the times required and will complete the expected number of hours.
2. If client is ill or unable to work for some other reason, client will notify the supervisor *before* the hour of expected arrival.
3. Client will participate in a work discussion group.
4. Client will follow supervisor's instructions while on the job. If a problem develops, it should be discussed in the work discussion group or with one of the group leaders individually. However, work must be finished for the day in spite of the problem.
5. If client is given a task that he or she is not sure how to do, client will ask the supervisor for directions.
6. If others are working in the same area, client will cooperate with them as necessary but will not interrupt their work with conversation or disruptive behavior.
7. Client will be put on probation for (a) failure to follow the guidelines or (b) one unexcused absence from work or group. After two unexcused absences, client will be suspended from the program. Readmission to the program may be negotiated.

______________________________
Client signature

______________
Date

*Fig. 5-9. Guidelines for Structured Client Work Program.*

(Fig. 5–9). The program is a dynamic one: When the vocational needs of the client change, his or her work assignment is changed accordingly.

All the clients participating in the program are required to attend a weekly 45-minute meeting of the work processing group. This group, which is co-led by an occupational therapist and a social work student, is a forum for discussion, role playing, and instruction. Once a month a state vocational rehabilitation counselor visits the group to become acquainted with the clients for future vocational potential in the community.

*Case Study**

Ralf is a 44-year-old man with chronic schizophrenia. He has a history of institutionalization from age 15 until six years ago, when he was deinstitutionalized to a group home and a sheltered workshop in the community. Ralf became very anxious and disorganized during this transition and within two months had failed at both placements. He was then moved to a nursing home, where he currently resides.

For the past six years Ralf has been participating in an activity-oriented day program for chronic mental health clients. He was referred to the Structured Client Work Program by day program staff because his performance in activity groups had been consistently good for over a year and because they felt he was ready to explore a

*This case study was written by Suzanne Poirier, M.S., OTR, Dr. Solomon Carter Fuller Mental Health Center, Boston, Massachusetts.

**Occupational Therapy Vocational Skills Evaluation**

Client: ______ Evaluator: ______

| | | Date | Date | Date | Comments |
|---|---|---|---|---|---|
| *Attendance:* | Is present except when excused for legitimate reasons (medical, vacation, etc.) | | | | |
| *Punctuality:* | Is ready to commence work at appointed time and works until designated time | | | | |
| *Appearance:* | Is clean, well-groomed, and appropriately dressed | | | | |
| *Cognitive Skills:* | Is able to undertand instructions | | | | |
| | Is able to organize task | | | | |
| | Is able to retain instructions | | | | |
| | Can concentrate on task being performed | | | | |
| | Demonstrates problem-solving abilities | | | | |
| | Demonstrates decision-making abilities | | | | |

| | | | | |
|---|---|---|---|---|
| *Interpersonal Skills:* Is able to ask for help appropriately | | | | |
| Can take initiative | | | | |
| Cooperates with supervisor | | | | |
| Demonstrates pride in work | | | | |
| Accepts supervision appropriately | | | | |
| *Task Skills:* Is able to work independently | | | | |
| Is able to follow through on task | | | | |
| Has good attention to details | | | | |
| Demonstrates work tolerance | | | | |
| Shows motivation and interest in task | | | | |
| Works with care and neatness | | | | |
| Rating: A1. Demonstrates strength<br>A2. Acceptable skill<br>B1. Problem specific to present task<br>B2. Adjustment needed<br>C1. Intervention needed | | | | |

*Fig. 5-10. Work behavior checklist. (Courtesy Cathi Wong-Bussetti, OTR.)*

worker role. Ralf had no previous work history except the short workshop placement mentioned above.

Prevocational evaluation revealed that Ralf was maintaining a stable daily routine organized within the day program–nursing home structure (Fig. 5–10). Although in this structure he was able to maintain a good level of task performance, he was hesitant to take risks and was "scared" of any new tasks or changes in routine. Within task groups he was cooperative and accepted supervision well. However, he was unable to ask for help or clarification when necessary. He could only say that this made him scared. His attention span, the quality of his work, his interest in activities,

*Fig. 5-11. Rating scale for establishing wage rates.*

**Vocational Skill and Production Rating Scale**

| Rating | Description |
|---|---|
| 100 | Meets or surpasses standards for business or industry. Approximately 100% of overall standard when compared with nonhandicapped workers at the work area. |
| 90 | Approaches average standards for business or industry and can work with minimal supervision. Approximately 90% of overall standard when compared with nonhandicapped workers at the work area. |
| 80 | Approaches average standards for business or industry but requires more than average supervision. Approximately 80% of overall standard when compared with nonhandicapped workers at the work area. |
| 70 | Below standards for business or industry but can work with average supervision. Approximately 70% of overall standard when compared with nonhandicapped workers at the work area. |
| 60 | Below standards for business or industry and requires more than average supervision. Approximately 60% of overall standard when compared with nonhandicapped workers at the work area. |
| 50 | Well below standards for business or industry. Approximately 50% of overall standard when compared with nonhandicapped workers at the work area. |
| 40 | Well below standards for business or industry. Approximately 40% of overall standard when compared with nonhandicapped workers at the work area. |
| 30 | Far below standards for business or industry. Approximately 30% of overall standard when compared with nonhandicapped workers at the work area. |
| 20 | Far below standards for business or industry. Approximately 20% of overall standard when compared with nonhandicapped workers at the work area. |
| 10 | Generally unacceptable. Approximately 10% of overall standard when compared with nonhandicapped workers at the work area. |
| 0 | Generally unacceptable. Productivity is inconsequential. |

and his relationship to other clients were all good. His goals, however, were vague: "I never really thought about me working. Maybe I could get a job and get off welfare."

After completing a simulated job application (see Fig. 5–8), Ralf was interviewed by the head of the maintenance department for a job that entailed mopping floors, polishing chrome, and washing woodwork in specific areas throughout the 12-story mental health center. Ralf, the job supervisor, and the occupational therapist together decided that Ralf should begin working two hours each morning. Ralf read and signed a contract that outlined the rules and regulations of the work program, including participation in a work processing group that met once a week. They agreed that he should continue in the day activity program for the remainder of the day.

The therapist and the job supervisor together set up criteria to measure Ralf's performance and established an individualized plan for instructing Ralf in his job. It was emphasized that Ralf needed success and positive feedback to feel a sense of competence. Because transitions would probably be problematic, it was also agreed that Ralf should increase his work time at his own pace.

Ralf quickly learned his work routine through individual instruction and by using maintenance department employees as role models. After four days he was able to work without direct supervision. At the end of the first two weeks his production was at 75 percent of a nonhandicapped worker's (Fig. 5-11). This increased steadily until at three months he had maintained 100 percent production for two hours per day for two weeks. Quality was consistently 100 percent. As his rate of production increased, his paycheck also increased to a ceiling of $1.45 per hour. During this time he received encouraging feedback from the job supervisor, the occupational therapist, and his peers in the work processing group.

At four months into the program, Ralf asked the occupational therapist during a work processing group meeting if she would let him work more hours. It was agreed after discussion that Ralf should negotiate this directly with his job supervisor. This made him anxious, but after two role-playing sessions, he successfully negotiated an increase in his hours to three per day. At the end of six months, he happily announced to the group that he had again negotiated an increase in hours to four per day and that this made him feel "like I can make decisions for myself and I'm my own person."

During the first weeks of the work processing group meetings, Ralf was quiet, participating passively. Gradually he began asking questions about banking and budgeting his paycheck and jobs available outside the mental health center. At the end of six months he had opened his first bank account, asked for individual help in budgeting from the occupational therapist, and contacted the state vocational rehabilitation counselor to explore possible jobs in the community. In addition, his goals became more focused: "I like working alone and I like my job in maintenance. I want to try working outside doing work on the grounds. If I work hard I'll bet I'll have a real job in less than one year."

## Forensic Psychiatry Programs

The forensic psychiatric institution presents a unique combination of goals and limitations for prevocational and vocational programs. By virtue of its patient population, it is usually a maximum security institution, not unlike a prison. However, it is also a hospital with an emphasis on restoring the mental health of its patients and shaping them into responsible citizens. Work-related occupational therapy programs in two such institutions are described here.

## CLIFTON T. PERKINS HOSPITAL CENTER*

### *Treatment Setting*

Clifton T. Perkins Hospital Center in Jessup, Maryland, is a forensic psychiatric institution. It serves approximately 240 male patients, 25 percent of whom are "pretrial," that is, court-committed patients charged with major crimes. Before a pretrial patient goes to court, the patient is examined to determine his competency to stand trial (whether he understands the charges and is capable of cooperating with the court) and his responsibility (whether he was suffering from a mental disorder that caused him to lack substantial capacity to appreciate the criminality of his conduct and/or conform his conduct to the requirements of the law) at the time the crime was committed. Fifteen percent of the population consists of penal transfers. These are patients who have become mentally ill while serving a jail or prison term. They remain institutionalized at the Center until their symptoms or behavior improves. Twenty percent of the patients come from other state hospitals. They are usually behavior or management problems causing danger to themselves or others. Approximately 4 percent are at the Center for observation and treatment for competency before standing trial. Finally, 50 percent have been declared insane by the courts (not guilty by reason of insanity) at the time of the commission of the crime; they are sent to Perkins until their behavior is no longer considered dangerous.

The average length of stay at the Center is 2½ years. Under the direct care of the hospital staff, patients are exposed to a multidisciplinary approach. They are seen regularly on their ward by a treatment team consisting of a psychiatrist, a clinical nurse, a nursing attendant, a social worker, a psychologist, and an occupational or activity therapist. This team evaluates the patient's strengths and weaknesses and attempts to coordinate a comprehensive program addressing those needs. Treatment includes drug therapy, verbal support groups, individual therapy, and activities. Occupational therapists screen patients observing characteristics such as hygiene, physical disabilities, perceptual problems, time use, cognition, and interests and assessing previous life situations. As a result further evaluation and treatment may be deemed appropriate.

The occupational therapy department is eclectic in its approach, taking into account the theories of Gail Fidler, Anne Cronin Mosey, Gary Kielhofner, and Claudia Allen [1]. The functional status of each patient is assessed in the hospital. Questions to be addressed include the following: How is he able to cope with stress, relate to others and his environment, and take care of his physical needs? What does he attend to? Can he follow written or verbal instructions? How complex? Does he have special interests? How realistic are those interests? What does he do during his unstructured time? Can he work in a group setting, or can he relate to only one person? What are his functional math skills?

*Most of this section was developed directly from information presented by Robin Klein, OTR.

*Evaluation*

All patients referred to the occupational therapy department undergo two hours of group testing. The first hour includes a questionnaire that assesses reality orientation, problem solving, time use, interests, perception, functional math skills, attention to written instructions, short-term memory, and leisure interests and identifies significant others. Reading and writing skills are also observed at this time. People who are functionally illiterate are questioned orally.

The second hour of the evaluation is task oriented. Patients are first given a model and instructed to reproduce it as closely as possible with the materials provided. This task addresses problem solving, sequencing, task organization, time management, fine motor skills, and the ability to follow verbal instructions. Patients are allowed 30 minutes to complete the project. Then a group task is presented. A large sheet of paper and several drawing media are placed on a table. The patients are instructed to plan, organize, and complete a mural as a group. They are allotted 30 minutes for the task. In this task each patient's ability to participate in a group is evaluated. The quantity and quality of contribution, the informal social interaction, the subject of the drawing, and its relation to the theme chosen by the group are all considered in this part of the evaluation.

The information extracted from the evaluation assists in developing a profile of the patient's functional abilities, interests, and values so that an individual treatment program can be formulated.

*Occupational and Activity Therapy Programs*

The hospital offers two interconnected departments: occupational therapy and activity therapy. The departments interface in patient treatment. However, the occupational therapist is solely responsible for evaluation and consults on activity therapy program development.

Patients are placed in an occupational therapy program according to their level of function. As skills develop and behavior changes, patients progress to the next higher level. The occupational therapy program's approach is similar to that of the hospital in that behavior and insight are the barometers of patients' readiness to move to less restrictive and more privileged environments. This progression eventually leads to a work release ward and finally to the community, at which point the patient is placed in a halfway house. After placement in a halfway house, the patient is followed for five years and must meet specific conditions or be subject to legal action.

The various occupational therapy programs attempt to address patients at every level.

In the *one-to-one* program the goal is to assist the patient who demonstrates an attention span limited to about five minutes. He may exhibit severe disorganization of thought processes; he may be unable to trust other patients or staff. The purpose of the therapy is to establish rapport through the introduction of simple familiar repetitive nonverbal tasks, such as playing cards, solving puzzles, drawing, listening to music and playing ball.

In *dyadic skills* the patient is introduced to the group therapeutic setting, which is structured into periods of 30 minutes and accommodates six patients. Games and tasks continue to be familiar and repetitive with the addition of verbal and nonverbal interactions between patients. Patients are paired, and activities are selected to elicit the sharing of materials. Verbalizing one's needs, decision making, and performance are encouraged.

The *project group* is task oriented. All craft activities and games are chosen by the therapist to maximize group participation and interaction. At this level the patient must be able to attend to an activity for an hour. Tasks are frequently novel, encouraging learning and exploration.

In *verbal problem and values clarification* patients are presented with verbal exercises and situations that stimulate discussion. Decision making, sharing ideas, and establishing personal norms are again encouraged. The emphasis here is on volitional development. Without this, interests and goals cannot exist since it motivates the pursuit of any vocation.

The *time management program* is for patients on the work release ward. One of the great difficulties for patients is the use of unstructured time. This problem often predates the patient's hospitalization. It continues throughout the course of hospitalization and can be exaggerated during the transition from a highly structured to an unstructured environment. Therefore, leisure planning and scheduling become an important focus. Simultaneously patients may attend a prerelease group centering on job hunting, interviews, money management, nutrition, grooming, apartment hunting, and homemaking. This group is continued when patients eventually move to the community halfway house.

In all groups activities are designed to be enjoyable, to stimulate self-activitation, and to foster "subcortical" learning.

Like occupational therapy programming, activity therapy programs are also on a grouped, graduated basis. Patients are initially placed in arts and crafts and gross motor activity groups and given on-ward cleanup duties. They progress to dining room cleanup and music therapy, then custodial services. At this level emphasis is on janitorial work skills taught via classroom and practical experience. This program runs six hours a day, five days a week for six months. In addition, workshop programs, which consist of contract projects such as separating cotton batting and assembling bingo cards, are available. These are the only programs that offer a small monetary compensation. As patients progress to the less restrictive work release ward, they are assigned to various departments (e.g., maintenance, dietary, and library services), where they learn different tasks through apprenticeship techniques. Patients are evaluated by staff members, who help determine readiness for working in the community. Most of the vocational programs are offered outside the hospital at other facilities. The emphasis within the hospital is on controlling behavior, improving insight, and developing the foundation skills necessary to survival in the community.

*Limitations of the Forensic Environment*

The forensic patient is often limited in what he can pursue prevocationally in the hospital. The security orientation of the hospital is extremely restrictive, with items made of materials such as glass, rope, metal, and wood often considered contraband or, if allowed, requiring close supervision. These restrictions narrow the variety of training that can be offered.

Cultural and educational considerations also play a part in vocational emphasis. The patient population at Perkins is of diverse origin (both rural and urban); many come from impoverished environments, and many are functionally illiterate. Other limiting factors are staffing and funding. (These limits are not exclusive to maximum security hospitals!)

A final limiting factor is the double stigma superimposed on all patients deemed "not guilty by reason of insanity." Not only are patients labelled "mentally ill," but they often have to cope with a "criminal" identification as well. Many of the patients are well known in the community because of media coverage of the criminal incident. This often interferes with obtaining work or entrance to training school. The occupational therapy department attempts to address this issue by role playing confrontations in groups.

Currently the occupational therapy department at the center is two years old. Patients who have been referred to the department are in either the early or late portion of their treatment course. Chronic patients require slow, steady incremental challenges to assimilate learning and build trust. Improvement is frequently minimal, and in some cases maintenance of present function is a realistic treatment goal.

*Case Study**

L. D. is a 27-year-old single man who was admitted in 1980 on charges of assault with intent to rape. The offense was committed at another hospital. When L. D. was 14 he was taken in to be raised by an aunt after the suicide of his father and the death of cancer of his mother. He was described as a poor student and was placed in special education classes from seventh through twelfth grade. He was active in sports and had many girl friends. At the age of 18 L. D. suffered a stroke, which resulted in right-upper-extremity hemiparesis with mild residual spasticity and atrophy, an ataxic gait, and some perceptual dysfunction. The patient was left dominant. He was hospitalized for one month at an acute-care hospital, then received outpatient therapy at a rehabilitation hospital. This therapy was discontinued after two months because of his irregular attendance. After his stroke his behavior changed dramatically. L. D. exposed himself in public, followed women soliciting sex, and was considered a nuisance by the neighborhood. He was employed for a short time but was fired because of his inability to concentrate on the job. Two weeks later he was persuaded

*This case study was provided by Robin Klein, OTR, Clifton T. Perkins Hospital Center, Jessup, Maryland.

by the family to go to a state mental hospital. At the hospital he attempted to rape a nurse.

After this offense, L. D. was sent to Clifton T. Perkins Hospital Center to be evaluated for competency and responsibility. He was diagnosed as having organic personality syndrome and was found competent to stand trial by all four state psychiatrists. He was adjudged not guilty by reason of insanity by the circuit court, which sent him back to Perkins for treatment.

The patient's course in the hospital was marked by emotional lability and impulsive agitated behavior. He was frequently observed pacing, talking to himself, using profanity toward staff, masturbating in the presence of female nurses, and provoking fights with other patients. Treatment with haloperidol (Haldol) and carbamazepine (Tegretol) was begun, with a resulting reduction in violent behavior.

The patient was referred to the occupational therapy department in 1981. Muscle testing revealed mild flexor spasticity in forearm, wrist, and fingers of the right upper extremity. Other motions in the right upper extremity were in the F+ to G− range. Mild sensory deficits were noted in sharp-dull discrimination on the volar surface of the forearm. The rest of his sensation was intact. No field cut was evident. Perceptual testing revealed mild deficits in figure-ground discrimination, constructional praxis, and position in space. The questionnaire revealed difficulty with written instructions, mathematics, short-term memory, spelling, and grammar. He was oriented to time, place, and person and completed the evaluation during the time allowed. In the tile coaster assembly task, the patient followed three-step verbal instructions correctly. He used his left (dominant) hand to manipulate the ¼-inch tiles and his right hand as a weak assist. The patient organized his project in a recognizable manner, and sequencing was accurate. He did not complete the task during the time allotted. L. D. performed on a parallel group level during the mural section of the evaluation. He did not contribute to the planning or implementation of the drawing. He observed others draw until most of the mural had been completed and then colored using broad strokes of a crayon in the area of the paper directly in front of him. Minimal verbal communication was noted.

L. D. reported that his employment history consisted of temporary janitorial work. He stated that his goals in the hospital are to "marry and get along with people on the outside." He listed his leisure interests as "games on the ward and baseball." The patient's description of a typical morning, afternoon, and evening outside the hospital was "I help take out laundry, bring back laundry, and sweep the floor," which was in actuality a description of his activities within the hospital. His response indicated deficits in reality testing and temporal awareness.

Treatment has been multifaceted. The patient exhibited psychological, organic, and motor deficits that impede skill, life role, and volitional development. The patient was initially placed in occupational therapy at the one-to-one level for one-half hour twice weekly. The goals were to maintain and improve right-upper-extremity function, increase compensation for perceptual deficits, improve written and oral communication skills, and increase leisure skill repertoire. His present role is as a patient rather than a worker (which is more age appropriate). His interests have been limited, and his day has been extrinsically structured (by the hospital). The primary occupational therapy used was card games, therapeutic exercises, Purdue Pegboard assembly, Frostig worksheets, programmed math and reading books, Nerf ball games, clerical tasks (collating and stapling), and strumming an autoharp. Treatment was slow and progressive. Initially the focus was on right-upper-extremity function with repetitive activities and exercises. As the patient learned to perform the tasks independently, he was advanced to writing exercises that incorporated reading and functional math problems. Exercises were then monitored periodically. Autoharp strumming and memorization of songs were added. Card games were used as a vehicle for learning new leisure skills and practicing communication skills by teaching the therapist new games. All tasks increased in complexity and challenge. Six months after treatment began it was noted on the ward that the patient had ceased masturbating, was less "playful," and had stopped getting into altercations with the other patients. In the arts and crafts activity group it was observed that he was able to handle delicate ceramic greenware with his right hand. He was also able to follow two- or three-step verbal instructions and maintained a steady work pace without encouragement. However, the patient consistently worked alone.

L. D. was advanced to the dyadic skills group three months later. He continues to participate in arts and crafts, and a gross motor gym group has been added to his program. All tasks in dyadic skills require sharing verbal information and materials with a partner. L. D. has not been spontaneous in this area; frequent structuring and encouragement by the therapist are required. Once he can incorporate social interaction with task organization and completion, he will progress to higher-level groups until he is capable of working in a simulated hospital job. Assuming his behavior continues to improve, he will eventually be ready for community placement.

## CALGARY GENERAL HOSPITAL FORENSIC PSYCHIATRY UNIT*

Calgary General Hospital, located in the city of Calgary, Alberta, Canada, offers another example of occupational therapy's involvement in forensic psychiatry. The psychiatric wing of the hospital consists of three inpatient units (maximum 67 patients) and the forensic unit (maximum 20 patients). The patients are remanded to the forensic unit for up to 30 days for one of several purposes: (1) for pretrial assessment of fitness to stand trial, (2) for presentence assessment to recommend possible psychiatric facilities and treatment follow-up, (3) for assessment for parole, and (4) for acute treatment. At the end of the patient's stay, the assessment team submits a letter to the court indicating whether or not the patient is fit to stand trial, with recommendations for immediate or future placement and presentence reports.

Although the primary goal of this unit is assessment, patients also undergo treatment and therapeutic intervention in the form of therapy groups concerned with life skills training, basic communications, sexuality, alcohol, and psychodrama. The occupational therapist leads an assertiveness training program, an art therapy group, and a workshop program besides participating in daily community meetings.

As a member of the assessment team, the therapist evaluates the patient's functional level before and since admission to the unit, that is, how the patient copes with activities of daily living. Typically used is the standardized Bay Area Functional Performance Evaluation,† which consists of a task-oriented assessment, a social interaction scale, and a written functional assessment form. In addition, the workshop program described in the following section is an integral part of the assessment. Utilized in the workshop is the Activity Therapy Evaluation (Fig. 5-12).

The workshop is a daily 1½-hour program run in conjunction with the recreational therapist. It provides activities that serve as assessment tools and

* Most of this section was written directly from information presented by Robert C. Schneider, OTR.

† Consulting Psychologists Press, Inc., 577 College Ave., Palo Alto, CA 94306.

| 1 Almost never<br>2 Occasionally<br>3 Half the time<br>4 Three-quarters of the time<br>5 Almost always<br>N/A Not applicable<br><br>Program/Date | | | | | | | | | | |
|---|---|---|---|---|---|---|---|---|---|---|
| A. LEVEL OF TASK DIFFICULTY | | | | | | | | | | |
| B. INTERPERSONAL/PSYCHOLOGICAL FUNCTION | | | | | | | | | | |
| 1. Appropriate appearance in relation to role, social group situation, age, sex | | | | | | | | | | |
| 2. Absence of nonproductive behaviors (rocking, playing with hands, repetitive movements, preoccupation) | | | | | | | | | | |
| 3. Expression of affect (spontaneous, clear, appropriate) | | | | | | | | | | |
| 4. Cooperative with group (verbal/nonverbal) | | | | | | | | | | |
| 5. Demonstrates ability to initiate, respond to, sustain verbal interaction | | | | | | | | | | |
| 6. Demonstrates ability to make own decisions | | | | | | | | | | |
| 7. Accepts authority, yet can state own opinion without aggression | | | | | | | | | | |
| 8. Demonstrates ability to compromise and negotiate | | | | | | | | | | |
| 9. Recognizes and acts on strengths and weaknesses | | | | | | | | | | |
| 10. Self-direction in unstructured setting and/or task | | | | | | | | | | |
| 11. Demonstrates awareness of others' needs/feelings | | | | | | | | | | |

| C. COGNITIVE/TASK SKILLS | | | | | | | | | | |
|---|---|---|---|---|---|---|---|---|---|---|
| 1. Reality orientation (place, person, time, situation) | | | | | | | | | | |
| 2. Attention span for activity duration | | | | | | | | | | |
| 3. Demonstrates ability to engage in structured activity without staff encouragement | | | | | | | | | | |
| 4. Follows oral directions | | | | | | | | | | |
| 5. Follows written directions | | | | | | | | | | |
| 6. Remembers instructions | | | | | | | | | | |
| 7. Concentrates despite distraction | | | | | | | | | | |
| 8. Appropriate pace in activity | | | | | | | | | | |
| 9. Tolerates frustration | | | | | | | | | | |
| 10. Able to organize task (plan, understand, perform) | | | | | | | | | | |
| 11. Can solve problems | | | | | | | | | | |
| 12. Assumes responsibility for own actions, thoughts, feelings | | | | | | | | | | |
| D. WORK BEHAVIOR | | | | | | | | | | |
| 1. Punctuality | | | | | | | | | | |
| 2. Neatness in activity | | | | | | | | | | |
| 3. Reliability (adherence to expectations) | | | | | | | | | | |
| 4. Demonstrates safety awareness | | | | | | | | | | |
| E. MOTOR SKILLS | | | | | | | | | | |
| 1. Demonstrates spontaneous reactions and reflexes | | | | | | | | | | |
| 2. Demonstrates adequate gross motor coordination for task (movement patterns, balance, proprioception) | | | | | | | | | | |
| 3. Demonstrates adequate fine motor coordination for task (hand manipulative skills, eye-hand coordination, perceptual motor coordination) | | | | | | | | | | |
| 4. Physical endurance for activity duration | | | | | | | | | | |
| F. ATTENDANCE | | | | | | | | | | |

*Fig. 5-12. Activity therapy evaluation, Calgary General Hospital.*

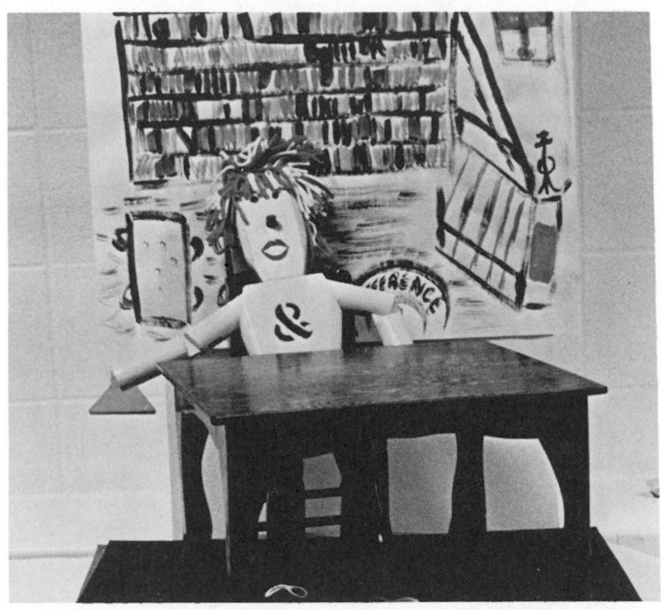

A

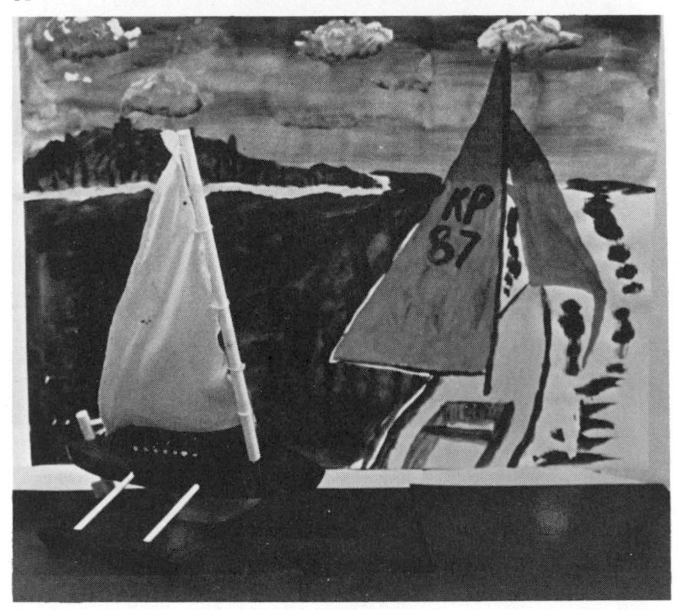


B

*Fig. 5-13. Toys constructed by patients in the Calgary General Hospital workshop. A: Puppet. B: Sailboat.*

promote skill development. Patients construct toys that are distributed to needy children in the Calgary community (Fig. 5-13).

As an assessment instrument

> [the] workshop functions as a means of patient assessment as observed through the activity process. This includes:
> 1. general task behaviors of frustration tolerance, level of concentration, motor coordination, decision making, judgment and problem solving;
> 2. interpersonal behaviors such as cooperation with others, level of independence, sociability or self assertion; and
> 3. work skills evaluation in areas of self responsibility, punctuality, motivation, initiative, dependability and quality of work produced, as well as some basic work history and attitudes towards work [33].

As a skill development tool, the workshop encourages goal attainment and achievement. It develops in the patient a sense of responsibility for his own behavior through fulfillment of a work contract (Fig. 5-14) and active participation. It facilitates the daily interaction with others and awareness of their effect on the work environment through daily participation and weekly discussion. By means of weekly goal setting, group discussion, and the encouragement of independent decision making, the workshop develops independent planning and goal achievement. It develops basic woodworking skills through instruction and demonstration by therapists, and it fosters self-esteem through realization of accomplishment, achieved again through weekly

*Fig. 5-14. Workshop contract used at Calgary General Hospital.*

WORKSHOP CONTRACT

Name: ______________________ Date: ______________

Please think carefully about whether involvement in this program would be helpful to you, and then fill in the appropriate space below:

(1) I agree to participate in the workshop and work for __________ of the five days of the week

*or*

(2) I would like to observe the program for one week __________

*or*

(3) I do not think it would be helpful for me because ______________

______________________________________

Goal for the week: ______________________________

______________________________________

*[For next week. . .]*

I achieved/did not achieve the above goal because ______________

______________________________________

______________________________________

Signature ______________

Witnessed ______________

group discussion, peer support of accomplishments, communication of the workshop achievements in community meetings, and positive feedback from therapists.

All patients meeting minimal criteria (the patient can tolerate a 45-minute structured group meeting and is not actively suicidal or a threat to the security of the unit) are eligible for entrance into the program and are expected to attend an orientation session. In the orientation session the following information is provided:

I. Introduction to therapists
II. Explanation of workshop program
  A. Meeting time and days of workshop
  B. Break schedule
  C. Purpose of workshop
    1. An assessment tool
    2. A treatment group
    3. An enjoyable activity
III. Explanation of shop guidelines
  A. Tool use
  B. Cleanup of materials
  C. Arrival time
  D. Notification of therapists if late for appointment
  E. Explanation of contract
IV. Explanation of work history form
V. Tour of workshop

In addition, the patient is asked to perform a short, simple activity to provide the therapist with a preliminary skill assessment.

The workshop program includes a weekly 1½-hour meeting of all the patients involved in the program for the past week. The meeting is conducted by the workshop coordinator, who also writes notes on the meeting for the following week. This coordinator, who is selected by the therapists, is a patient who has been involved in the workshop program for at least one week and who demonstrates the capacity to coordinate the meeting.

The weekly meeting is an important aspect of the treatment process, providing for personal and group problem solving. It offers an opportunity to discuss achievement (or nonachievement) of goals. Patients develop awareness of others through sharing ideas and contributing project accomplishments to the group. During the meeting conflicts between patients and staff are worked out. Patients determine their personal goals for the following week and sign a contract for the following week (see Fig. 5-14). Other areas explored in the group include the patient's potential in the job market and possible avenues of career training while the patient is in prison (e.g., classes and training programs). The group may also help the patient understand his behavior and attitudes and their relationship to his ability to hold a job.

Low self-esteem and difficulties accepting authority and endeavoring to overcome alcohol addiction are major problems among the patients in the forensic unit at Calgary General. Participation in the workshop program has facilitated working through these issues.

*Evaluation*

The therapist assesses the patient's progress in the workshop program and all activity groups via the Activity Therapy Evaluation (Fig. 5-12). This evaluation is derived from the evaluation of the same name of the activity therapy department of Sheppard and Enoch Pratt Hospital, Towson, Maryland, as well as from Claudia Allen's work on cognitive disabilities [1].

The department uses Claudia Allen's hierarchy of cognitive *levels of task difficulty* (Table 5-1) to select and design activities that correspond to the patient's level of ability[1]. All activities have been analyzed using Allen's task analysis for cognitive disability (Table 5-2) and then graded on a scale of 1 to 5. These levels correspond directly to Allen's levels 2 to 6, that is, Calgary's level 1 corresponds to Allen's level 2, Calgary's level 2 corresponds to Allen's level 3, and so on. Allen's level 1 has been eliminated because the "reflexive" patient, that is, the patient who appears unaware of his external environment, would not attend occupational therapy but would be in constant nursing care. The following are examples of tasks for patients at the various levels:

In *Level 1* the patient sands and paints (with one color of his choice) a previously constructed toy. The toy is simple and without difficult corners. The patient works in a minimal-stimulation area.

In *Level 2* the patient does straight crosscut sawing. An example is a boat project for which the patient cuts several blocks of wood, sands, and paints. Therapist shows the patient an unpainted sample, performs some shaping of the hull, and assists the patient in stacking deck sections (see Fig. 5-13).

In *Level 3* a model stunt plane is an ideal project. The patient is shown a sample product, is given a pattern to trace, and performs rounded and angled cuts. The patient then shapes, sands, glues, and paints the airplane in a two-color scheme.

In *Level 4* the patient is given a choice of several simple patterns for a car. The patient performs all parts of the task except drilling holes for wheels, for which he may need assistance. Variations in color and other options are available.

In *Level 5* the patient may choose to draw an original plan for a toy. Limitations are set as to the size of the toy and the type of materials available.

*Sections B through E* of the evaluation (see Fig. 5-12) provide *other measures* of performance through the therapist's observations in the areas of interpersonal and psychological function, cognitive and task skills, work behavior, and motor skills. Progress is measured by an increased score within specific performance areas and by successful completion of increasingly difficult tasks.

*Table 5-1. Levels of Cognitive Disability*

| | *Level 1: Reflexive* | *Level 2: Movement* | *Level 3: Repetitive Actions* |
|---|---|---|---|
| Attention | Patients do not seem to be able to focus their attention or screen out external stimuli | Patients attend to their own postural movements | Patients attend to the effects their own motor actions have on the environment |
| Goal Selection | Patients are conscious and reflexes are functional; they may or may not be able to eat and drink | Chance body movements create an interesting result, which patients attempt to repeat | Chance movements cause a perceived environmental result, which they repeat many times |
| Imitation | No imitation is observed | Patients can approximate gross body movements if they are familiar schemes; therapist may imitate patient's movement | Patients can imitate therapist when their own familiar schemes are demonstrated |
| Tangible Objectivity | Patients are subjective; do not seem to be aware of people or objects in the external environment | Patients watch with transient awareness people and objects that are moving | Objects and people are understood in terms of patient's own motor actions; external causes are not understood |
| Time | There is no behavior to indicate that patients can mark the passage of time | Attention is focused for a very limited period; patients require continual direction | Patients can focus their attention on tasks that have repetitive actions; can remember and anticipate a series of events based on their own actions |

Table 5-1 (continued)

| *Level 4: End Product* | *Level 5: Variations* | *Level 6: Tangible Thought* |
|---|---|---|
| Patients can focus their attention to complete a task; an end product that can be visually perceived; sustains attention | Patients seek novelty through variations in their actions and end products; perceptual cues are used to adjust motor actions | Patients begin to think about possibilities before physically testing the result; visual images guide motor actions |
| Patients can use several familiar schemes to achieve an end product | Overt trial and error is used to discover a new means of achieving the goal | Covert trial-and-error-problem solving occurs; images are used to test solutions to problems |
| Actions that expand their familiar schemes can be imitated, one scheme at a time; errors are not corrected | A series of schemes can be imitated and remembered; new schemes can be imitated and learned | Patients can imitate therapist when therapist is no longer present |
| When an object can be seen, patients are aware that it has its own movement, causing its own effect | Patients explore the potential of other objects and people | Patients begin to infer the cause of a change; they may need to validate the cause |
| Patients can anticipate future events based on an interpretation of signs, using the actions of others | Time is measured by the hours and days required to produce the novelty | Through the use of images, patients can separate themselves from the immediate present and project themselves into the past or future |

Source: From C. Allen [1].

*Table 5-2. Task Analysis for Cognitive Disability*

| | *Level 1: Reflexive* | *Level 2: Movement* | *Level 3: Repetitive Actions* |
|---|---|---|---|
| *Patient characteristics* | | | |
| Attention to | Internal thoughts and feelings with little awareness of external stimuli | Patients enjoy planned postural movements | Energy is invested in doing simple tasks with repetitive actions |
| Attention span | Transient, generally less than 1 minute | Average 5–20 minutes; patients are distracted by movement and sound and need frequent redirection | Average 15–30 minutes; continuous refocusing of attention is required |
| *Therapist's directions* | | | |
| Imitation | Looks at demonstrated directions but does not imitate them | Gross body movements; you may need to guide the movement physically | Patients will follow demonstration when their familiar schemes are used |
| Verbalizations | May respond to one-word verbs such as "eat" or "chew" | Reinforce demonstration with a few simple nouns and verbs | Reinforce demonstration with repeated simple nouns and verbs |
| Number of directions | One direction, repeated | One direction, repeated | One direction, repeated |
| *Task selection* | | | |
| Structure of the activity | Most important tasks are eating and drinking | Familiar, repetitive gross body movements | Tasks with one repeated step or scheme |

| | | | |
|---|---|---|---|
| Predictability | Familiar foods and fluids | Familiar body movements | Repetitive actions with a uniform effect upon the environment |
| Choice provided | When possible, recognize individual food preferences | Therapist plans the movements and may respond to patients' suggestions or actions | Limited to two or three items to avoid distractions |
| Tools | Fingers and hands, rather than utensils | Objects that are associated with gross body movements, e.g., jump ropes, soft balls | Generally patients do better with their hands; some use of familiar tools |
| Storage of materials and projects | Obtained for the patients | Taken care of by therapist | Taken care of by therapist |
| Preparation by the therapist | Food packages and cartons may need to be opened for patients | Plan movements and obtain any needed equipment | Lay out supplies in advance; do any preliminary and/or finishing steps that are not repetitive or not familiar |
| *Setting* | Reduce the number of stimuli when possible | Open space | Clutter-free |

Table 5-2 (continued)

| *Level 4: Goal Directed* | *Level 5: Variations* | *Level 6: Tangible Thought* |
| --- | --- | --- |
| Patients focus on visual sample of an end product | Overt trial-and-error problem solving; patients are interested in doing similar tasks, which permit variations in their actions | Covert trial-and-error problem solving; energy is directed toward using images to plan an action |
| If interrupted, patients can refocus their own attention in order to achieve their goal; average task should be completed within 30–45 minutes | Attention may be sustained while external stimuli are present; tasks may take two or more sessions to complete | Within normal limits |
| Patients can imitate moderately novel demonstrations that expand familiar schemes | Patients can learn through serial imitation so that a number of steps may be demonstrated; unfamiliar steps may be introduced and through practice will be learned | Patients can learn through delayed imitation so that demonstrated directions may be retained over a period of time; through use of images, simple diagrams or familiar written directions may be followed |
| Use simple nouns and verbs, avoiding discussions or open-ended questions | Adjectives and prepositions may be used in explaining variations | Use of images may be encouraged when materials to be worked with are present |
| One direction for each step; wait until each step is completed before giving the next direction | Two or more directions may be given at one time | Two or more directions may be given at one time |

| | | |
|---|---|---|
| Simple quick tasks with a visual end product, bright colors, and two-dimensional shapes; avoid childish connotations with adults | Activities that permit variation; the effects of one's actions can easily be seen and corrected | Activities that permit variation in selecting and planning steps |
| Potential errors should be easily corrected by the therapist | Patients must be able to physically perceive the effect their actions have on objects and end results | Patients must be able to predict the effect their actions will have on objects and end results |
| Avoid confusion by limiting the decisions and materials; provide opportunity for exact replication of sample | Several choices in materials, tools, and activity selection may be provided; demonstrate and clarify variations | Several choices in materials, tools, and tasks can be provided and discussed |
| Familiar objects; no power tools | Simple tools that are a linear extension of the hand or arm are the must successful | Patients can learn how to use unfamiliar machines and tools |
| Patients can place and/or find materials when clearly visible or very familiar | Patients can search for things in probable locations and can place or find things in labelled drawers or cabinets | Patients can follow verbal directions to place or find materials |
| Lay out supplies in advance, provide an exact sample of the finished product, and do the steps that require unfamiliar tools or schemes | Sample of the finished product need not be exact; patterns and procedures must be supplied by therapist | Materials, designs, and/or pictures must be present for covert problem solving |
| Other patients working on the same task | People, music, and clutter can be present | Free access to materials and supplies |

*Case Study**

A. A., a 61-year-old married male, was admitted to the forensic unit on transfer from a city court in Alberta, Canada, where he was facing several charges related to alleged sexual indiscretions with children. The charges leading to his admission to the forensic unit were his first contact with the legal system.

A. A. was at first quite wary of the unit and appeared overwhelmed by his situation. He initially appeared depressed, with social isolation, crying episodes, and a decreased appetite, but seemed to adjust to the unit in a few days.

A. A. is a farmer with an eighth-grade education. He appeared older than his stated age. He was oriented to time, person, and place and was not psychotic on initial contact.

On the third day after admission, the occupational therapist approached the patient to involve him in the workshop, explaining the program and its contribution to the forensic assessment. In the initial session, the patient demonstrated low self-esteem ("I can't do anything, I'm just a farmer") and stated that he had had minimal experience in working with wood. Nevertheless he was cooperative and agreed to "try" to attend the workshop.

In the following sessions it was evident that A. A. had had woodworking experience. With initial help from the therapist in deciding on a project, A. A. designed a doll chair. Although progressing successfully, he continued to voice self-deprecating comments and required reinforcement from the therapist for his short-term accomplishments. A. A. also experienced fine motor tremors and required occasional assistance in following a straight edge with a pencil. His goal for the following week was to have the pieces of the chair cut, glued, sanded, and ready for staining.

In the following week the patient consistently attended the workshop program. He became more bright and spontaneous. His self-esteem increased, as noted in his work independence and fewer self-defeating comments. The patient also became more definite in his decision making. In the weekly workshop meeting he stated that he had accomplished his goal from the previous week and gave others some woodworking suggestions.

Although continuing to exhibit a fine motor tremor, A. A. was able to handle a saw effectively and cut a fine line. He continued with the project, sanded and stained it, and painted on two coats of varnish.

While waiting for the varnish to dry, A. A. designed a table to match the chair. He designed the table on paper, transferred the design on to x-ray paper to make a permanent pattern, and used the pattern effectively to cut pieces of wood for the table. He completed this table before discharge from the unit. His approach to the final product demonstrated forethought, constructive problem solving on detailed work, and a tolerance for dealing with the frustration that occurs daily in a workshop on a locked unit.

In early workshop sessions A. A. was demanding of the therapist's attention and demonstrated helplessness and inability to perform. However, this receded as the patient involved himself in his project. He grew less dependent and his skills became more noticeable. As his work progressed, he received encouragement and compliments from other workshop participants. They would ask A. A. for ideas, and he freely gave suggestions and demonstrated the use of various tools.

A. A. was involved in psychological testing for three days but attended 17 of 20 offered workshop sessions.

A. A. was found fit to stand trial by the forensic team. The occupational therapy workshop program provided the following information to assist in this decision:

*This case study was prepared by Robert C. Schneider, OTR, Calgary General Hospital, Calgary, Alberta, Canada.

1. The patient does not appear to be psychotic (i.e., no hallucinations or delusions noted).
2. Although he appeared depressed initially, his progress, increased socialization, increased motivation, and active involvement suggest that his mood would not affect his appreciation of the trial.
3. Although parkinsonian movements hinder his fine motor abilities, the tremors do not affect his functional performance.
4. The patient does not appear to have an organic brain condition or to be mentally retarded to a degree that would affect his comprehension of the trial.
5. The patient appears to possess adequate problem solving, decision making, and foresight to instruct counsel and assist in his own defense.
6. The patient seems to posses adequate frustration tolerance and control of his impulsiveness to tolerate the length of the trial and not to decompensate while awaiting trial.

Additional information on the patient's overall work and interpersonal skills in occupational performance was gained through observation.

The patient's discharge diagnosis (according to the format outlined in the Diagnostic and Statistical Manual*) was as follows:

Axis I. Paraphilia—pedophilia
Axis II. No diagnosis
Axis III. Questionable Parkinson's disorder
Axis IV. Psychosocial stressor moderate IV
Axis V. Adaptive functioning good III

A. A. was found guilty of his offenses and received a sentence of three months in the city jail system.

### Correctional Institutions

Work-related programs in correctional institutions are diverse, reflecting the goal ambiguity that exists in correctional philosophy. While rehabilitation is the avowed objective of incarceration, in reality funding priorities reveal a greater commitment to protecting the public from the offender and to maintaining order within the institution. For example, in 1979 only 1.5 percent of the total costs of incarceration in the United States went for work-related programs [11].

A brief review of the types of work-related programs will provide a framework for discussing occupational therapy's place in these facilities. There are two general categories of work-related programs: institutionally based and community-based.

#### INSTITUTIONALLY BASED PROGRAMS

Most work-related programs in prisons are institutionally based. In most instances such programs are designed, implemented, and evaluated solely

*American Psychiatric Association. *Diagnostic and Statistical Manual of Mental Disorders* (3rd ed.). Washington, D.C.: APA (1700 Eighteenth St., N.W., Washington, D.C. 20009), 1980.

by correctional administration and staff. Others, however, involve community members in both curriculum design and instruction. The use of instructors from local educational institutions facilitates training that more closely resembles the type received in the community. In some instances, offenders released before completing such training may have the opportunity to do so when released. A third type of institutionally based program is designed to provide workers for the maintenance of the correctional facility or for prison industries. Historically, prison industries were created to offset the high cost of institutional operations and to provide job training while giving inmates opportunity to earn money while incarcerated. In reality, prison industries are often low paying and have little carry-over to community jobs. For example, it was not until recently that the manufacture of license plates, a common prison job, was also done commercially outside correctional facilities.

In 1975 the Law Enforcement Assistance Administration piloted the concept of combining realistic work opportunities with useful skill training. Entitled the Free-Venture Project it required that

> representatives of industry be involved in the planning and implementation of the institutional industrial program. The project also requires that market surveys be conducted as a part of the planning process, equipment and training be comparable to that in industry, and job placement services be provided to offenders returning to the community. The program must replicate the community work environment as closely as possible. [11]

In one program inmates were trained as and became computer analysts for large firms while imprisoned. These inmates, upon discharge, were hired by the same firms [11, 15].

Another effort to provide institutionally based programs is the school district concept. Instructional services are designed and administered through collaborative agreements between correctional institutions and state or local education agencies [11].

### COMMUNITY-BASED PROGRAMS

In community-based programs, which are less common, the inmates are released from the institution for a portion of the day to obtain on-the-job training or job-related training in a community facility. Work release and halfway house programs are two types of community-based programs.

#### *Work Release Programs*

Work release programs afford the inmate the opportunity to work outside the correctional setting. Although in the 1970s work release regarded as a promising reform, public resentment toward the presence of sentenced offenders in the community curtailed its expansion. Potter observes that except in a handful of states work release has never really caught on: "Seldom are more than 10 percent of a state's inmates involved in work-release programs. Most often, the proportion is 1 or 2 percent" [31].

## HALFWAY HOUSE PROGRAMS

Halfway house programs give inmates an opportunity to gain on-the-job training while residing in minimum-security institutions within the community, thus providing a gradual transition from institutional life to society. An inmate is typically eligible for placement in a halfway house within six months of release or when serving a sentence of less than a year.

Blackmore estimates that 2,200 prerelease or halfway houses are in operation in the United States, 600 of them housing adults. These centers house from 30,000 to 40,000 offenders. Fifty-one percent of all federal prisoners are released to these programs. These persons have lower unemployment rates, better job attendance records, and higher earnings than do those released directly from prisons into the community [11]. However, Penner [29] notes that "only those programs that combine realistic job-training with placement in worthwhile jobs appear to have any effect upon recidivism."

## OCCUPATIONAL THERAPY IN CORRECTIONAL INSTITUTIONS

Gross, an occupational therapist who worked for two years with female inmates while doing her dissertation [15], notes

> Prevocational programs for prisoners need to be based upon the type and needs of the population, which is mostly poor, urban, very inadequately educated, young and male. In order to enter the vocational system, they would need exposure to learn about vocational areas and skills, actual practice in social and vocational arenas and then the opportunity for this to be put into practice when they were discharged. Those programs where employers have a commitment to hiring them or where inmates work for wages and learn real job skills and requirements while incarcerated would be helpful.

Corrections is an area in which occupational therapy can provide a useful service, particularly in work-related programming. Although our profession's literature at present sparsely describes this role, I and others believe that this is an area of practice that may develop more fully in time [10, 29, 30].

Correctional institutions typically have a number of security levels or classifications. These custody and security policies for any given facility may drastically affect the modalities of therapy and the extent to which occupational therapy services are provided. The therapist's role varies depending on the type of facility. Facilities for the juvenile offender may emphasize rehabilitation in areas such as activities of daily living, social skills, and the development of compensatory strategies. When appropriate, sensory integrative therapy may also be provided. In adult facilities, commonly segregated for men and women, occupational therapists can "assist in the maintenance of life-task performance; provide leisure-time activities; provide opportunities for social and cognitive development; and can work collaboratively with job training program personnel to assess and develop work habits and assist in the development of desired vocational and employability skills" [29].

It is essential for any therapist entering this area of practice to have a realistic set of expectations. In reviewing the literature on this subject, Penner [29] has formulated conclusions particularly relevant to the development of occupational therapy programs:

1. The conditions that seem to have the greatest correlation with avoidance of recidivism are availability of family or other social group support after release; stable job prospects; and aging.
2. Regardless of what occurs in the prison, programs are likely to have little effect on the conditions to which inmates return; some recidivism may be seen as inevitable.
3. Prisons exist primarily to punish. Inmates are not likely to view prisons as existing for their benefit, and are likely to reject anyone's claims that they do exist for their benefit.
4. It may be difficult if not impossible to ascertain the prisoner's desire for change, especially if there is any possibility that parole contingencies are attached to outcomes of the occupational therapy program.
5. Lasting behavioral change in an inmate will occur only if the inmate truly desires to change.

## WASHINGTON STATE SPECIAL OFFENDER CENTER*

One of the few examples of occupational therapy's role in corrections is at the Washington State Special Offender Center, which is located 20 miles northeast of Seattle, Washington. It is a maximum-security prison housing 144 men. The typical offender comes from an impoverished population and has little or no work history and few or no work skills or positive work habits. The center comprises four 36-cell units with an occupational therapy clinic on each unit. There is one full-time occupational therapist. Occupational therapy plays an important role in evaluating the inmates and providing them with the opportunity to learn essential work-related behaviors and attitudes such as attention span and task tolerance, acceptance of and ability to follow instructions, and increased motivation before job placement.

### *Evaluation*

Ideally each inmate is seen briefly within the first three days of admission. Evaluation, which lasts approximately one hour, occurs over the next few days. It is designed to assess several key areas of the individual's general functional and developmental levels: (1) basic living skills and activities of daily living, (2) cognitive and perceptual processing, (3) sensory integrative functioning, (4) work tolerance, (5) work-related skills, (6) avocational and leisure skills, (7) general coordination, (8) aptitudes, (9) hand dexterity, and (10) mental status.

The evaluation involves completing simple tasks such as writing, drawing, copying, following directions, and handling small objects, as well as gross motor and frustration tolerance tasks. In addition the therapist explores the inmate's self-care and homemaking abilities, decision making, interests, time

*Most of this section was written directly from information provided by Sandra Palmer, OTR.

management skill, and memory. Observations are made as to the person's general behavior and interactions with the therapist.

*Work-Related Programs*

All work-related programs at the Special Offender Center are institutionally based, with three basic types of work stations: on-unit jobs, off-unit jobs, and "sheltered" jobs. Whenever possible, on- and off-unit jobs are arranged to simulate jobs in the community. The inmates are required to fill out applications, go through an interview process, complete written performance evaluations, receive training and supervision, await job openings, and cope with layoffs.

The emphasis of all the jobs is on building positive work habits and attitudes, self-esteem, community skills, and general job awareness. Participation in the work programs is required to advance within the treatment programs. In addition, practical training in job seeking—interviewing skills and job searching methods—is provided.

*On-unit jobs* are general operational tasks necessary to the maintenance of the unit. There are 20 to 25 jobs available on each unit, ranging from low-level janitorial tasks to more complex and independent work such as tier (unit) laundryman or porter. Other jobs include inmate meal server, bi-unit (two-tier) supervisor, recreation aide, and occupational therapy aide. Wages are variable up to a maximum of $30 per month. Inmates are allowed to hold more than one job; however, their maximum earnings remain fixed.

To be eligible for an *off-unit job*, the inmate must (1) require medium and/or high custody, (2) be active and successful in the unit programs, and (3) have no disciplinary infractions for a specified period. These jobs require higher functional abilities such as the ability to work independently, follow complex instructions, and accept supervision appropriately. Off-unit positions include laundry aide, maintenance aide, janitorial aide, plumber's aide, electrician's aide, and kitchen aide. At present there are 20 jobs; however, new ones are always being created.

*Sheltered jobs* at the Special Offender Center are similar to jobs in a sheltered workshop, although the center does not have a sheltered workshop per se. Investigations are being made into appropriate types of contracts and products suitable to the facility's limited space. Of interest are simple assembly and sorting tasks that can be graded for complexity.

Many of the inmates are transferred from the center to work-release facilities. These function like halfway houses and provide an opportunity for inmates to continue to learn and expand vocational skills.

In summary, Palmer [28] notes:

> Occupational therapy can play an active, contributing role to an individual's rehabilitation, adjustment and successful return to the community. Occupational therapy can provide a supportive, common link with community life by aiding in the personal

growth and development of each individual, through guided activities. Individuals participating in occupational therapy have the opportunity to build needed experiential background to deal with the community and society in general.

*Case Study**

Brett is a pleasant-looking, tall, blond young man of 23. He speaks in a quiet though clear voice and speaks calmly about most issues.

Brett has been involved with the social correctional systems of the state since age 8. At that time his parents were killed in an automobile accident, and Brett was placed in a foster home. He was able to remain at the same school in which he had started that year. His teachers repeatedly reported that Brett had difficulty paying attention in class and always seemed to be making up stories. He reportedly had no close friends and was most often alone at school and at home. Numerous referrals to the school district psychologists and communication specialists resulted in many confusing reports. No agreement was ever reached, but impressions included childhood schizophrenia, attention deficit disorder, traumatic adjustment reaction, and autism.

By the time Brett was 16, he was no longer in school. He had been suspended for creating disturbances in his classes several times and had finally been expelled. His foster parents (Brett's fourth placement) felt unequal to dealing with what they termed Brett's moodiness. On the recommendations of the school district, they attempted to enroll Brett in an alternative school for emotionally disturbed students. Brett refused to attend and withdrew further into himself. During this time he was on probation for numerous counts of drunkenness, disorderly conduct, and shoplifting.

Brett began staying out late and drinking quite heavily. He received money from a trust established from his parents' estates but was never able too make any budgeting decisions. He either gave his money away, bought alcohol, or made impulsive purchases.

The offense for which Brett is currently incarcerated is taking a motor vehicle without permission (joyriding). The charges were reduced from grand theft, auto, because of his close relationship to the car's owners, former foster parents. He had previously been in prison for two counts of burglary in the second degree and one count of indecent liberties. He served three years of a seven-year maximum sentence. Brett was on parole for about six months before being arrested for this current offense.

When Brett had served only six months of his current sentence (he was scheduled for release in less than eighteen months), he proved unable to remain within the general prison population at the Washington State Corrections and Training Center. He reportedly had been raped on numerous occasions and had been victimized in other ways. He was kept in protective custody.

During his final months at the corrections center, cell mates and staff reported Brett's ritualistic motions and habits. His cell walls were covered with drawings and patterns associated with satanic cults. He was periodically heard talking to himself in two different voices. Brett committed many infractions—having alcohol in his cell and being under the influence of intoxicants. Brett was observed to exhibit bizarre and self-mutilating behavior. After inflicting a three-inch laceration on his left leg that required stitching, he was transferred to the Washington State Special Offender Center (SOC) as a prisoner in need of immediate stabilization.

During the 30-day initial evaluation period, Brett was diagnosed by the members of the treatment team as being severely disturbed. He claimed to have two souls living within him: one Jesus the Savior, the other a warlock named Bodar. While he admitted that he drank a great deal and that he needed the alcohol, he stated that his drinking was not a problem and that he was not an alcoholic. He felt that alcoholics drink

* This case study was provided by Sandra L. Palmer, OTR, Washington State Special Offender Center, Monroe, Washington.

without reason, and he had a reason: "Bodar tells me to do awful things to people, and the booze keeps him quiet so I can hear the good things that Jesus is saying to me."

Brett agreed to take medications prescribed for him and to participate in the various aspects of programming offered on the admissions unit. He soon became involved in group therapy, individual therapy, therapeutic recreation, and occupational therapy.

The recreation staff was soon able to involve Brett in activities and continued to include him whenever possible. They attempted to increase his social skills, develop alternative leisure interests, and work on group belonging and cooperative play through sports and games.

In occupational therapy he was given a series of short-term tasks and crafts to establish reality orientation, provide success experiences, and increase his decision-making skills. His social skills were reinforced, his self-care was stressed, and a therapeutic trust relationship was established. The occupational therapist was able to extend Brett's group tolerance, attention span, and instruction following above minimum levels. Brett soon began showing more emotion and animation. He complained less often that Bodar and Jesus were bothering him.

Within six weeks of his admission, Brett was progressing well and the medications were controlling his delusions and hallucinations. At this point Brett had become motivated to change his behavior and stated that he felt happier without the two souls fighting over him. He was transferred to a long-term treatment unit.

In the new unit Brett became an active participant in his own treatment plan, showing rapid progress. He continued his involvement in occupational therapy and recreation with increasing goals and expectations. He began attending education classes to complete his GED requirements. He expressed more often his desire to plan for the future and learn skills to keep himself from decompensating badly again. He requested whatever job training could be offered him. He had already shown capability and was learning work habits as an on-unit janitorial aide. During his time on the treatment unit Brett had moved upward through the program privilege levels and was entitled to apply for off-unit work.

Brett made application to the classification committee for a change in his custody status—an advance from maximum security (his status since his commission to the department of corrections) to medium custody, which is required to leave the unit without escort or to work off-unit. Once his custody status was changed, he made application to work on the building's maintenance crew. He was interviewed and placed on a waiting list for the next available position. In about two weeks Brett was called to work with the building's plumber.

Brett proved to be an enthusiastic crew member and continued to improve in the areas of work habits, instruction following, and problem solving. Even though he was showing progress in these areas, he continued in occupational therapy groups to reinforce his existing skills, increase social skills, increase acceptance of female authority, and provide for continuing success experience. Within three months Brett was working three to four hours each afternoon; he received good evaluations from his job supervisor each month.

At about this time the occupational therapist and Brett's primary therapist both began noticing increasing anxiety and a quickness of temper not usually seen as Brett's behavior pattern on the treatment unit. Brett also began refusing to attend school and occupational therapy groups. His job supervisor reported that Brett was "almost working too hard, and is reluctant to return to the unit." In individual therapy sessions Brett's therapist uncovered several incidents of homosexual harassment of Brett by another inmate. Brett had been unwilling to report this because he felt it might affect the way staff saw his progress and placement alternatives. Once the investigations of these matters were concluded, Brett resumed active and progressive movement through the program's treatment objectives.

Brett shortly became eligible for restricted minimum custody and began working in the kitchen as an aide and dishwasher. He worked in this position for about a month before the department of corrections qualified him for minimum custody, which allowed him to begin preparations for release within the next eight months.

Brett was interviewed and selected for inclusion in the Reintegration Program (RIP). During the six weeks (48 to 60 hours), of the RIP, he was given a community skills refresher course and instruction and assignments preparing him to deal with a work release setting. Topics included bus schedules, work release rules and procedures, behavioral expectations, medications, state agencies, public assistance, mental health follow-up, and job interviewing skills.

On completing the RIP, Brett was transferred to a work release center associated with SOC. This center provided follow-up to the skills and psychotherapeutic issues developed during his six-month stay at SOC. Brett was maintained at the work release center on a limited-movement basis for a few weeks to allow him to adjust to being out of prison and to phase into the community. Group therapy sessions were continued during this time to help him deal with the expected anxiety and behavior difficulties of a new setting. He was given additional help in learning to look for work and exploring educational areas of interest.

Brett was interviewed and tested by a local community college for their specialized adult basic education programs. It was determined that this would be the best course of action to enable Brett to avoid decompensation or return to alcohol or to reoffense. Brett enrolled in school and became an avid participant. At the same time he took part in the school's vocational exploration and testing programs.

Assuming he continues to progress and commits no infractions or new criminal activity, Brett should complete his final months of incarceration at the work release center. He would then be eligible to ask the Board of Prison Terms and Paroles for release on parole according to an approved plan.

## Programming for Adults with Neurophysiologic Problems

Occupational therapists working with persons with physical or neurologic disabilities practice in a variety of facilities—inpatient and outpatient hospitals, rehabilitation centers, insurance companies, state institutions, private practice. For these therapists, many variables must be addressed in planning work-related programs. These variables include not only the physical and neurologic ramifications of the disability, but also its psychosocial impact, all too often overlooked. The person unable to pursue his or her present vocation or perhaps any vocation may become anxious and may suffer a loss in self-esteem, self-image, motivation, and status within both the family and society at large. Whenever these issues arise, they must be addressed in therapy. When working with those with an acquired dysfunction, for example, quadriplegia, right hemiplegia, head injury, back injury, or amputation, the therapist must be aware of the individual's feelings toward work before the insult or accident as well as the person's present feelings.

Throughout this chapter you will find descriptions of innovative programming and assessment for clients with physical and/or neurologic disabilities.

But first I will briefly discuss some ramifications of specific dysfunctions with respect to work-related programming.

The employment potential of a person with a spinal cord injury "is not necessarily correlated with the injury and its residual manifestations. A person with a debilitating injury is able to return to work if he or she is motivated, possesses employable knowledge and skills, is offered reassurance from family and friends, and is able to find a job" [10]. It is important that in addition to finding a job the person be given a chance to be successful. In this chapter and the Appendix to Chapter 6, you will read of such persons acquiring training and entering successfully into the field of computers.

For the hemiplegic "the effect on vocational potential can be serious, depending on skills previously attained and the impairment of intellectual functions. Return to previous vocation depends in large measure on the type of job the patient was doing, the patient's status in the company, the understanding of the employer, and the patient's ability to regain employable skills" [10].

The head-injured individual offers a complex challenge to developing work-related programs and assessments. These persons are more likely to be hindered by cognitive, behavioral, and social difficulties in performance than by physical deficits. "The level of pretrauma intellectual functioning and achieved educational level help in regaining vocational potential" [10]. Programming should provide head-injured patients with opportunities to work on familiar skills with multiple steps and repetition of instructions. In addition a time for practice and defined outcome criteria are important [17].

The person with congenital neurophysiologic problems for example, cerebral palsy or mental retardation, presents a different therapeutic picture. Many of these clients have had little or no exposure to work-related skills, behaviors, and habits; thus programming must be planned to facilitate acquisition of these items.

Much activity in the area of work-related evaluation for the individual with physical and/or neurologic dysfunction has been evident in recent years. Terms such as *work tolerance screening*, *work capacity evaluation*, and *situational assessment* have become familiar among therapists. These assessments will be discussed in detail within this chapter.

The therapeutic setting offers a wealth of in-house resources in evaluation development. Equipment available to the therapist such as computers, typewriters, carpentry power tools, and calculators may serve a dual purpose in providing an evaluation and training tool to the clients.

Whatever evaluation is used should provide information that will facilitate the development of programs to teach clients new skills, behaviors, and habits; to train them in the use of adaptive equipment (when necessary); and to develop alternative job opportunities.

**Drivers' Training Program**
BRAINTREE HOSPITAL'S
COMPREHENSIVE DRIVER EDUCATION PROGRAM

It is estimated that 1,500,000 employable disabled persons are unemployed because of lack of transportation. Braintree Hospital's Comprehensive Driver Education Program for the physically disabled is based on the premise that restriction of mobility is a serious problem that limits an individual's vocational, educational, social, and recreational opportunities and ultimately an independent life-style.

Extensive research and investigation, particularly of accident reports, have revealed that most disabled persons can be licensed as safe, competent drivers. However, the lack of essential medical input in commercial driving schools has kept many from succeeding.

Braintree Hospital's program, which is an extension of the rehabilitation process, provides clinical evaluation of the disabled client's driving potential. When indicated, on-the-road training in specially modified vehicles is also part of the program. Braintree Hospital patients, as well as school-based clients, may refer themsleves or be referred by a physician, rehabilitation counselor, or other health care professional. Referrals are most timely when the client has completed any active therapy programs and has attained his or her maximum functional potential.

At the time of the referral medical history, seizure history, a list of current medications, and discharge summaries from completed therapy programs are requested. This information is used to determine the client's appropriateness for the pre-driving evaluation and assists in answering questions such as Is the program timely with respect to the client's disability and rehabilitation progress? and Is driving a realistic goal for this client?

To date, clients with the following disabilities have participated in the program:

1. Cerebral vascular accidents
2. Traumatic brain injuries
3. Traumatic spinal cord injuries
4. Progressive neuromuscular disorders such as multiple sclerosis and muscular dystrophy
5. Amputations
6. Congenital defects such as spina bifida and cerebral palsy
7. Developmental disabilities such as mental retardation and minimal brain dysfunction

Program components include (1) A predriving evaluation completed by an occupational therapist, (2) An on-the-road evaluation, and (3) A physical medicine evaluation and medical certification letter to the Massachusetts Registry of Motor Vehicles.

*Clinical Predriving Evaluation*

The predriving evaluation has been designed to determine the client's driving potential through the assessment of his or her (1) physical skills, that is, range of motion, muscle strength, coordination, mobility, transfer skills, reaction time, and endurance; (2) perception; (3) congnition; (4) vision; (5) language skills; and (6) need for adaptive driving equipment and vehicle modification. The evaluating therapist also determines if additional therapy is needed before the client begins to drive.

When driving is contraindicated by the evaluation results, the following options are available:

1. Therapeutic intervention for remediation of residual deficits, for example, muscle strengthening, cognitive retraining
2. Recommendation for reevaluation of current medications, for example, for spasticity
3. Recommendations for equipment needed to transport the client safely as a passenger

When the evaluation results demonstrate that the client has the potential to drive, further recommendations may include a 30-hour classroom drivers' education program or an on-the-road training program in a specially modified vehicle. The amount of on-the-road training that the client will require depends on the complexity of the adaptive driving equipment and the client's prior driving experience, endurance, and ability to integrate new learning. The following indicates the average amount of drivers' training recommended for clients with various disabilities:

| *Disability* | *Amount of Training (hours)* |
|---|---|
| Spinal cord injury | 20–30 |
| Lower-extremity amputations | 10 |
| Cerebral vascular accidents | 10 |
| Traumatic head injuries | 15–20 |
| Congenital defects | 20 |

Besides classroom and on-the-road training, continued therapy for transfer training, wheelchair management, and muscle strengthening; specialized adaptive driving equipment that compensates for physical deficits (e.g., left foot accelerator, steering knob) (Fig. 5-15); or handicapped plates may be recommended. These plates, obtained from the Registry of Motor Vehicles, enable the client to use designated handicapped parking spaces, thereby increasing his or her independence.

*On-the-Road Evaluation*

The two-hour on-the-road evaluation is completed only when the client's performance during the predriving evaluation demonstrates borderline deficits

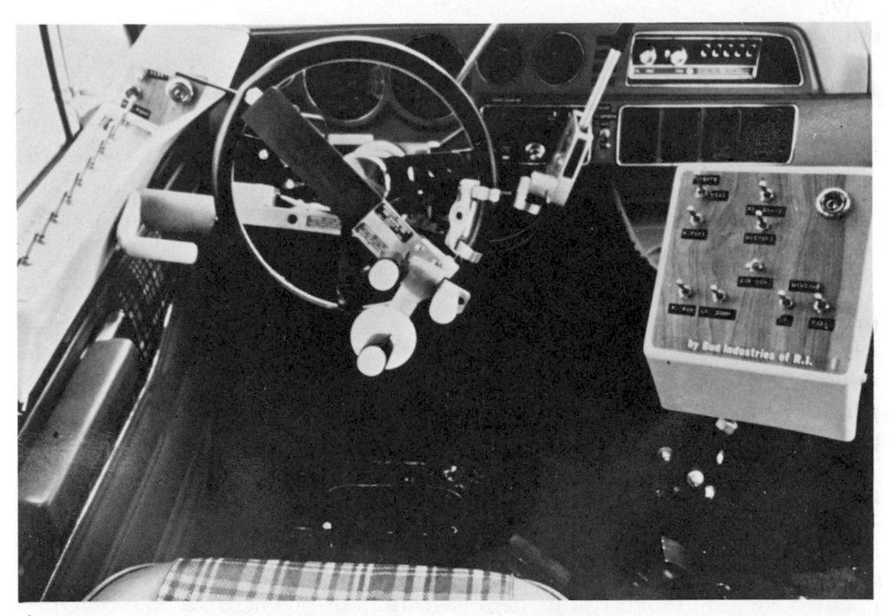


A

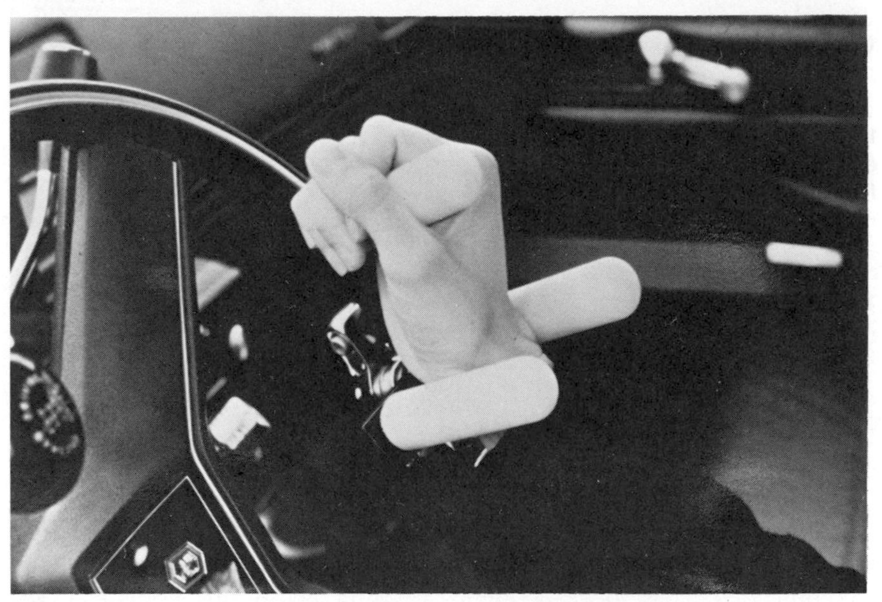

B

*Fig. 5-15. A. Adaptive driving equipment and vehicle modification for a van. B. Close-up of adaptive hand device. (Courtesy of Braintree Hospital.)*

in cognitive, perceptual, or visual skills. Before the evaluation, the predriving evaluator and the driver trainer plan functional tasks or situations that can be simulated in the vehicle to evaluate further the client's cognitive processing, attention span, impulsivity, reaction time, visual scanning, and depth perception.

The on-the-road evaluation is not a driving lesson but rather an assessment used to supplement clinical findings and determine if the client can return to driving.

*Physical Medicine Evaluation and Medical Certification Letter*

When all the evaluation components have been completed, a physician reviews them with the therapist and writes a letter explaining the results of the evaluation to the Registry of Motor Vehicles. This letter is sent to the medical affairs branch of the registry and recommends either a return to driving or suspension of the client's operator's license. In addition adaptive equipment needed for driving is summarized, and license restrictions are recommended. The final step for obtaining a valid operator's license, completion of the road competency test, is the client's responsibility.

*Results*

Braintree Hospital's Comprehensive Driver Education Program has been in existence since 1977. During this time it has seen much success and an increased need for its services. In 1981 the program evaluated 120 clients; in 1982, 135. The program's combination of thorough clinical evaluation and individualized driver's training has enabled 100 percent of the clients who complete the training to obtain a valid license. A license enables the disabled client to utilize fully the skills acquired through the rehabilitation process. This hospital-based driving program helps strengthen the link between rehabilitation and independent living.

Following are two case studies from the Braintree Hospital program and a list of companies that supply adaptive driving equipment.

*Case Study 1**

D. M., a 23-year-old woman, was involved in a motor vehicle accident that resulted in head injury, left eye blindness, multiple fractures, and coma for four weeks. Acute hospitalization lasted 2½ months and included status post tracheostomy and gastrostomy. When medically stable, D. M. was transferred to a brain injury unit for rehabilitation. After 4½ months, she was discharged and went home to her family for 24-hour supervision. As an outpatient D. M. received occupational, physical, and speech therapy for an additional 6 months. Current medications include phenytoin sodium (Dilantin), 200 mg per day, for seizure prevention. D. M.'s neurologist provided an on-medication agreement stating that she had been seizure-free since the time of the accident. State law requires that an 18-month seizure-free period be established before one can return to driving.

*This case study was provided by Holly T. Ehle, OTR, Braintree Hospital, Braintree, Massachusetts.

On completion of therapy D. M. worked as a secretary in a supervised job that had been arranged by her state vocational rehabilitation counselor in preparation for returning to competitive employment.

Before her motor vehicle accident, D. M. had had five years of driving experience. She also reported having successfully completed the classroom driver education safety course.

A predriving evaluation was completed 24 months after injury. Physical, visual, perceptual, and cognitive skills were evaluated with regard to D. M.'s ability to drive.

Physically, D. M.'s upper extremities demonstrated a functionally adequate active range of motion and generally fair muscle strength. The right upper extremity demonstrated normal muscle tone with below-average coordination. However, her left upper extremity demonstrated minimal hypertonicity, with associated reactions. Her left-upper-extremity tremors increased when she was frustrated, anxious, or angry, although overall coordination was minimally impaired. Therefore, her left arm was considered to be nonfunctional for driving. As a result, she would need to steer using her right hand with the aid of a steering knob and power steering.

D. M.'s right lower extremity demonstrated a functional active range of motion and muscle tone, fair muscle strength, and slower-than-average reaction times. The left lower extremity demonstrated increased hypertonicity with the presence of associated reactions and clonus and therefore was considered to be nonfunctional for driving. Because of these deficits, D. M. would be restricted to operating a car equipped with power brakes and an automatic transmission.

D. M. could walk independently without assistive devices. She entered and exited a car independently.

D. M.'s visual acuity was corrected to within Registry of Motor Vehicles requirements. The speed and accuracy with which she was able to scan her environment was impaired but within normal limits. D. M. suffered traumatic blindness in her left eye. The registry ruling on one-eyed vision states that the field of vision must be at least 135. D. M.'s visual field met registry standards at 155. Depth perception was minimally impaired. Night vision and glare recovery were severely impaired. As a result, D. M. would be restricted to daytime driving. Color vision and traffic color recognition were within normal limits.

Perceptually, D. M. demonstrated below-average spatial relation skills; however, figure-ground discrimination and auditory memory were functional. Visual memory was minimally below passing standard. Her speed of visual processing was one-third slower than average. However, her accuracy was functional when she was asked to alternate between two stimuli. Her behavior during the clinical evaluation included periods of impulsivity and low frustration tolerance.

The clinical predriving evaluation with the head-injured client is limited; identified deficit areas must be further assessed on the road. D. M.'s performance on the road demonstrated perceptual and behavioral impairments that interfered with her ability to drive safely. The most serious deficit was her slowed mental processing, exhibited by her impaired ability to adapt to and solve problems demanding quick, accurate responses. She was unable to control her frustration, anxiety, and impulsivity as was clearly demonstrated when she uncontrollably withdrew her hands from the steering wheel. D. M. acknowledged her behaviors but was unable to realize their implications with regard to safe driving.

On the basis of the clinical predriving evaluation and the on-the-road assessment, it was recommended that D. M. remain a passenger and not drive. It was also recommended that D. M. remain a passenger and not drive. It was also recommended that her license be suspended and not renewed. Various alternative activities were suggested to assist D. M. to develop the necessary predriving skills. D. M., her family, and her vocational counselor were informed that D. M. would be eligible for reevaluation if major progress could be demonstrated.

*Case Study 2**

At age 15 B. J. sustained a C6 spinal cord injury in a diving accident. A spinal fusion, C5 through C7, was surgically performed for neck stabilization. He received rehabilitation at a regional spinal cord injury unit. During rehabilitation he had difficulty with spasticity in his legs, which resulted in a right hip dislocation. He had surgical correction of his right hip and tendon releases for spastic abductors. After six months of rehabilitation he was discharged to his home, where he functions from an electric wheelchair and receives assistance from his family. The home was modified for electric wheelchair accessibility, including ramping and bathroom modifications.

B. J. returned to high school and hopes to attend college after graduation. He plans to study computers with the goal of full-time employment in business. The state vocational rehabilitation commission referred B. J. for an evaluation of driving potential and adaptive equipment needs.

B. J. did not have driving experience before his spinal cord injury. He completed classroom drivers' education at high school. B. J. depends on private wheelchair van companies for all transportation.

A predriving evaluation was completed 18 months after injury. Physical, cognitive, perceptual, and visual skills were evaluated in terms of B. J.'s potential to drive safely and of his adaptive driving equipment needs.

B. J.'s arms demonstrated the physical strength, active range of motion, sensation, coordination, and reaction times necessary for learning effective driving of a van with full hand controls. Specifically, the right arm demonstrated the abilities necessary to steer with reduced-effort power steering and a tri-pin steering device. His left arm demonstrated the abilities necessary to accelerate and brake with a right-angle–type hand control mounted on the left side of the steering column. A left wrist splint was needed for driving, to provide a secure interface with hand control and to maximize left arm strength. All driving functions had to be modified for activation with either right or left arm.

B. J.'s legs were nonfunctional for driving tasks because of the lack of voluntary movement. Full seat belting including shoulder, chest, lap, and leg belting was recommended. B. J.'s legs had to be secured away from conventional floor gas and brake pedals because of his spasticity. Since B. J. required assistance for all transfers, he had to drive from his electric wheelchair with a wheelchair tie-down system. His dependence on an electric wheelchair for mobility necessitated a specially modified van with an automatic wheelchair lift.

All cognitive and perceptual skills evaluated were within functional limits for learning to operate a van. Drivers' training was recommended to maximize these skills and to prepare for the registry road test.

All visual skills were evaluated with prescription lenses, and the results were within registry requirements.

The following actions were taken by the evaluating therapist:

1. A medical certification letter was mailed to the medical affairs branch of the registry, providing clearance for B. J. to begin drivers' training in a specially modified van.
2. Twenty-five hours of drivers' training was recommended for B. J. to learn safe use of adaptive driving equipment and to prepare for the registry road test.
3. On successful completion of the road test, B. J. would receive a restricted driver's license.
4. Because of B. J.'s permanent physical disability, handicapped plates were recommended for his specially modified van.

*This case study was provided by Karen Haggerty-Weake, OTR, Braintree Hospital, Braintree, Massachusetts.

The following restrictions would appear on B. J.'s driver's license:

1. Automatic transmission
2. Power steering
3. Power brakes
4. Steering device
5. Full hand controls
6. Hand-operated parking brake
7. Hand-operated dimmer switch

The state vocational rehabilitation commission assisted with payment for drivers' training and adaptive equipment. After 25 hours of training in his modified van, B. J. successfully completed the registry road test and has become a licensed driver.

## ADAPTIVE DRIVING EQUIPMENT COMPANIES

1. Action Mobility Products and Services, Inc.
   1925 Tenth Ave.
   Lake Worth, FL 33461
   (800) 432-1459

2. Robert Alba's Breakthrough Vehicles
   46 Pond St.
   North Easton, MA 02356
   (617) 238-2513

3. Terry Bilbrey's Handicapped Vans
   215 S. Locust
   Champaign, IL 61820
   (217) 398-1053

4. Drake-Scruggs Equipment, Inc.
   2000 S. Dirksen Pky.
   P. O. Box 2549
   Springfield, IL 62708
   (212) 753-3871

5. Drive-Master Corp.
   16-A Andrews Dr.
   West Paterson, NJ 07424
   (201) 785-2204

6. Falcon Equipment Specialist
   57 Tunxis St.
   Windsor, CN 06075
   (203) 688-7597

7. Freewheel Vans, Inc.
   16002 W. Fourth Ave.
   Golden, CO 80401
   (303) 278-2972

8. Handicap Mobility
   235 Central Ave.
   Needham Heights, MA 02194
   (617) 449-0682

9. Handicapped Driving Aids of Michigan, Inc.
   4020 Second
   Wayne, MI 48184
   (313) 595-4400

10. Handicapped Specialities, Inc.
    3727 S. Walnut
    Muncie, IN 47302
    (317) 288-1441

11. Haveco (Handicap Vehicle Conversion Co.)
    1223 N. Cameron St.
    P. O. Box 2227
    Harrisburg, PA 17105
    (717) 238-5535

12. Midwest Mobility Systems
    15587 Forest Blvd. N.
    Hugo, MN 55038
    (612) 426-1211

13. Northeast Kustom Kreations
    Mobility Equipment for the Handicapped
    D. and V. Girard
    Varney and S. Main St.
    Manchester, NH 03102
    (603) 622-0282

14. Owl Mobility Equipment
    650 Kennedy Rd.
    Lexington, KY 40505
    (606) 254-0576

15. Rehabilitation Equipment Co., Inc.
    1054 Evans Ave.
    Akron, OH 44305
    (216) 633-0072

16. R & R Van Lift
    1126 Old Covington Hwy.
    Conyers, GA 30207
    (404) 483-0767

17. Sylacauga Handicapped Equipment
    3426 Taladega Hwy
    Sylacauga, AL 35150
    (205) 249-3717

18. United Lift
    P. O. Box 607
    Stoughton, WI 53589
    (608) 873-9607

**Rehabilitation Centers**

LIBERTY MUTUAL MEDICAL SERVICE CENTER

Liberty Mutual Insurance Company, the country's largest underwriter of workers' compensation, has been a forerunner in the field of providing rehabilitation for the industrially injured (Fig. 1-1). Its outpatient facility, the Liberty Mutual Medical Service Center, provides two types of rehabilitative services: a clinic and a rehabilitation center.

The clinic, which was first opened in Boston in 1913, provides outpatient treatment for minor industrial injuries (e.g., dislocations, burns, punctures, sprains). Treatment is available five days a week during typical working hours (8:30–4:30).

The rehabilitation center was founded in 1943 to provide rehabilitation (including occupational therapy) after more serious injuries, including all types of hand injuries, back and neck injuries, extremity fractures and amputations, and other orthopedic problems. Comprehensive rehabilitation is provided for workers' compensation policyholder employees, both locally and nationally. Liberty Mutual believes that an intensive program of rehabilitation will enable an injured person to return to work sooner, thus reducing the human and economic costs of disability.

*Evaluation*

Occupational therapy is one of the main components of the rehabilitative process. On admission to the center the therapist provides the patient with a complete occupational therapy evaluation (Table 5-3).

*Table 5-3. Occupational Therapy Evaluation*

| *Evaluation Category* | *Example* |
|---|---|
| Range of motion (ROM) | Standard ROM measurements<br>Can the patient bend over, stoop, sit, and reach all work surfaces? |
| Sensation | Must any precautions be observed because of limitation in sensation? |
| Strength, endurance | What amount of weight can be lifted, pushed, carried? Is endurance for repetitive activity limited? |
| Sitting and standing tolerance | What is the patient's tolerance for sitting and standing activities? |
| Edema | Standard measurements |
| Psychosocial | How did personality characteristics influence behavior in the evaluation situation? How does this person relate to co-workers, supervisors? |
| Medical history | Review of injury and treatment |
| Functional | Is the patient independent in self-care and mobility? |
| Job history | Does the patient feel able to do his or her former job? What motions, mechanical adaptations are required? How much repetitive lifting is required? |
| Body pain chart | Where are the areas of subjective bodily complaints? |
| Adaptive equipment needs | Does the patient need adaptive equipment to facilitate returning to his or her former job or to function more easily at home? |

An average evaluation involves three to six hours of testing, in either a single session or multiple sessions; thereafter, short-term and long-term goals and treatment plans are established. The following is a brief example of the results of an evaluation of a patient with a below-elbow amputation of the dominant hand:

1. Short-term goals
   a. To increase range of motion of shoulder and elbow
   b. To increase bilateral strength of upper extremities
   c. To increase use of affected upper extremity
2. Long-term goals
   a. To develop effective use of prosthetic device
   b. To maximize independence in activities of daily living (ADL)
   c. To return to work place where bilateral upper-extremity use may be required

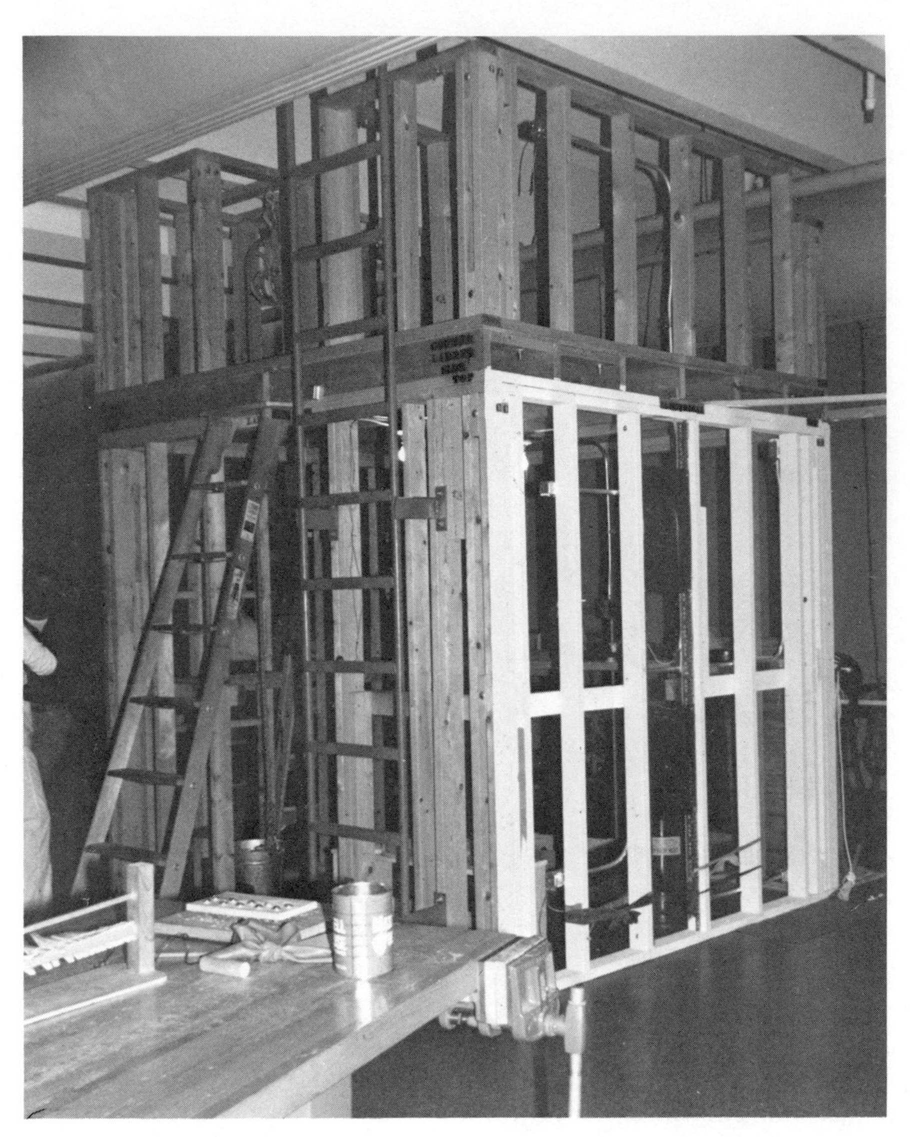

A

3. Treatment
   a. Upper extremity exercise with and without resistance, using a computerized work simulator
   b. Issuance and instruction in use of necessary adaptive equipment
   c. Therapeutic craft activities (e.g., leather craft, copper tooling, woodworking) to facilitate use of affected upper extremity (may necessitate adaptive aides to facilitate independence in projects)
   d. Prosthetic training
   e. Work simulation (as appropriate)

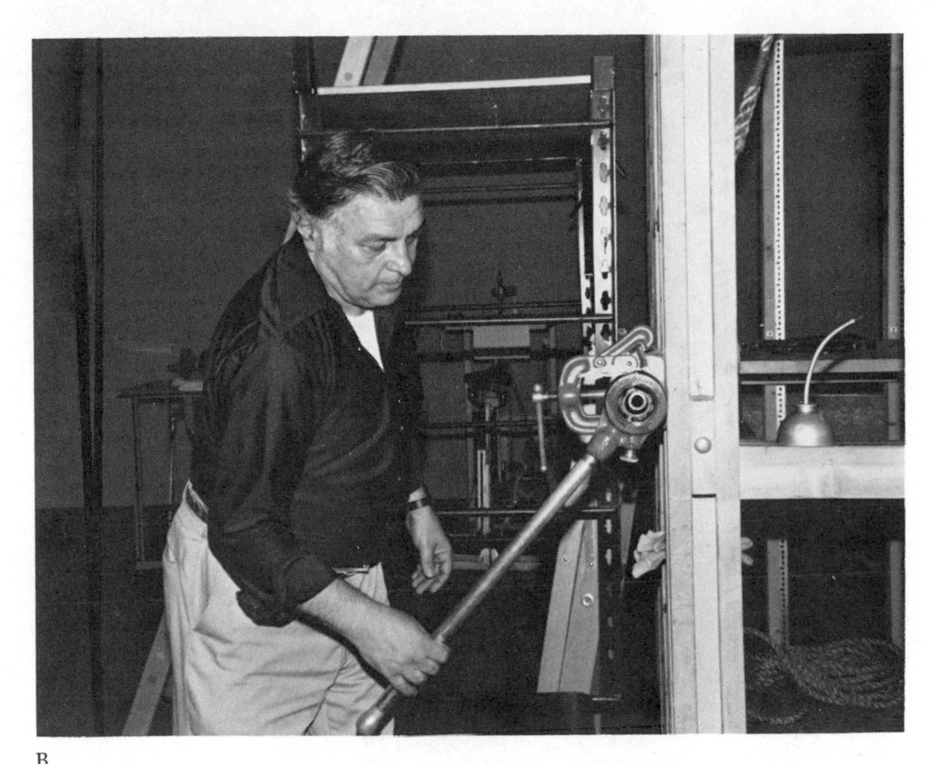

B

*Fig. 5-16. A: Multiwork station that resembles a section of a two-story house under construction. B: Client doing construction work at the work station.*

*Innovative Program Elements*

The occupational therapy program at the Liberty Mutual center offers several innovative elements.

At the *multiwork station*, a work station resembling a section of a two-story house under construction (Fig. 5-16) is used to help patients test their ability to return to strenuous work. It enables them to develop their capacity to handle some of the more physically demanding tasks associated with jobs such as climbing ladders, staging, lifting heavy or large objects, working overhead, using heavy wrenches, pipe cutting and threading, electrical wiring, tiling, siding, and painting.

A cross-section of a *truck cab* (Fig. 5-17) is used to simulate the job of a truck driver. The cab has been modified to offer adjustable resistance on the steering wheel, clutch, and stick shift. In conjunction an audiotape or videotape is used to simulate the auditory and visual dimensions of actual driving situations.

When the patient has upper-extremity injury, a *computerized work simulator* (Fig. 5-18) may be used. This is an instrument that consists of two primary components mounted on a pedestal base: (1) A passive variable-

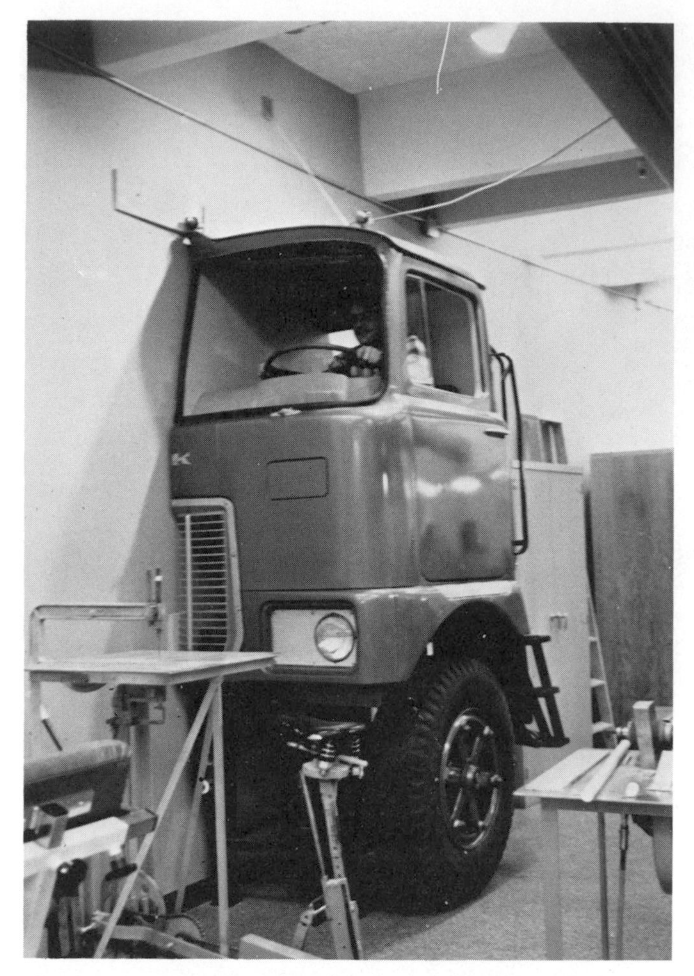

*Fig. 5-17. Cross-section of truck cab used for job simulation.*

resistance assembly from which a shaft protrudes. Attachments such as a power grip and steering wheel fit onto the shaft. (2) A computer control panel that indicates the time and distance that the patient has exercised at a level of resistance determined by the therapist. A readout prints the above information as well as additional data about force, workload, and other variables.

A *lifting-lowering device* operated by compressed air enables the patient to lift or retrieve boxes of weights from levels deemed appropriate by the therapist.

Materials handling equipment including loading platforms, two-wheel trucks, conveyor rollers, and other items is available to simulate actual work conditions and increase patient tolerance of work.

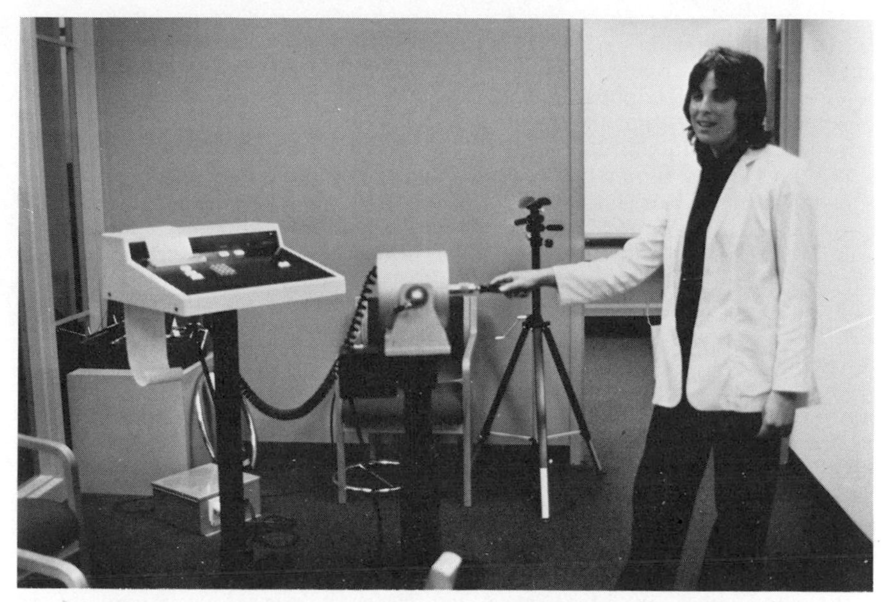

*Fig. 5-18. Therapist demonstrating use of computerized work simulator.*

*Case Study 1**

K. J. is a 38-year-old man who was admitted to the Liberty Mutual Medical Service Center for rehabilitation following a lower-back injury. Admission to the center took place 3½ months after an L5 diskectomy to correct a ruptured disk. The patient had sustained his injury while repairing a crane during his work as a mechanic of construction equipment.

On admission K. J. reported numbness and tingling in his left lower leg and pain in the left buttock and across the lower back. These symptoms increased with activity.

Observation revealed a short, muscular man in no acute distress. He stood symmetrically without evidence of scoliosis, kyphosis, lordosis, or pelvic obliquity. However, the patient demonstrated increased weight bearing on the left lower extremity during standing. He walked quickly and with a symmetrical arm swing, but with a slight deviation in gait. Although no limp was present, the left leg rotated externally to a greater degree than did the right leg. He could stand for one hour, but only if he was able to place one leg and then the other on a low footstool. He had a sitting tolerance of one hour when seated in a chair with a back and using a pillow at the lower back and a footstool. He could squat and perform an activity for a maximum of two to three minutes. He climbed a vertical ladder using a smooth reciprocal pattern.

A functional evaluation disclosed a few limitations in ADL. He was unable to drive for more than 30 minutes. He was unable to vacuum, mow the lawn, or repair his car. He was able to perform all other ADL.

Before a treatment program was implemented, a job description was secured to devise a job simulation treatment program and to help determine readiness to return to work. As an on-site job evaluation was not possible because of distance, the job description was obtained from the patient. K. J.'s work as a mechanic of large equipment required that he be able to assume a variety of postures and perform several

*This case study was provided by Karen Lindau, M. S., OTR, Liberty Mutual Medical Service Center, Boston, Massachusetts.

motions for various periods of time: standing, pushing and pulling very resistive levers, lifting 50- to 100-pound objects, squatting, kneeling, climbing stairs and ladders, and maneuvering in and out of awkward or confined spaces. After the therapist had obtained the job description, the therapist and patient jointly devised a treatment program that would simulate the motions and postures his job required. Treatment activites would include crafts performed in a standing position, pulling and pushing a short lever on the computerized work simulator, lifting a weighted box, laying tile while squatting and kneeling, climbing ladders, and "wriggling through" the exposed framework of the multiwork station. He was also given both upper- and lower-extremity exercises to perform. It was felt that if the extremities were strengthened his back would be required to assume less stress. Upper- and lower-extremity exercises included use of the bicycle saw, the bucket hoist, and the inclined sander. K. J. was also instructed in proper body mechanics and was evaluated for the need for adaptive equipment.

On admission K. J. had physician's orders for occupational therapy, physical therapy, and recreation therapy. He initially attended occupational therapy twice a day. A graded approach to treatment, gradually increasing time and weights and overall strenuousness of activities was followed. The more strenuous activities included more difficult climbing and activities performed in a squatting position. Monitoring and instruction in body mechanics took place throughout treatment. In the meantime, he was encouraged to engage in increasingly strenuous activities at home.

K. J. participated in the rehabilitation program at Liberty Mutual for one month, at the end of which he and the medical staff felt that he was ready to return to work. By the time of discharge, K. J. was attending occupational therapy three times per day for a total of approximately 2½ hours per day. He was not limited in any ADL, including mowing the lawn, repairing his car, or driving. He did continue to have mild residual discomfort during some activities. However, he felt that the discomfort was not severe and was something he "could live with." K. J. was discharged back to his attending physician to be followed by our rehabilitation nurse. As recommended by our physician and therapy staff, he returned to work shortly after discharge. We remained available in the event the patient encountered any difficulties following return to work.

### *Case Study 2**

J. M. is a 47-year-old woman who had worked as a light parts process checker for A. Co. for 10 years. On June 20, 1983, she was walking in the corridors of A. Co. toward the lunch area when she slipped on a floor mat and fell onto her right dominant hand, fracturing her right fourth metacarpophalangeal joint (MP). She was placed in a long arm cast for four weeks. When the cast was removed, however, J. M. found that she had pain at the volar aspect of her right ulnar wrist area. J. M. attempted to return to work in September, three months after her accident. She found, however, that the manual activities required for her job increased her right wrist pain. In November of 1983, J. M. saw a hand surgeon who injected cortisone into this area to relieve the pain. This treatment proved to be unsuccessful. On May 30, 1984, J. M. underwent removal of the pisiform bone because of degenerative changes in the joint between the pisiform and triquetrum bones.

On July 2, 1984, J. M. began attending Liberty Mutual Medical Center in Boston every day as a full-time patient, commuting from her home in the greater Boston area. The rehabilitative program at Liberty Mutual included occupational therapy, physical therapy, and recreational therapy.

*This case study was provided by Sara Hargreaves, M. S. OTR, Liberty Mutual Medical Service Center, Boston, Massachusetts.

In occupational therapy, J. M. was initially evaluated for range of motion, strength, sensation, social and emotional status, and function in terms of her work environment and ADL. Physical evaluation revealed limitations of right wrist dorsiflexion, volar flexion, and ulnar and radial deviation. The right shoulder had pain and decreased range of motion in flexion, abduction, and horizontal abduction and adduction (frozen shoulder secondary to protection of injured hand). The right hand grasp was evaluated at one-quarter the strength of the left. Wrist strength was measured at F+ to G− on manual muscle testing. Otherwise the right upper extremity was G− to G overall on initial examination. J. M. filled out the body pain chart, noting pain in the ulnar wrist area, especially when ulnarly deviating and flexing her wrist. The right hand appeared edematous.

Preliminary job evaluation revealed the following: J. M.'s job as a light parts process checker for A. Co. requires fine to gross manual dexterity in working with small tools and small to large objects. Tools used includes large and small screwdrivers, nut drivers, masking tape, and wire cutters. Power grip, precision, and piecework are required. J. M. stated that she prepares metal parts to be chromated by other workers. She wires the metal parts together which requires an ulnar flexion of her right dominant wrist, and places them on brass hooks. Other requirements include tightening screws and nuts of various sizes. At the initial interview J. M. indicated strong motivation to return to work but was unsure whether she could indeed perform her job without pain. Evaluation of J. M.'s psychosocial status revealed that she lives in her own home with her husband and daughter, who offer a good amount of physical and emotional support. She appeared cooperative and motivated to work on her treatment program. ADL evaluation revealed that J. M. was able to perform self-care activities but with moderate difficulty. Problems included pushing down with the palm of her hand when getting out of the bathtub, hygienic wipe with toilet activity, and picking up small objects. J. M. compensated for these activities with her left hand. ADL requiring ulnar flexion (e.g., meal preparation, washing dishes, crocheting, crewelwork, writing) were severely hampered.

Goals initially were to increase the range of motion of the right wrist, the strength of grasp and pinch of the right hand, and the strength and endurance of the entire right upper extremity. The treatment plan included hand and shoulder exercises, tool use on a hand machine with measured force of resistance, hoisting, lifting small to large weighted objects, and projects requiring hand dexterity including ADL and workbench activities. J. M. performed with good motivation and cooperation on a gradually increasing resistance program, which appeared to increase the strength and range of motion of the right upper extremity. To increase knowledge of actual work requirements, an on-site job evaluation was performed on July 25, 1984. Results of the on-site job evaluation were as follows:

*Workbench measurements*

Desk height is 32 inches; a ¾-inch pipe 19 inches above the workbench runs the length of the workbench and is used for hanging the objects being wired.

*Manual dexterity requirements*

1. Masking, which involves pushing and pulling small rubber and Teflon plugs into holes with long-nose pliers.
2. Wiring small metal parts together with aluminum wire and then wiring these parts to copper hangers suspended from the 19-inch-high pipe. Upper-extremity force is required to push these hangers onto and off the pipe for chromating.
3. Cutting four or five thicknesses of aluminum wire with wire cutters.
4. Pulling aluminum wire from large rollers with resistance of up to 60 pounds.
5. Tightening small screws using a jeweler's screwdriver.

*Summary of on-site evaluation*

J. M.'s job requires almost constant upper-extremity elevation of about 100 degrees or less while working. Twisting motions of the hand (wrist flexion and extension and ulnar and radial deviation) appear necessary for about 90 percent of her working day, although actual work varies with production requirements.

The patient's tool box and supply of wire and metal parts for wiring were brought back for use during job simulation activities. To simulate her workbench, ¾-inch pipe was placed 19 inches above a table 32 inches high.

J. M. initially performed simulations of her job requirements for 10 minutes at a time. She also performed hand and upper-extremity exercises, hand craft activities, ADL, and tasks on the computerized work simulator in occupational therapy as well as receiving physical and recreational therapy. In two weeks J. M. had progressed to performing one-half hour of work simulation without pain four times a day interspersed with her other treatment programs. By the second month J. M. progressed to performing four hours of work simulation without pain. By the third month other exercises and activities in occupational, physical, and recreational therapy were excluded, and J. M. performed a successful week of full-day work simulation. J. M. confidently returned to work on December 28, 1984, able to perform her job requirements as well as her ADL and self-care activities without pain.

## ALFREDA REHABILITATION UNIT

The Alfreda Rehabilitation Unit is another example of a short-term, outpatient care facility providing treatment for the client with acute and chronic physical problems such as peripheral nerve lesions, fractures, back disorders, strokes, and sports, hand, and head injuries. It differs from the Liberty Mutual Medical Service Center in that the unit is state financed and affiliated with the Queen Elizabeth Hospital located in Royal Park, Australia.

The unit's objective is to enable clients through rehabilitation to achieve the optimal level of work performance and life-style in a relatively short period of time. The rehabilitation program aims at providing comprehensive education in health maintenance and preventive health care—diet, recreation, stress management, exercise [7, 8].

Occupational therapists are integral staff members in this multidisciplinary approach to rehabilitation that involves physicians, physical and speech therapists, social workers, and physical education and trade skill instructors. Although the role of occupational therapy is diverse, it entails assessment and treatment of each client as an individual. Dean, Cox, and Auricht [12], occupational therapists at the unit, have described their role as having major emphasis: (1) direct client contact, (2) community health promotion, (3) occupational therapy administration, and (4) education and research.

### *Direct Client Contact*

Client *assessment* at the unit takes two forms: initial assessment to determine the goals of therapy within the rehabilitation program (Figs. 5-19 and 5-20), and ongoing assessment to monitor progress.

*Fig. 5-19. Form used in initial client assessment at Alfreda Rehabilitation Unit.*

DISABILITY: ONSET:

OCCUPATION:

HISTORY:

SOCIAL SITUATION:

HOME CONDITIONS:

TRANSPORT:

FUNCTIONAL ABILITY:

*Mobility:*

| | |
|---|---|
| Posture | Squatting |
| Lie to sit | Kneeling |
| Sitting tolerance | Rolling |
| Sit to stand | Walking |
| Standing tolerance | Lifting |

*Trunk:*

| | |
|---|---|
| Forward flexion | Side flexion |
| Extension | Twisting |

*Results of Lower Back Function Questionnaire:*

UPPER LIMB FUNCTION: (use upper limb assessment for more detail)

LOWER LIMB FUNCTION:

| | *Left* | *Right* |
|---|---|---|
| *Hip* | | |
| *Knee* | | |
| *Ankle* | | |
| *Strength* | | |
| *Sensation* | | |

ACTIVITIES OF DAILY LIVING:

*Personal:*
*Domestic:*

LEISURE ACTIVITIES, HOBBIES:

COMMUNICATION:

PERSONALITY, MENTAL STATE, ATTITUDES:

EDUCATION:

WORK HISTORY:

PRESENT WORK SITUATION:

*Name of Employer:*

*Contact Person:*

*Length of Employment:*

*Job Description:*

| GOALS: | OT PROGRAMME: |
|---|---|

Fig. 5-19 (continued)

The following *specific therapy* is provided:

1. Prescribed activities to improve function in specific areas
2. Back care: individual back care education (given to clients with back injuries and also as a preventive measure to those "at risk"), using visual aids, models, and supervision of workshop activities to reinforce postural awareness and good working habits; graded lifting program to reinforce correct lifting techniques and increase endurance and confidence; group back care sessions, conducted as a health promotion project, using visual aids and models
3. Joint preservation techniques for arthritis clients, using visual aids, demonstrations, and suggestions of aids and adaptations
4. Upper limb assessment and retraining, using standardized tests, remedial equipment, and activities
5. Sensory assessment and retraining
6. Assessment and retraining of higher cortical function (including perception and cognitive functions)
7. Splinting
8. Assessment or review of activities of daily living; when appropriate, instruction on methods of increasing independence and on use of aids

The work-related activities of the occupational therapy program include the following:

In *work assessment* general assessment of the worker's abilities and an assessment of the worker's abilities on specific tasks are carried out.

In *work simulation* activities that simulate the client's work situation are given when possible.

*Counseling* on suitable alternative employment areas and *training* in job application skills and interviewing skills are provided.

*Fig. 5-20. Lower back function questionnaire.*

**Lower Back Function Questionnaire**

Date: ________________

Name: ______________ Age: ________

How long have you had back pain? _____ years _____ months _____ weeks

How long have you had leg pain? _____ years _____ months _____ weeks

*PLEASE READ BEFORE COMPLETING THE QUESTIONNAIRE:*

This questionnaire has been designed to give information as to how you function in everyday life with your back condition. Please answer every section, and mark in each section only the *ONE* box which applies to you. We realise you may consider that two of the statements in any one section relate to you, but please *just mark the box which most closely describes your* condition.

*Section 1—Personal Care* (washing, dressing, etc.)

☐ I can look after myself normally.
☐ I can look after myself but I am slow and careful.
☐ I need some help but manage most of my personal carc.
☐ I need help every day in most of my personal care.

*Section 2—Lifting* (Think in terms of everyday things such as a 2-kg bag of sugar, etc.)

☐ I can lift heavy weights, for example ________________
☐ I cannot lift heavy weights off the floor, but can manage if they are conveniently positioned, e.g., on a table.
☐ I can lift light to medium weights, for example ________________
☐ I can lift light to medium weights if they are conveniently positioned.
☐ I can lift very light weights, for example ________________

*Section 3—Walking*

☐ I can walk any distance.
☐ I can walk for about 1 hour.
☐ I can walk for about 30 minutes.
☐ I can walk for about 15 minutes.
☐ I can walk for about 5 minutes or less.

*Section 4—Sitting*

☐ I can sit in any chair as long as I like.
☐ I can sit in certain chairs as long as I like.
☐ I can sit for about 1 hour.
☐ I can sit for about 30 minutes.
☐ I can sit for about 15 minutes.
☐ I can sit for about 5 minutes or less.

*Section 5—Standing*

☐ I can stand for as long as I want.
☐ I can stand for about 1 hour.
☐ I can stand for about 30 minutes.
☐ I can stand for about 15 minutes.
☐ I can stand for about 5 minutes or less.

*Section 6—Sleeping*

☐ I sleep the same as before I had my back condition.
☐ My sleep is sometimes disturbed by my back condition.
☐ My sleep is often disturbed by my back condition.
☐ My sleep is always disturbed by my back condition.

*Section 7—Sex Life*

☐ My sex life is not affected.
☐ My sex life is slightly restricted.
☐ My sex life is moderately restricted.
☐ My sex life is severely restricted.
☐ My sex life is absent.

*Section 8—Social Life*

☐ My social life is the same as it was before I had my back condition.
☐ My back condition has no significant effect on my social life apart from limiting my more energetic interests, e.g., dancing.
☐ My social life is restricted and I do not go out as often.
☐ My social life is restricted to my home.

*Section 9—Travelling* (by your usual means of transport, i.e., car, bus, motorbike, bicycle)

☐ I can manage journeys anywhere.
☐ I can manage journeys of about 2 hours.
☐ I can manage journeys of about 1 hour.
☐ I can manage journeys of about 30 minutes.
☐ I can manage journeys of about 15 minutes or less.

*Section 10—Pain Management*

☐ I can cope with the pain I have without having to use painkillers.
☐ Even when the pain is bad I manage without taking painkillers.
☐ Painkillers give complete relief.
☐ Painkillers give some relief.
☐ Painkillers give very little relief.
☐ Painkillers give no relief.

*Section 11—Pain Intensity*

Put a cross on the line to indicate your level of pain when

I am at my best. |————————————————|

No pain ... Pain so severe I would consider suicide

I am at my worst. |————————————————|

How I feel at this moment. |————————————————|

Fig. 5-20 (continued)

In *work simplification and application of ergonomics* individualized education is given, using visual aids, handouts, and, when necessary, demonstration or supervision. Ergonomic principles are applied to make the work situation as safe and efficient as possible.

To foster *communication with the employer* the therapists communicate with the client's employer (1) to minimize misunderstandings that may arise between employer and employee, (2) to promote an understanding of the rehabilitation process, (3) to negotiate suitable return to work conditions (this may be graded on a part-time basis to allow redevelopment of confidence, endurance, and skills), and (4) to discuss matters arising from work site visits. Ideally, the therapist communicates with the client's immediate boss, because a higher-level manager may have limited contact with the client.

*Visits to the client's work site* are arranged by the occupational therapist; other members of the rehabilitation team may also participate. The purpose of such visits is (1) to assess the client's work (Table 5-4); (2) to advise on

*Table 5-4. Topics Covered in Work Site Visit*

- Physical environment
    - Lighting
    - Noise level
    - Dust, fumes
    - Housekeeping, e.g., obstacles on floor, adequate storage areas
    - Type of building, e.g., under cover, open to weather
    - Architectural barriers, e.g., steps, ladders
    - Flooring or ground surface
        - Slippery
        - Uneven
        - Duckboards available
    - Temperature
        - Cold
        - Hot
        - Air conditioners
        - Heaters
    - Situation of toilets, lunchrooms
    - Access
- Safety
    - Signs
        - Large
        - Appropriate
        - Different languages
    - Fire extinguishers
    - Safety officer
    - Education sessions, e.g., on lifting techniques
    - Surfaces on floor, benches
    - Guards on machinery
    - Lifting devices
    - Availability of earplugs, safety shoes, spectacles
    - Protective clothing
    - State of repair of equipment

Table 5-4 (continued)

Psychological and social work environment
- Attitude of employers
- Attitude of workers
- Stress
  - Bonus systems
  - Other workers relying on client
- Isolated (working alone)
- Able to hold conversations with others
- Music
- Concentration required
- Responsibility
- Initiative
- Situation of lunchrooms; tea and lunch breaks
- Peer group
- Opportunity for change
- "Rehabilitation corner" (generally detrimental to separate handicapped worker from his usual work environment; better to modify usual work)

Actual job demands
- Range of movement, mobility
- Tolerance, endurance
- Weights lifted, moved
- Repetition
- Work positions
- Variety of work
- Frequency of breaks
- Time limits
- Shift work
- Communication
- Relying on others or vice versa

Considerations
- Will employer accept part-time return to work?
- Does client need to be "passed fit" by the industry's medical officer?
- Negotiate part-time return to work initially if possible, and if Alfreda staff feel this would be most beneficial to client
- Will employer modify job if necessary?
- Is job able to be modified?
- Are appropriate alternative duties (rather than "lighter" work) available?
- Will modified work affect rates of pay?
- Will other workers accept injured worker on modified duties?
- Attitude of unions?
- Confidentiality: Alfreda staff are acting on behalf of the client; it is generally prudent to say little or be as positive as possible about the client's programme
- Previous work history, attendance record
- Promotions?
- Time off
- Client's attitude regarding return to work

Source: Courtesy P. Dean, R. Cox, and R. Auricht [12].

possible modifications to work; (3) to advise on suitable alternative duties; (4) to develop an understanding of the rehabilitation concept among the employers, supervisors, and co-workers; (5) when necessary, to supervise the return-to-work process; and (6) when appropriate, to make follow-up contact to review the employee's progress.

The *client is introduced to skills* such as typing or welding to assess his or her potential in specific skills and, when further training is required, to guide the client into relevant community facilities.

*General life-style programming*, in the Alfreda Unit, emphasizes the development of general fitness through the use of an individualized graded activity program. Stress management—including relaxation training, techniques in time management, and coping and self-awareness exercises—is also taught. The client is encouraged to attain or to maintain a positive attitude toward the future. Therapists provide counseling on options for work and leisure and experience in selected activities to promote the development of skills. Adaptation to residual disability is encouraged. The occupational therapist may also communicate with family and significant others to foster an understanding of the client's situation and to encourage the family to assist in the client's rehabilitation. Supporting the client and family in adapting to role changes and other alterations to life-style is another function of the therapist. The therapist may also explore and teach the planning and organization of leisure time. When appropriate, clients are encouraged to participate in voluntary work or community groups. Therapists also report relevant information about the client to the treatment team and participate in case conferences. Finally, discharge or separation and follow-up review are planned with treatment team.

*Community Health Promotion*

When unit resources are available, the occupational therapist and the physical therapist present a back care seminar in one community.

*Occupational Therapy Administration*

Occupational therapists at the Alfreda Unit perform the following administrative duties:

1. Communication with other staff members such as the trades instructor and the assistant trades instructor
2. Ensuring an adequate range of activities to achieve objectives (e.g., communicating with instructors regarding design and adaptations to equipment and choice and supply of materials)
3. Communication with regional administrative staff regarding workshop staff coverage, the purchase of equipment and materials, and participation in staff meetings and supervisors' meetings
4. Public relations, that is, disseminating information about the unit to visiting individuals and groups
5. Arranging for specialist community speakers to address unit clients

6. Providing statistics on occupational therapy services to regional administration and committees

*Education and Research*
The occupational therapy department provides in-service training and ongoing education and occupational therapy student affiliates to the unit. When funding is available, the therapists also conduct research into the importance of occupational therapy at the unit [12].

## INSTITUTE OF REHABILITATION MEDICINE*

The Institute of Rehabilitation Medicine (IRM), New York University Medical Center, is a 150-bed comprehnsive rehabilitation center for severely disabled adults and children. Its occupational therapy department comprises many specialized units, one of which is the prevocational evaluation area. The therapist's case load in this area includes both inpatients and outpatients; the most common disabilities are spinal cord injuries, cerebral vascular accidents (CVAs), and traumatic brain injuries.

Staff vocational counselors refer patients to the prevocational area for evaluation. Concurrently, occupational therapists provide functional information on the patient. Specific criteria for patient referral have been developed for the major disabilities (Table 5-5).

The patient's program varies according to individual needs and interests. Work samples and tests are included in the following areas:

1. Clerical evaluations including bookkeeping, accounting, and business school work samples and TOWER tests; computer operator evaluation
2. Computer programming evaluation: aptitude testing (IBM test) and BASIC language instruction
3. Electronics evaluation (Heathkit assembly)
4. Drafting evaluation (TOWER series and mechanical drawing texts); computer graphics introduction
5. Mechanics evaluation: engine model assembly, carburetor assembly
6. Sheltered workshop and factory assembly: variety of standardized manual dexterity tests such as Purdue Pegboard, Pennsylvania Bimanual Work Sample, Minnesota Rate of Manipulation Test, TOWER workshop assembly tasks

A microcomputer has been used in the prevocational area since 1980. It has been useful as an evaluation and training tool for most patients. Specifically, a patient's potential to enter the programming field can be assessed by instructing the patient in BASIC and subsequently having him or her write and run original programs. Academic software is used to evaluate the potential for high school and college training. Many CVA hemiplegics have computer experience from their former jobs. Thus the microcomputer using

*This section was developed from information provided by Dorothy Milner, OTR.

*Table 5-5. Criteria for Patient Referral for Prevocational Evaluation*

| *Patient Group* | *Goals* | *Criteria* |
|---|---|---|
| Quadriplegics | | |
| High-level | To return to school or work | Cervical traction has been removed and sitting posture is upright<br>Assistive devices such as balanced forearm orthoses have been used in OT<br>Use of a mouthstick for typing, painting, and turning pages has been started in OT<br>Patient has expressed the wish to develop skills related to school or work |
| Low-level | To return to school or work | Sitting posture is upright<br>Patient has expressed the wish to develop skills related to school or work |
| Hemiplegics | To return to work or the evaluation of existing skills for a new vocation | Cognitive and perceptual deficits are minimal; learning potential and carry-over are fair<br>Deficits in attention span and concentration are minimal; potential for improvement is evident from response to activities in OT clinics<br>Dominance retraining has been initiated in OT; handwriting is fairly legible<br>Functional Communication Profile scores with input from speech therapists regarding reading, writing, and arithmetic ability<br>Evidence of patient's denial, which may interfere with testing, may be present<br>Prevocational screening test is completed; submit test results with referral |
| Patients with traumatic brain injury | To return to competitive or noncompetitive employment | Visual and spatial orientation is present<br>Attention and concentration abilities are fair<br>Manual dexterity with one or both hands is fair<br>When higher-level skills are present, include criteria for hemiplegics |

The Functional Communication Profile (FCP) was devised in 1969 by Martha Taylor Sarno, M.S., Director of Speech Therapy at the New York Institute of Rehabilitation Medicine. The Profile is a speech therapy test based on studies of premorbid functioning. The therapist obtains a percentile score of functional language (100% being the highest score). Depending on the results of the evaluation, a prevocational therapeutic referral may be appropriate.

standard business software becomes a viable assessment tool for them. Occupational therapists at IRM are researching computer interfaces for high-level quadriplegics and other severely disabled persons who may not be able to use the conventional keyboard. (Fig. 5-21).

Quadriplegic patients are referred to the prevocational area to develop communication skills and independence in performing desk-top work such as typing; writing; using a tape recorder, telephone, calculator, and computer. In addition the therapist constructs out of any low-temperature plastic material finger loop writing devices and typing fingers for C5 or C6 and lower-level quadriplegics to facilitate increased independence in page turning and using a telephone, typewriter, and other push-button equipment (Fig. 5-22).

Paraplegics with normal hand function are referred to prevocational evaluation for a general skills assessment in their interest areas, such as electronics, drafting, and mechanics.

The occupational therapist and the home-planning consultant collaborate to plan home and office modifications for the spinal-cord-injured patient and others who may need a special setup.

CVA patients and brain-damaged patients are given the prevocational screening test before referral for a full OT evaluation. (Fig. 5-23). This test was developed to determine a baseline work competency level. These patients are then evaluated to determine their ability to return to their former jobs or to less demanding vocations.

Patients from the pediatric service are referred to the prevocational area by the vocational counselor to assist with high school curriculum planning. Disabilities in patients from this service include spinal cord injuries, spina bifida, cerebral palsy, and other congenital and acquired disabilities. The assessment tools are geared to the teenaged population and include academic testing.

*Case Study 1**

PREVOCATIONAL EVALUATION

Mr. C., a 30-year-old C5 quadriplegic, attended the prevocational area one hour a day from June 20 to October 8, 1984. Injured in a truck accident last winter, Mr. C. is realistic about his vocational future. He can no longer be a truck driver and hopes, instead, to open a small sporting goods business, which would be popular in his hometown in upstate New York.

Initially, Mr. C. was dependent on bilateral balanced forearm orthoses for activity. As endurance and strength improved, he could type and write without them, using dorsal wrist extension splints and vertical holders.

Equipment needs and basic store planning became the responsibility of the prevocational and home-planning services. Table heights, accessible display cases, and convenient placement of all necessary equipment were taken into consideration. The evaluation of a suitable cash register (cash box) and printing calculator as well as other necessary equipment needs was accomplished. Prices were submitted to the insurance company.

Mr. C. was conscientious and well motivated throughout the evaluation, often finding solutions to problems on his own, given the basic equipment.

*This case study was prepared by Dorothy Milner, OTR, Institute of Rehabilitation Medicine, New York, New York.

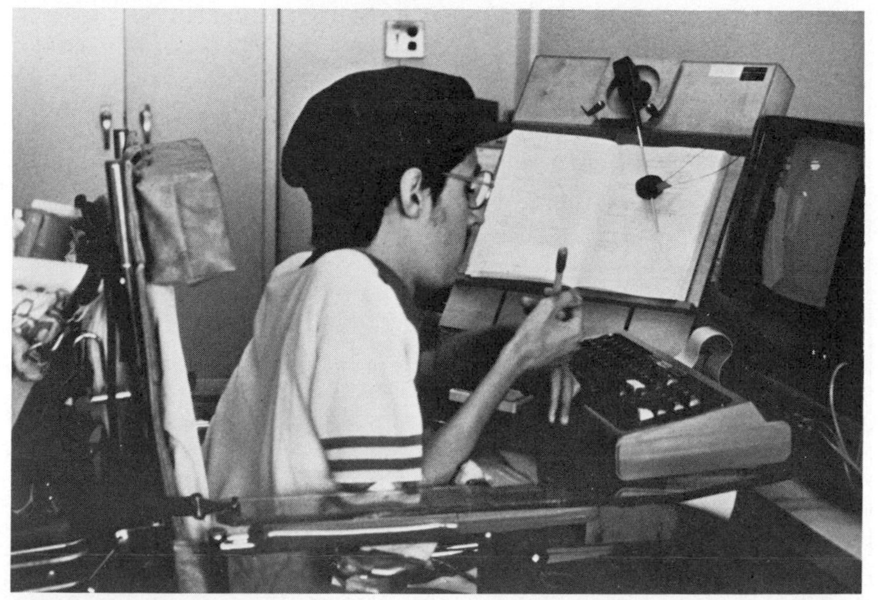

A

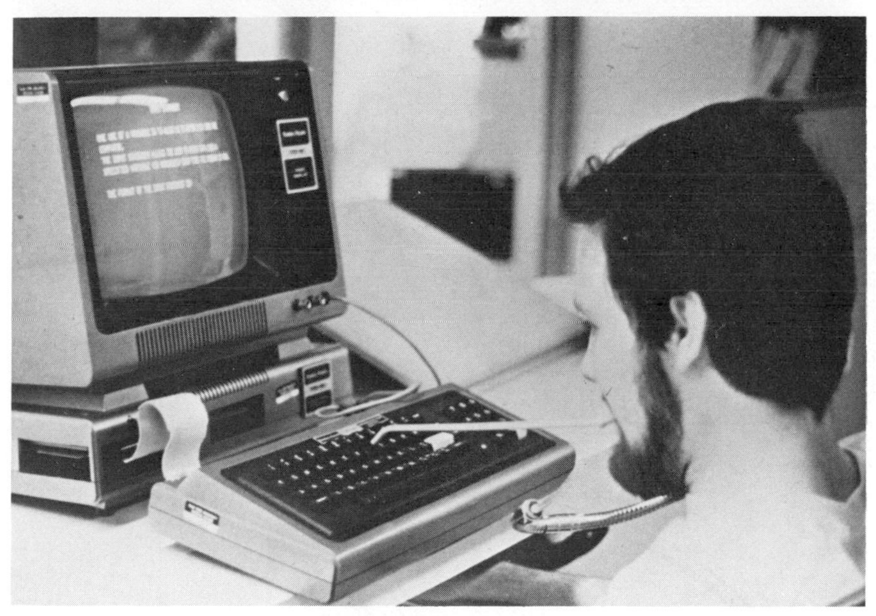

B

*Fig. 5-21. A. Muscular dystrophy quadriplegic using chin mouthstick in his fingers with the computer and an electronic page turner. B. C3 quadriplegic using microcomputer with mouthstick.*

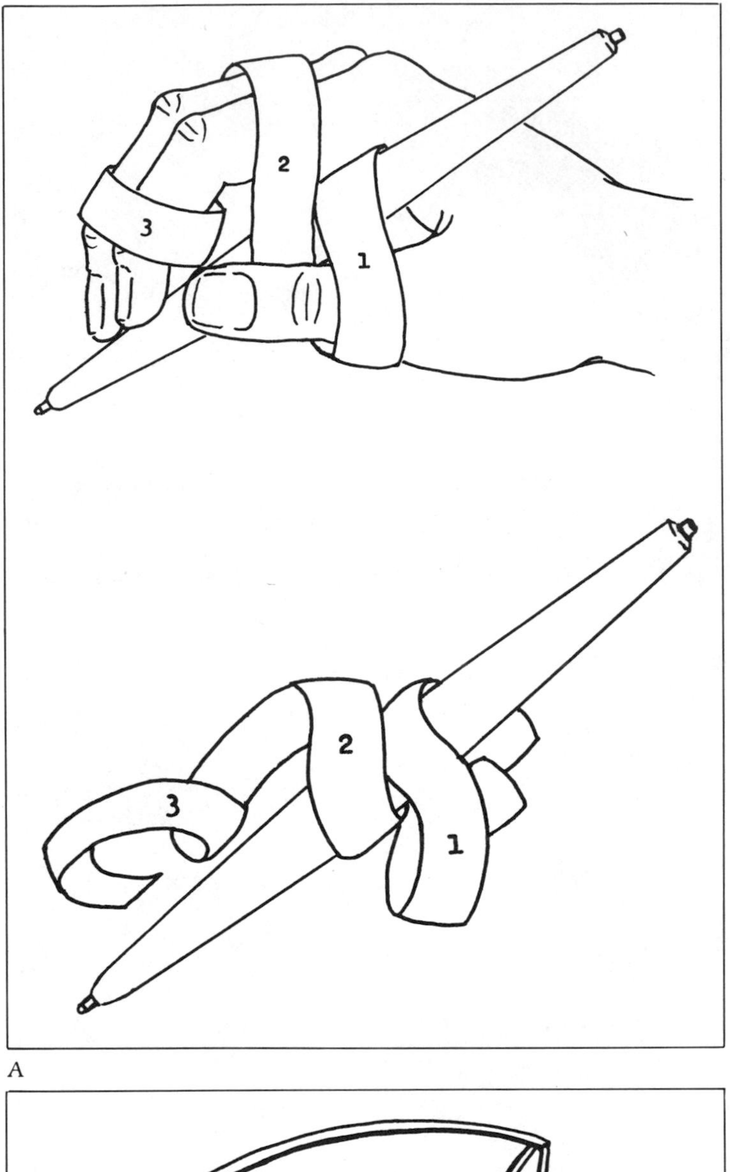


A

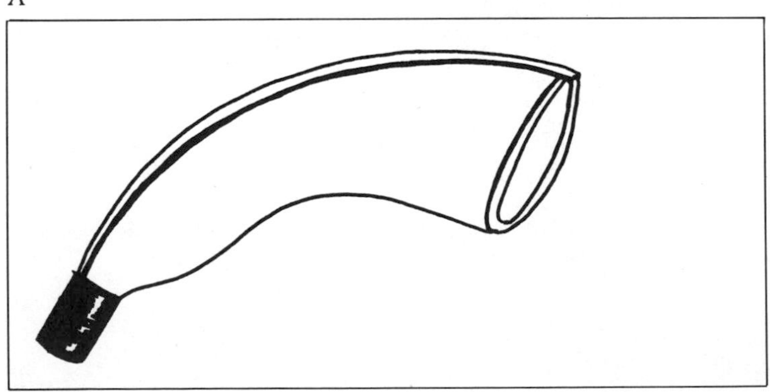

B

*Fig. 5-22. Devices developed for quadriplegics by Dorothy Milner, OTR. A: Finger loop writing device, made out of any low-temperature plastic material. B: Typing finger, made from any low-temperature plastic material.*

*Fig. 5-23. Prevocational screening test used at the Institute of Rehabilitation Medicine. (Used with permission.)*

1. 74 + 83   35 + 78   $10.00 − 8.57   8 × 17 =   5 × 11 =   24 ÷ 12 =   150 ÷ 15 =

2. A store purchased 450 balloons for $67.50 and sold them for 20¢ each. What was their profit?

3. Number the names in alphabetical order: Matthew Gold
   Susan Goodman
   Jennifer Jacobs
   Mary Jones
   Louise Dunn

4. If you bought a hamburger for 89¢, how much change would you receive from $1.00?

5. Write the telephone extension listed for Dr. Rusk using the Medical Center Directory.

Some of the items below are circled, some are underlined, some have boxes around them, and others have checkmarks or initials behind them. You are to find each item that is underlined or has initials after it. Put an X through these items with your pen.

| | | |
|---|---|---|
| Jon Jacobs✓ | OT | Gold |
| September | Camping | Statue of Liberty |
| Stoneham Zoo KJ | Lacla | Geranium |
| Four | February MG | Time |
| Boston University | Art | OTR |
| Logan Airport | Washington | Canary LG |
| Kentucky KG | Carpentry | Photography✓ |
| June 21 LD | Dr. | Work |
| Flowers | G. Green | Lisa Grace |
| JPSA | Computer✓ | Television |

*Time:* ________________

________________

continued

If the two dollar amounts are the same, circle the S (for same). If they are different, circle the D (for different).

| | | | | |
|---|---|---|---|---|
| 1. | $43.99 | $43.99 | S | D |
| 2. | $27.02 | $27.02 | S | D |
| 3. | $83.62 | $93.62 | S | D |
| 4. | $4875.73 | $4885.73 | S | D |
| 5. | $43.70 | $43.70 | S | D |
| 6. | $5297.09 | $5927.09 | S | D |
| 7. | $379.58 | $36.68 | S | D |
| 8. | $23.29 | $23.39 | S | D |
| 9. | $906.06 | $906.06 | S | D |
| 10. | $90.20 | $70.02 | S | D |
| 11. | $6395.58 | $6396.58 | S | D |
| 12. | $73.82 | $37.82 | S | D |
| 13. | $57.03 | $57.03 | S | D |
| 14. | $573.29 | $572.29 | S | D |
| 15. | $9206.72 | $9206.72 | S | D |
| 16. | $345892.01 | $345892.01 | S | D |
| 17. | $6540095.00 | $6540095.00 | S | D |
| 18. | $6910103. | $6910103. | S | D |
| 19. | $6430325.99 | $6403325.99 | S | D |
| 20. | $97934.78 | $97934.78 | S | D |

Time: ___________

Fig. 5-23 (continued)

Please complete the application form at the bottom of the page using the information in the following letter:

25 Johnson Drive
Northborough, MA 01867
January 1, 1985

McDonald's
111 Needham Street
Newton, MA

Dear Sir:

I am interested in applying for a position as a cashier at your store. I am 18 years old, single, and a high school graduate. I worked as a cashier at a summer camp for two months during the summer of 1984, and enjoyed the work very much.

I would appreciate your sending me an application form.

Sincerely,

Erica Osborn

Erica Osborn

APPLICATION

Name of applicant ______________________________

Address ______________________________
(street number) (street) (city) (state)

Telephone ____________________

Age ____________________ Height ________ Weight ________

Marital status ____________

Date of application ____________

Previous experience ______________________________

______________________________

Time: ____________

Fig. 5-23 (continued)

Answer the following questions using the sample check and stub below:

1. What day was the check written? ______
2. What is the amount of the check? ______
3. To whom is the money being paid? ______
4. Whose account will the money come from? ______
5. Where is the bank located? ______
6. What is the number of the account? ______
7. What is the number of this check? ______
8. What is the balance in this account after the check is paid? ______

NO. 604 $ 275
March 5 19 85
PAY TO Learning Prep School
FOR

| | DOLLARS | CENTS |
|---|---|---|
| BAL. BRO'T. FOR'D. | 500 | — |
| (ADD DEPOSITS OR SUBTRACT ANY CHARGES.) | | |
| | | |
| NEW BALANCE | 500 | — |
| AM'T. THIS CHECK | 275 | |
| BAL. CAR'D. FOR'D. | | |

604

March 5 19 85 53-164/113

PAY TO THE ORDER OF Learning Prep School $ 275. 00/100

two hundred and seventy five — 00/100 DOLLARS

BayBank | Merrimack Valley
BayBank Merrimack Valley, N.A.
Massachusetts

FOR

Karen Jacobs

0604

continued

*Case Study 2**

PREVOCATIONAL EVALUATION

Mr. J. a 49-year-old right hemiplegic with severe receptive-expressive aphasia, initially attended the prevocational area on May 8, 1984. Having suffered a CVA three years ago, he came to the institute primarily for vocational services. Attendance is regular, three days a week for one-hour sessions. As a former plumber's assistant, he has followed a program in the following areas: (1) recognition of word similarities, matching; (2) simple arithmetic skills such as making change; and (3) evaluation of one-handed skills, including assembly tasks, carpentry, electronic wiring, and use of hand tools.

Mr. J.'s right upper extremity is nonfunctional. He walks with a cane and is independent in self-care activities. He can follow only demonstrated instructions and imitates models for copying.

Mr. J's aphasia has affected his calculation ability. He can add two digits; however, his speed is nonfunctional, and his answers are not consistently correct. Subtraction, multiplication, and division are impossible for him. He cannot make monetary change.

*This case study was provided by Dorothy Milner, OTR, Institute of Rehabilitation Medicine, New York, New York.

Compare the two checks to each other. They should be identical. Circle any differences you find on the bottom check:

account number
048 0 087829
No. 113
53-117
113
March 1 19 85
PAY TO THE ORDER OF Learning Prep School $ 65. 30/100
sixty five 30/100 DOLLARS
Arlington Trust company
Lawrence
Massachusetts
Karen Jacobs
⑆011301170⑆

account number
048 0 087829
No. 113
53-117
113
March 1 19 85
PAY TO THE ORDER OF $ 65. 30/100
sixty five 30/100 DOLLARS
Arlington Trust company
Lawrence
Massachusetts
Karen Jacobs
⑆011301170⑆

continued

Mr. J. can match names, a functional skill for a job in mail sorting. His speed is slow but should improve with continued practice.

One-handed hand skills are good. He has excellent dexterity with his nondominant left hand. Specific hand skill testing results are as follows:

1. Hand tool dexterity test (use of pliers, wrench, screwdriver): slow speed but demonstrates good use of tools
2. Doorlock (TOWER): average speed with one hand; no errors
3. Plug jack assembly (TOWER): use of putty as a stabilizer; average speed with one hand; no errors
4. Washers and pins (TOWER): some difficulty noted closing pin with ten washers on it
5. Nuts and bolts: Theraplast as stabilizer; fair speed with one hand

6. Electronic wiring: good dexterity noted; has difficulty reading schematics for color of wire needed; learning ability good after repetition
7. Small carpentry assembly: unable to use hammer and nails without maximum assistance

Mr. J.'s drafting skills are limited to copying simple forms and shapes. He measures accurately and draws neatly; however, his aphasia affecting reading and arithmetic preclude further training in this area.

In summary, Mr. J. displays good hand skills and a potential for learning new and unfamiliar tasks. Speed improves with repetition and increased familiarity with the required job. He cannot read or write, but he can follow demonstrated one-step-at-a-time instructions.

*Case Study 3**

PREVOCATIONAL EVALUATION

Mr. D., a 50-year-old right-dominant right hemiplegic, was evaluated in the prevocational area from January 23 to April 2, 1984. After his CVA in December 1983, he contracted meningitis, which left him deaf bilaterally. Before his illness Mr. D. had worked as an electronics maintenance engineer with a major broadcasting company. He is considered an expert in the field of cathode-ray oscilloscopes, and his employers offered their assistance with the evaluation, eager to have him return after his rehabilitation program.

Mr. D.'s primary concern initially was dominance retraining, that is, left-handed writing. He learned the basic techniques easily and practices on his own. He exhibited exceptional coordination with his left hand during various assembly tasks and learned one-handed stabilization techniques without difficulty.

Mr. D. was evaluated in basic electronics, building a small Heathkit radio. He proved that he can solder safely with one hand and managed the small parts and wiring involved with amazing facility. He had no problems in reading both written and schematic instructions. Final tuning of the radio was impossible for him because of his hearing loss.

At this stage of the evaluation, his employers were asked to assist us. They delivered malfunctioning oscilloscopes for Mr. D. to repair. Mr. D. proceeded with this task eagerly and performed as well as expected.

Because of Mr. D.'s loss of hearing, certain communication problems relating to his job were anticipated, as were the functional limitations caused by his CVA. Mr. D. will never be able to walk; he must use a wheelchair. He is independent performing his job tasks, except for reaching and lifting heavy objects. His employers agreed to a three-month probationary period of employment, with final decision as to his being rehired to be made after that time.

## Centers for Work Capacity Evaluation

Work capacity evaluation (WCE), developed over the last several years at Ranchos Los Amigos Hospital, Casa Colina Hospital for Rehabilitative Medicine, and Downey Community Hospital, is a new area of specialization within occupational therapy that is gaining national attention. More comprehensive than the traditional vocational evaluation offered by occupational therapists and vocational evaluators, it has the principal distinction of focus on the active development of the patient-worker's potential rather than the current

*This case study was provided by Dorothy Milner, OTR, Institute of Rehabilitation Medicine, New York, New York.

functioning assessed in the traditional static model. Briefly defined, WCE is a comprehensive process which focuses upon the measurement and development of the evaluees' potential for work. It includes evaluation of feasibility for employment, physical and emotional work tolerances, and assessment of aptitudes, temperament, and vocational interests. It is more than an evaluation process in that it often provides services that are intended to improve the evaluee's potential. These services are generally termed "work hardening." [23]

WCE "goes beyond the evaluation of the patient's current work tolerance to the prediction of the patient's potential in these areas" [23]. It is an aggressive approach to rehabilitation" in that it expects and promotes improvement in patient function over a relatively short period of time" [23].

Work tolerance screening (WTS) is the primary evaluation component of WCE.

> As an intensive evaluation of an individual's ability to sustain work performance, Work Tolerance Screening can be offered as a stand-alone evaluation service or integrated into a comprehensive Work Capacity Evaluation program. Work Tolerance Screening measures work performance factors that are more basic to work *output* than factors such as work skills, aptitudes, or interests. While information about these latter factors is certainly useful in predicting the ability of a person to sustain work output, they are clearly secondary in importance to factors such as the individual's ability to lift and carry objects, sit or stand for prolonged periods, or work with hand tools on an ongoing basis.
>
> Work Tolerance Screening as a stand-alone service is a one-hour to three-hour evaluation in which selected critical demands of work are simulated in a controlled setting. This work simulation allows the evaluee to demonstrate his or her own unique response to these work demands. The availability of this information can be of great benefit to the evaluee and to the professional with whom he or she is working in the development of an appropriate vocational goal. It can help determine whether he or she can return to the usual and customary occupation or perform the work demands of a new job that is being considered [24].

The information presented thus far on WCE and WTS is but an overview of this area of specialization. I refer you to texts by Leonard N. Matheson [23] and by Matheson and Linda Dempster Ogden [24] for in-depth discussions.

The following three examples of occupational therapy programs utilizing CE will facilitate a better understanding of this new area. The first is a program at Downey Community Hospital, one of the centers that helped to develop the evaluation. The next two centers use the evaluation in private practice specializing in hand rehabilitation: Hand Therapy and Rehabilitation Associates, and Hand Rehabilitation Specialists.

## DOWNEY COMMUNITY HOSPITAL*

Downey Community Hospital is a 171-bed non-profit hospital located near major industry in the greater metropolitan area of Los Angeles. The Downey

*Most of the section on Downey Community Hospital was written by Karen S. Schultz, M. S., OTR.

Hand Center has existed since 1974 and is part of the rehabilitation services provided by the hospital. In 1979 it was found that a gap existed between the optimal level of function a patient could achieve in the hand clinic setting and the level of function required to return successfully to work. Using a model found successful at Rancho Los Amigos Hospital, occupational therapists Kay Golgi and Lois Barber, L. N. Matheson, and physician Garry Brody, together with the hospital administration, collaborated on the planning and implementation of a work hardening unit to fill this void in rehabilitation services. The program has gained an outstanding reputation and consistently receives referrals from physicians, therapists, insurance companies, and vocational counselors. While upper-extremity rehabilitation is a specialty, the work hardening center has expanded to serve a wide variety of diagnostic groups including back-injured and head trauma patients.

The Downey Community Hospital Work Hardening Center provides a program of maximal reconditioning before return to work or to optimal occupational role. Rather than exercise, graded work samples such as shoveling gravel or assembling nut and bolt units are used in three-to-six hour treatment sessions (Fig. 5-24). The therapists can simulate a specific task or job and evaluate a client's specific activity tolerance (Fig. 5-25). The information regarding a client's work tolerance can then be shared with the physician, the client, the vocational counselor, and the employer.

The principal goal of work hardening is to return a person who has experienced a decrease in function to his or her previous occupation or to an optimal occupation if the residual level of dysfunction precludes return to usual and customary work. In support of this global goal are several subgoals:

1. To provide optimal physical reconditioning for work (maximize range of motion, strength, stability, endurance)
2. To increase the client's confidence in his or her ability to return to work or to productive activity
3. To identify problems that may require adaptation of a goal occupation or may alter the choice of goal occupation
4. To maintain or reintroduce the worker role to the client
5. To provide optimal psychosocial and cognitive reconditioning before return to productive activity

Clients who require a program with the above-stated goals are appropriate candidates for work hardening. On admission to the program each client receives a thorough intake evaluation including a physical status evaluation (range of motion, strength, sensibility), a functional tolerance evaluation, and a review of future job or activity demands at either the usual and customary work or at a new vocation (Fig. 5-26). The program is geared to bring a client from his or her current level of function to a level that will permit gainful employment or purposeful activity. When a client reaches this level of function, discharge is recommended and a report is provided to the client and to his or her physician. A client may be discharged if he or she is unable to use the facility appropriately. A client is also recommended for discharge when a plateau is reached and no further gains are made in a one-to two-week period.

Bridging the gap between medical rehabilitation and vocational rehabilitation, the occupational therapist makes a unique contribution. He or she can evaluate the client for specific parameters of physical functioning and can perform an activity analysis of the client's goal task or job. With this information, the therapist can design a graded work hardening program of work simulation to increase the client's ability to perform critical tasks. The ability to identify specific skills and then translate these skills into functionally relevant—and therefore vocationally relevent—information is key to returning an injured person to his or her optimal occupational role.

*Case Study**

George, a 23-year-old right-dominant man, was employed as a telephone cable splicer at the time of his injury. On May 25, 1983, he fell 28 feet from a ladder and sustained a fracture-dislocation of his right elbow and multiple fractures of his right wrist as well as other orthopedic injuries to his lower extremities. He underwent open reduction and internal fixation (ORIF) of his right elbow and right wrist.

George began a hand therapy program 4½ months after his injury, after prolonged immobilization in various casts. At six months after injury he was evaluated for the work hardening program. At this time his grip strength had plateaued at 40 pounds, and his maximum active and passive wrist extension was 20 degrees. George was unable to grip forcefully with his fingers and simultaneously maintain wrist extension; his wrist collapsed into flexion. A program of work samples including woodworking, block wall assembly, pipe tree assembly, and a simulated cable-splicing activity was initiated in conjunction with progressive wrist splinting and aggressive resistive exercise of the entire upper extremity, with emphasis on the wrist extensors. It was noted that the wrist extensors were caught in scar at the ORIF site at the wrist and thus could not achieve their optimal excursion. A program of vibration and vigorous massage of the scar was added. George was discharged to return to work on January 25, 1984, after two months of work hardening. His grip strength was 58 pounds; his active wrist extension, 45 degrees. He was able to demonstrate good hand balance when forcefully gripping and could maintain wrist extension with strong finger flexion. The client was confident of his ability to return to his usual and customary work. In his program he had lifted and carried objects similar in size and weight to those used in his previous job. He had also used tools that required the same types of grip and pinch required in his usual and customary work. George resumed work as a cable splicer for the telephone company.

## HAND THERAPY AND REHABILITATION ASSOCIATES†

Hand Therapy and Rehabilitation Associates was founded in 1976 in Los Gatos, California, by Thelma Wellerson Hook. It comprises two divisions: the hand service (the original practice) and a newly established vocational division, the work evaluation unit.

*This case study was provided by Karen S. Schultz, M. S. OTR, Downey Community Hospital, Downey, California.

†The information presented on Hand Therapy and Rehabilitation Associates was written by Thelma Wellerson Hook, M.A., OTR.

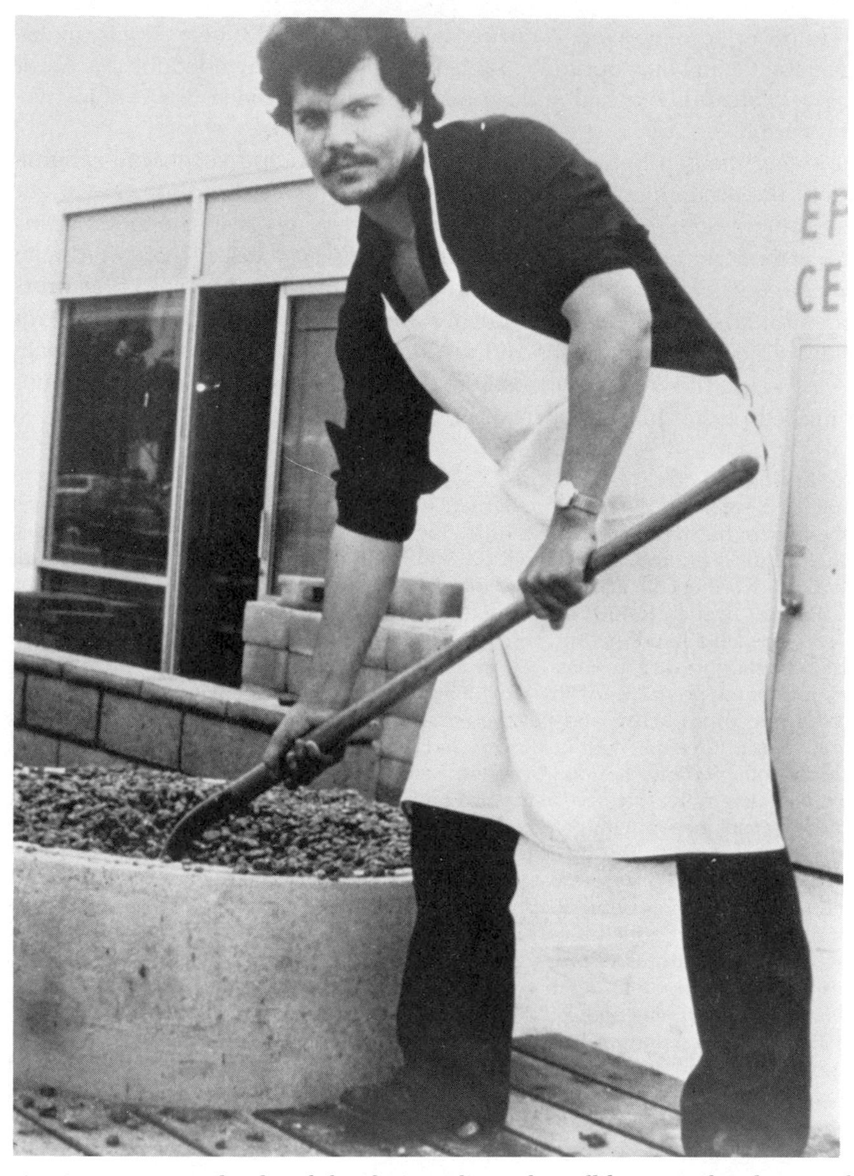

*Fig. 5-24. An example of work hardening. Client who will be using shovel in usual and customary work as a mold maker builds tolerance for this task by shoveling gravel. (Courtesy of Karen S. Schultz, M.S., OTR.)*

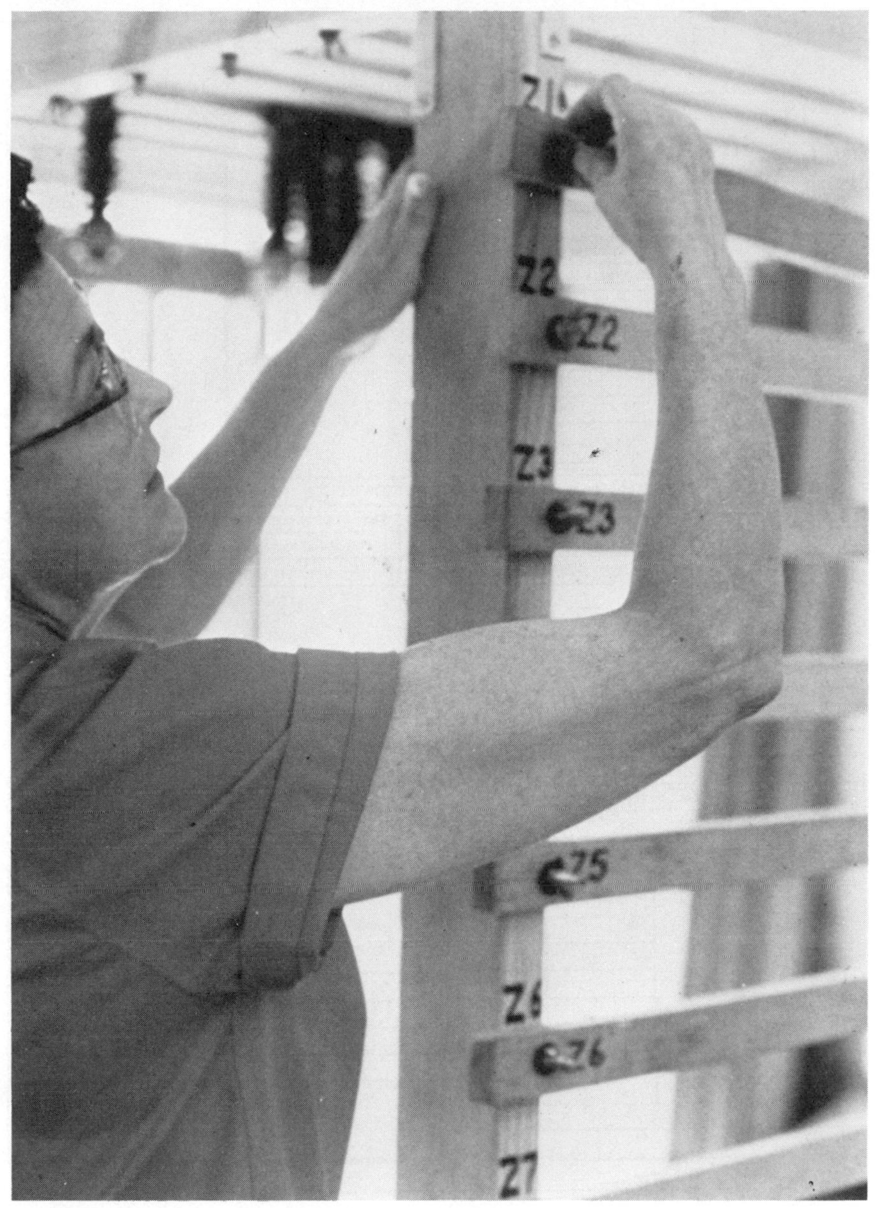


*Fig. 5-25. Client performs work sample that evaluates the ability to manipulate objects at various planes of the body. (Courtesy of Karen S. Schultz, M.S., OTR.)*

WORK HARDENING

WORK CAPACITY EVALUATION

UPPER EXTREMITY

DOMINANCE L R
INVOLVED L R

EVALUATOR
DATE

| / | RANGE OF MOTION |
|---|---|
| | Joint exam attached |
| | Significant limitations present |
| | L R Limitations: Scapula |
| | L R Limitations: Shoulder/Arm |
| | L R Limitations: Elbow/Forearm |
| | L R Limitations: Wrist |
| | L R Limitations: Fingers |
| | L R Limitations: Thumb |

FINGER PADS FROM PALMAR CREASE: if touch use +

L I____cm M____cm R____cm L____cm
R I____cm M____cm R____cm L____cm

FINGER TOUCH PALM: if touch, use+, if not use

L I____cm M____cm R____cm L____cm
R I____cm M____cm R____cm L____cm

DISTANCE THUMB TIP FROM FINGER PADS:

L I____cm M____cm R____cm L____cm
R I____cm M____cm R____cm L____cm

DISTANCE THUMB TIP FROM HEAD OF 5th MC

L____cm R____cm

| ✓ | STRENGTH/ENDURANCE |
|---|---|
| | Muscle exam attached |
| | L R Limitations: Muscle Strength |
| | L R Limitations: Endurance |
| | L R Cocontraction |

| GRIP (JAMAR), (lb) | | LEFT | RIGHT |
|---|---|---|---|
| I = Narrowest<br>Comments: | I | | |
| | II | | |
| | III | | |
| | IV | | |
| | V | | |
| PALMAR PINCH (lb) | | | |
| LATERAL PINCH (lb) | | | |
| F/A Circumference | | | |
| Hand Volume | | | |

L R

SENSIBILITY

AMPUTATED ■ IMPAIRED ⁙ ABSENT ▨

| | |
|---|---|
| | Detailed exam attached |
| | L R Limitations: Functional Sensibility |
| | L R Limitations: Protective Sensibility |
| | L R Paresthesias (Describe): |
| | L R Limitations: Stereognosis |
| | L R Limitations: Proprioception |
| ✓ | OBJECTIVE SENSIBILITY |
| | L R Limitations: Color |
| | L R Limitations: Turgor |
| | L R Limitations: Rugal Folds |
| | L R Limitations: Skin Temperature |
| | L R Limitations: Sweat |
| ✓ | SUBJECTIVE SENSIBILITY |
| | L R Limitations: Sharp/Dull |
| | L R Limitations: Light Touch |
| | L R Limitations: Texture |
| | L R Limitations: Temperature |

PATIENT

*Fig. 5-26. Forms used in upper-extremity work capacity evaluation at Downey Community Hospital. (MP = metacarpophalangeal; PIP = finger proximal interphalangeal; DIP = finger distal interphalangeal; IP = interphalangeal.)*

UPPER EXTREMITY EVALUATION

INITIAL________ FINAL________

TESTER________________

CLIENTS NAME________________________ DATE________________

INVOLVED R L — ACTIVE RANGE OF MOTION — DOMINANT R L

LEFT SIDE

| SHOULDER | INVOLVED | NORMAL |
|---|---|---|
| FLEXION | | 0-180 |
| ABDUCTION | | 0-180 |
| INT. ROT. | | 0-80 |
| EXTERN. ROT. | | 0-60 |

| ELBOW | INVOLVED | NORMAL |
|---|---|---|
| FLEXION | | 0-150 |
| EXTENSION | | 150-0 |
| PRONATION | | 0-80 |
| SUPINATION | | 0-80 |

| WRIST | INVOLVED | NORMAL |
|---|---|---|
| FLEXION | | 0-70 |
| EXTENSION | | 0-60 |
| ULNAR DEV. | | 0-30 |
| RADIAL DEV. | | 0-20 |

| FINGER | MP | PIP | DIP |
|---|---|---|---|
| NORMAL | 0-90 | 0-100 | 0-70 |
| INDEX | | | |
| MIDDLE | | | |
| RING | | | |
| LITTLE | | | |

| THUMB | | |
|---|---|---|
| MP | | |
| IP | | |
| CM ABD. | | |
| CM ADD. | | |

| MANUAL MUSCLE TEST |
|---|
| |
| |
| |
| |
| |

RIGHT SIDE

| SHOULDER | INVOLVED | NORMAL |
|---|---|---|
| FLEXION | | 0-180 |
| ABDUCTION | | 0-180 |
| INT. ROT. | | 0-80 |
| EXTERN. ROT. | | 0-60 |

| ELBOW | INVOLVED | NORMAL |
|---|---|---|
| FLEXION | | 0-150 |
| EXTENSION | | 150-0 |
| PRONATION | | 0-80 |
| SUPINATION | | 0-80 |

| WRIST | INVOLVED | NORMAL |
|---|---|---|
| FLEXION | | 0-70 |
| EXTENSION | | 0-60 |
| ULNAR DEV. | | 0-30 |
| RADIAL DEV. | | 0-20 |

| FINGER | MP | PIP | DIP |
|---|---|---|---|
| NORMAL | 0-90 | 0-100 | 0-70 |
| INDEX | | | |
| MIDDLE | | | |
| RING | | | |
| LITTLE | | | |

| THUMB | | |
|---|---|---|
| MP | | |
| IP | | |
| CM ABD. | | |
| CM ADD. | | |

| MANUAL MUSCLE TEST |
|---|
| |
| |
| |
| |
| |

Fig. 5-26 (continued)

*Hand Service*

The hand service is a private, medically oriented hand therapy and rehabilitation practice that serves private, industrial, and hospital-based physicians in northern California. Its offices are located in an urban area in Santa Clara County, a location central to hand surgeons, orthopedic surgeons, plastic surgeons, rheumatologists, and other practicing physicians in northern California.

The sole purpose of this medically prescribed treatment program is to treat industrial and private patients with traumatic hand injuries and hand dysfunctions. The program is designed to assess the special needs of each patient. An individualized therapeutic program is prescribed by the referring physician. Each member of the staff is committed to returning the patient to his occupation and accustomed life-style as soon as medically feasible.

The hand service program includes continuous intensive hand evaluations and tests. Some examples of the specialized therapeutic programs are (1) reduction of edema, (2) scar care, (3) therapeutic exercises, (4) custom fabrication of dynamic or static splints, (5) prosthetic evaluation and training programs for upper-extremity amputees, (6) joint protection techniques, (7) activities of daily living, and (8) physical evaluation abilities or on-the-job assessment. All of these programs assist the physician in restoring the injured hand to functional capacity and in determining the patient's readiness to return to work.

*Work Evaluation Unit*

As an adjunct to the highly successful hand therapy division, a separate vocational division was established in November 1982. This work evaluation unit is a private practice, non-medically-oriented office. It serves industrial, government, and private rehabilitation counselors, consultants, claims adjustors, nurses, self-insured company administrators, casualty adjustors, applicants' attorneys, benefits managers, and corporate industry in northern California.

The work evaluation unit is located near the hand therapy division in an urban area adjacent to the high-technology industry of the Santa Clara Valley.

The primary purpose of the work evaluation unit is to assess traumatic hand injuries and hand dysfunctions of industrial and private clients, whose injuries may or may not be classified as permanent and stationary. The program is designed to provide information to the referring agent, and to the client, on the client's physical ability to meet specific job requirements and occupational goals. A comprehensive written report with specific recommendations is given to the referring agent. The work evaluation unit increases the client's motivation to work and assists in his or her rapid return to employment, which results in reduced corporate costs.

Staffed by therapists with training in occupational therapy, guidance, and personnel work as well as in hand therapy and vocational rehabilitation, the work evaluation unit offers the following programs and services: work tolerance screening, work capacity evaluation, work hardening, job analysis, on-the-job assessment, job site modification, and corporate consultation.

*Work tolerance screening* takes from two to four hours, and the ratio of supervision is one to one. The screening assesses the client's hand and extremity physical abilities by measuring range of motion, muscle strength, grip strength, pinch strength, edema, tolerance to hot and cold, and sensation limitations. In addition there is a limited appraisal of the client's physical ability to use the injured hand and upper extremity on a minimum number of nonspecific job samples and tests. These require fine and gross manipulation of tools and equipment and hand and arm range of motion under load.

*Work capacity evaluation* is an individualized planned program lasting one to seven six-hour days. The ratio of supervision is one to four clients. The evaluation assesses the client's hand and upper extremity physical abilities, as described under Work Tolerance Screening, with the additional goal of an in-depth appraisal of the client's ability to use the injured hand and upper extremity at work. Numerous systems are used to make this assessment. These include standardized evaluations such as (1) the Wide Range Achievement Test, (2) the Raven Progress Matrices, (3) the Gates-McKillop-Horowitz Reading Diagnostic Test, (4) Work Evaluation Systems Technology (WEST), (5) the Purdue Pegboard, and (6) the Minnesota Rate of Manipulation Test; standardized such as the TOWER system or work samples especially developed to simulate jobs indigenous to the Santa Clara Valley industrial area; and situational assessment, exemplified by observation of the client's performance on the job for a limited time. The goal is to observe the client using the injured hand and arm in a realistic work situation. The job situation is chosen on the basis of a client's real, or perceived, occupational goal.

*Work hardening* is an individualized physical conditioning and training program in half-day sessions lasting for a period of two weeks. The ratio of supervision is one to six clients. The purpose of work hardening is to build up the physical ability to meet the demands of the work day. The modalities are work tasks. The tasks, amount of work time, and resistance are graded throughout the duration of the program.

*Job analysis* is a systematic description of the work performed by the client before or after injury. The goal of this assessment is to aid the referring agent in understanding the job skills that are required of the injured employee. This analysis is provided on an hourly basis.

*On-the-job assessment* evaluates a client's work endurance, stamina, tolerance to pain, and physical performance on a given job. The objective of this service is to observe the client at work, analyze the actions required of the client's injured hand or arm, and analyze the client's physical ability to perform those actions within the context of industrial performance and standards. The assessment, provided on an hourly basis, includes recommendations for placement in a specific job and consideration of physical limitations in job placement.

*Job site modification* is a service that anlyzes the job, the client, and the place of work. The objective of this service, which is also provided on an hourly basis, is to determine what changes in the job, client, and work place will enable the worker to perform the job satisfactorily. The analysis includes recommendations for either client or job site modification. Such recommendations may include use of ergonomic principles, fabrication of adaptive equipment designed especially for the individual client, instruction for the client in compensatory body mechanics, and modification of job skills and equipment that will enable the client to meet industrial standards.

*Corporate consultation* is available to industry on a company-wide basis. The goal of this service is to aid in the prevention of on-the-job injuries to the employees' hands and upper extremities. Through evaluation of jobs and recommendations for changes, corporate costs can be reduced.

### *Case Study 1**

Diagnosis 1. Primary diagnosis is not available from medical histories
2. Frozen shoulder, right
3. Flexion contracture, right elbow
4. Causalgia, right upper extremity

Surgery 1. Manipulation of right shoulder and elbow August 17, 1983
2. Stellate blocks (medical history available reports three)

Date of Injury: August 7, 1979
Date Last Worked: 1980
Occupation: Machine operator, pill packaging

Date of attendance: December 9, 1983

#### OBJECTIVES OF REFERRAL

The client was referred for a half-day work tolerance screening with the following objectives:

1. To determine physical ability of right arm and hand
2. To determine physical ability of right arm and hand in performance of former job
3. To determine physical ability of right arm and hand in clerical work

#### PAIN

The client reported pain in right middle, ring, and little fingers and numbness in all three digits. The client stated that the numbness is constant.

The client also complained of pain and burning from the right neck area through the right shoulder blade and down the right arm. This occurs when the neck is flexed approximately 10 degrees after working for approximately 50 minutes.

#### SENSATION

Two-point discrimination testing shows normal sensibility in all digits (Fig. 5-27). EMG report was not available to evaluator.

#### EDEMA

The water displacement test for measurement of swelling in the right hand had the following results: right, 345 ml of water displacement; left, 310 ml.

#### RANGE OF MOTION

Dominant right hand; injury on right. There is loss of range of motion in the right shoulder (Fig. 5-28) as compared to the left:

* This case study was provided by Thelma Wellerson Hook, M.A., OTR, Hand Therapy and Rehabilitation Associates, Los Gatos, California.

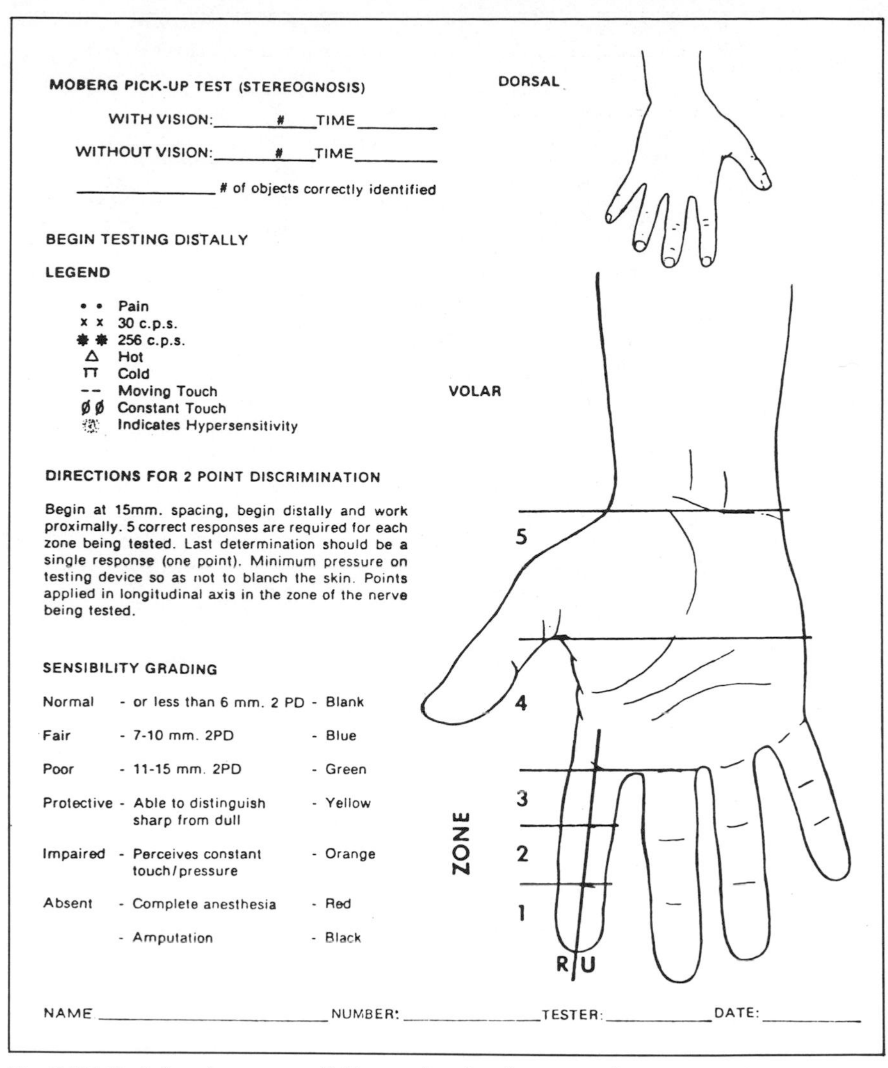

MOBERG PICK-UP TEST (STEREOGNOSIS)

WITH VISION:________#____TIME________

WITHOUT VISION:________#____TIME________

____________ # of objects correctly identified

BEGIN TESTING DISTALLY

LEGEND

- • • Pain
- x x 30 c.p.s.
- ✱ ✱ 256 c.p.s.
- Δ Hot
- ΠΤ Cold
- -- Moving Touch
- Ø Ø Constant Touch
- ⁂ Indicates Hypersensitivity

DIRECTIONS FOR 2 POINT DISCRIMINATION

Begin at 15mm. spacing, begin distally and work proximally. 5 correct responses are required for each zone being tested. Last determination should be a single response (one point). Minimum pressure on testing device so as not to blanch the skin. Points applied in longitudinal axis in the zone of the nerve being tested.

SENSIBILITY GRADING

| | | |
|---|---|---|
| Normal | - or less than 6 mm. 2 PD | - Blank |
| Fair | - 7-10 mm. 2PD | - Blue |
| Poor | - 11-15 mm. 2PD | - Green |
| Protective | - Able to distinguish sharp from dull | - Yellow |
| Impaired | - Perceives constant touch/pressure | - Orange |
| Absent | - Complete anesthesia | - Red |
| | - Amputation | - Black |



NAME____________ NUMBER:____________ TESTER:____________ DATE:____________

*Fig. 5-27. Peripheral nerve sensibility evaluation (cps = cycles per second; 2PD = two-point discrimination).*

| | |
|---|---|
| Abduction (away from the body to the right) | – 10 degrees |
| Flexion (away from the body forward) | – 40 degrees |
| Extension (away from the body behind) | – 10 degrees |
| Internal rotation (hand to middle back) | – 11 degrees |
| External rotation (hand behind neck) | – 55 degrees |

There is loss of range of motion in the right elbow extension as compared to the left:

| | |
|---|---|
| Extension (straighten elbow all the way) | – 30 degrees |
| Flexion (hand to shoulder) | Normal |

NAME ______ No. ______ ( Right Major)

Circ. (inches) Biceps ___ / ___ Wrist ___ / ___

Forearm ___ / ___ Hand ___ / ___

MOTIONS: Report as a fraction (injured/uninjured) in degrees of Active Motion

| Shoulder: | | Forearm | |
|---|---|---|---|
| Abd. | 70/90 / | Pron. | / |
| Flex. | 0-140/0-180 / | Sup. | / |
| I R. | 34/45 / | | |
| E R. | 35/90 / | Wrist DF | 65 / 75 |
| Ext. | 50/60 / | PF | 73 / 73 |
| Add. | / | RD | 25 / 30 |
| | | UD | 30 / 40 |

Elbow: Ext. 140/180 /

Flex. 60/60 /

Thumb: (ABD. 50 / 56 (degrees)

(ADD. Tip misses head of 5th MC. ___ / ___ inch

Report as a fraction inj./uninj.

| | | Proximal | Middle | Distal | Finger tips miss palm: inches | | |
|---|---|---|---|---|---|---|---|
| Thumb | (Ext | | XXXXXXXX | | | | |
| | (Flex | 40/40 | XXXXXXXX | 85/76 | | | |
| Index | (Ext | | | | | | |
| | (Flex | 80/80 | 103/102 | 63/70 | T | | |
| Middle | (Ext | | 173/180 | | | | |
| | (Flex | 80/80 | 105/105 | 64/78 | T | | |
| Ring | (Ext | | 176/180 | | | | |
| | (Flex | 80/83 | 110/112 | 60/65 | T | | |
| Little | (Ext | | | | | | |
| | (Flex | 83/85 | 113/112 | 64/71 | T | | |

Grip (dynamometer readings) 8444

Right Inj. Uninj. Left

07/12/08/11/12/ 35/53/35/31/24

/

/

| Pinch | Right Inj. | Uninj. Left |
|---|---|---|
| Thumb-Index | 8.5 | 16 |
| Lateral | 13 | 18 |
| Jaw Chuck | 5.5 | 19 |

In case of bilateral disability state estimated normal as ABD. 140/160 (EN 180).

MEASUREMENTS NOT SHOWN ARE CONSIDERED NORMAL

All measurements should be made in accordance with the standard method as described in the book "Evaluation of Industrial Disability."

*Fig. 5-28. Range of motion, grip strength, and pinch strength measurements of client with frozen right shoulder, flexion contracture of right elbow, and causalgia of right upper extremity.*

There is loss of range of motion in the right wrist as compared to the left:

| | |
|---|---|
| Dorsiflexion (raise cocked fist) | − 10 degrees |
| Plantar flexion (drop hand down) | Normal |
| Radial deviation (move hand to the left) | − 05 degrees |
| Ulnar deviation (move hand to the right) | − 10 degrees |

All digit range of motion is within normal limits.

GRIP STRENGTH

The norm group for the client is women aged 45 to 49 years. The client is well below the tenth percentile for grip strength on the right for women of her age group, and at the tenth percentile on the left for women of her age group (Fig. 5-29).

NAME ______________ No. ______ (Right Major)

Circ. (inches) Biceps ____ / ____ Wrist ____ / ____

Forearm ____ / ____ Hand ____ / ____

MOTIONS: Report as a fraction (injured/uninjured) in degrees of Active Motion

Shoulder: Abd. ____ / ____ Forearm Pron. ____ / ____

Flex. ____ / ____ Sup. ____ / ____

I R. ____ / ____

E R. ____ / ____ Wrist D F 45 / 55

Ext. ____ / ____ P F 45 / 50

Add. ____ / ____ R D 05 / 30

U D 30 / 45

Elbow: Ext. ____ / ____

Flex. ____ / ____

Thumb: (ABD. 52 / 60 (degrees)

(ADD. Tip misses head of 5th MC. T / T inch

Report as a fraction inj./uninj.

| | | Proximal | Middle | Distal | Finger tips miss palm: inches | | |
|---|---|---|---|---|---|---|---|
| Thumb | (Ext | | XXXXXXXX | | | | |
| | (Flex | 60/59 | XXXXXXXX | 60/60 | | | |
| Index | (Ext | | | | | | |
| | (Flex | 90/90 | 91/90 | 64/67 | T | | |
| Middle | (Ext | | | 145/180 * | | | |
| | (Flex | 95/96 | 85/90 | 74/70 | T | | |
| Ring | (Ext | | | | | | |
| | (Flex | 90/90 | 93/91 | 62/62 | T | | |
| Little | (Ext | | | 163/180 | | | |
| | (Flex | 90/90 | 92/86 | 53/60 | T | | |

Grip (dynamometer readings) 8444

*Swan Neck Childhood Injury

Right Inj. Uninj. Left

15/32/26/31/27/45/65/60/51/49

| Pinch | Right Inj. | Uninj. Left |
|---|---|---|
| Thumb-Index | 12 | 19 |
| Lateral | 20.5 | 25 |
| Jaw Chuck | 16 | 20 |

In case of bilateral disability state estimated normal as ABD. 140/160 (EN 180).

MEASUREMENTS NOT SHOWN ARE CONSIDERED NORMAL

All measurements should be made in accordance with the standard method as described in the book "Evaluation of Industrial Disability."

*Fig. 5-29. Range of motion, grip strength, and pinch strength measurements of client with bilateral Colles' fractures.*

PINCH STRENGTH

Palmar pinch (fingertip to thumb tip) was at the tenth percentile on the right and at the ninetieth percentile on the left. Three-point pinch (as in holding a pencil) was at the fiftieth percentile on the right and above the ninetieth percentile on the left. Lateral pinch (as in turning a key) was at the seventy-fifth percentile on the right and above the ninetieth percentile on the left.

FILING TEST

A TOWER filing test was given to test the ability to alphabetize names with 4" × 6" index cards and a file box. The task was explained orally with an interpreter and a demonstration was given.

RESULTS

1. No difficulty in alphabetizing; average speed and accuracy.
2. Complaints of numbness in right middle, ring, and little finger after 1 hour 26 minutes seated at standard desk chair (18 inches floor to seat) and desk (height 28 inches). Chair height was changed to 14 inches from floor to seat. The client asked to continue the task.
3. After working 15 minutes at the new chair height, the client complained of her right neck, shoulder, and arm hurting and burning. The client asked to continue the task.
4. Chair height was changed to 19 inches. The client complained of "bent neck" making arm go to sleep. Chair height was changed to 17 inches. There were no further complaints at this height. The client asked to continue the task.
5. Total working time was 2 hours 25 minutes with one break.

ATTITUDE

The client was cooperative and pleasant. She demonstrated motivation to continue given tasks. The client speaks clear and concise English. She was able to interpret for the evaluator when help was needed in instructing another non-English-speaking client.

The evaluator discussed with the client and her rehabilitation counselor the possibility of obtaining another opinion from a member of the American Society of Hand Surgeons concerning the alleviation of pain and the possibility of increased range of motion in the client's right arm and hand. The client stated that she no longer wants to participate in a medical program. She said she wants to return to her former job or to some form of work within her present physical limitation.

ASSESSMENT SUMMARY

1. The client complains of pain, numbness, and a burning sensation in the right upper extremity and hand that interfere with her functional capacity to work at a clerical table.
2. The client has loss of range of motion in the right shoulder in abduction and flexion that contributes to her right shoulder pain and to her discomfort when she is working at a standard desk. The loss of range of motion in elbow extension and wrist ranges is not such as to prohibit functional use of the elbow and hand at desk tasks.
3. The grip strength is at the tenth percentile but does not prohibit functional ability in clerical tasks.
4. The pinch strength ranges from the tenth percentile to the seventy-fifth percentile and is sufficient for functional use of pinch in clerical tasks.
5. The client was able to work for 2 hours 25 minutes with one authorized break. However, there were numerous complaints of pain, numbness, and burning.
6. The evaluator feels that because the client has not worked for three years she would benefit from a work hardening program of three weeks or a work capacity evaluation of five days before proceeding with a vocational evaluation.
7. The evaluator was unable to address the physical ability of the client's right arm and hand as a machine operator in pill packaging owing to lack of a job description. An evaluation on the job is needed for further determination.

RECOMMENDATIONS

1. Consultation with a member of the American Society of Hand Surgeons for possibility of alleviation of pain and increase in range of motion if the client so desires
2. A work capacity evaluation of five days or a work hardening program of three weeks to increase the client's potential for employment; both of these in clerical skills
3. On-the-job evaluation of the client in machine operator, pill packaging, position

*Case Study 2**
Dates of Attendance: May 2–6, 1983

OBJECTIVES OF REFERRAL
The client was referred by her vocational rehabilitation counselor for a five-day work capacity evaluation to assess the following:

1. Physical capacities as they relate to drafting tasks (Note problem areas.)
2. Physical capacities as they relate to computer aided design (CAD), which is performed largely at a terminal
3. General physical tolerances (This information will be used in broad vocational exploration.)

PAIN
The client stated on initial contact that she experienced pain in the knuckle of the right thumb when she used a pencil; numbness day and night in the right middle, ring, and little fingers; and a "hot poker" feeling in the middle of her palm day and night. During the evaluation the client did not complain of the above, but instead of pain in the lower back from "sitting too long" and a "rubber band pulling at the right shoulder and forearm" when the work was flat. She reported that her right wrist and thumb and the base of her left thumb on the radial side hurt.

RANGE OF MOTION
There is a decrease in right index finger touch to palm of −½ inch and a decrease in range of motion in straightening out the index finger (Fig. 5-30). The minimal loss of range of motion does not interfere with function in either traditional drafting or CAD.

GRIP STRENGTH
The grip strength of the client's right hand is below the tenth percentile for women aged 50. That of the left hand is at the fiftieth percentile.

PINCH STRENGTH
Palmar pinch (as in picking up a pin) is below the tenth percentile in the right and left hands. Three-point pinch (as in holding a pencil) is at the tenth percentile in both hands. Lateral pinch (as in turning a key) is at the twenty-fifth percentile in both hands. Muscle strength is within normal limits in all areas.

SENSATION
Sensation is normal (two-point discrimination is 4 mm in all fingers).

EDEMA
Measurements increased during the course of five working days: right hand, from 395+ to 405+; left hand, from 360+ to 390.

MAY 2
*Equipment and Tools*
Manual pencil sharpener, sandpaper, two pencils with carbon lead, T square, triangle, roll of drafting paper, scissors, drafting board with top tilted at 7 degrees, table height 29½ inches, chair height 25 inches with back support.

*This case study was provided by Thelma Wellerson Hook, M.A., OTR, Hand Therapy and Rehabilitation Associates, Los Gatos, California.

Date 5-2-83

NAME ______ No. ______ (Right Major)
Circ. (inches) Biceps ______ / ______ Wrist ______ / ______
Forearm ______ / ______ Hand ______ / ______

MOTIONS: Report as a fraction (injured/uninjured) in degrees of Active Motion

Shoulder: Abd. WNL / ; Flex. 140/145 / ; I R. WNL / ; E R. WNL / ; Ext. 52/40 / ; Add. /

Forearm Pron. / ; Sup. /

Wrist D F 63/62 / ; P F 63/67 / ; R D 25/20 / ; U D 40/30 /

Elbow: Ext. 180/180 / ; Flex. 30/30 /

Thumb: (ABD. 65/69 / (degrees)
(ADD. Tip misses head of 5th MC. T / T inch

Report as a fraction inj./uninj.

| | | Proximal | Middle | Distal | Finger tips miss palm: inches Right | | |
|---|---|---|---|---|---|---|---|
| Thumb | Ext | | XXXXXXXX | | | | |
| | Flex | 70/74 | XXXXXXXX | 60/60 | | | |
| Index | Ext | 160/180 | | 167/180 | | | |
| | Flex | 74/84 | 102/100 | 66/70 | -1/2 | T | |
| Middle | Ext | 160/180 | 175/175 | | | | |
| | Flex | 77/95 | 107/100 | 71/75 | -1/4 | T | |
| Ring | Ext | | | | | | |
| | Flex | 85/95 | 100/95 | 65/65 | T | T | |
| Little | Ext | | | | | | |
| | Flex | 91/85 | 94/85 | 65/70 | T | T | |

Grip (dynamometer readings)

Right Inj. / Left Uninj.
10/30/19/18/17 / 19/17/17/17/11

| Pinch | Injured Right | Left |
|---|---|---|
| Thumb-Index | 2.5 | 5 |
| Lateral | 10 | 8.5 |
| Jaw Chuck | 7 | 6 |

In case of bilateral disability state estimated normal as ABD. 140/160 (EN 180).

MEASUREMENTS NOT SHOWN ARE CONSIDERED NORMAL

All measurements should be made in accordance with the standard method as described in the book "Evaluation of Industrial Disability."

*Fig. 5-30. Range of motion, grip strength, and pinch strength of client with arthritis. (WNL = within normal limits.)*

*Work Sample*

The client was requested to produce 12 geometric figures from TOWER drafting test 5. The scale was 1 inch to 4 inches. The client completed the task 15 minutes before lunch break. After break she completed five figures in 13 minutes.

*Results*

The client reported at the end of the day that her left hand and wrist were beginning to hurt and that her back bothered her. She was told to try the option that had been offered her of working while seated, and it was found that sitting alleviated the back pain.

*Time*

11:20 A.M. to 12:00 noon; 1:00 to 3:00 P.M.

MAY 3

*Equipment and Tools*

Electric eraser (1¼ lbs.), erasing shield, dust brush, drafting board (top tilted at 10 degrees, table height 29½ inches, chair height 22 to 25 inches with no back support, masking tape, square scissors (1" x 1") 36 minutes, hexagon scale (1" × 1") 36 minutes.

*Work Sample*

The client was asked to repeat TOWER test. Standard time is 2 hours 7 minutes. The client completed the test in 59 minutes, in superior time range.

The client used the electric eraser with her right hand and the erasing shield with the left. She lifted masking tape with the thumb and index finger of right hand. She held the scissors in her right hand and pushed forward to cut against the static edge of the scissors. She used the dust brush with her right hand.

*The Results*

The client complained that the 25 inch chair height bothered her lower back. The chair was lowered to 23 inches.

*Time*

8:35 A.M. to 4:10 P.M. with 70 minutes for lunch and two 10-minute breaks.

MAY 4

*Equipment and Tools*

Drafting table with top at 65 degrees, 24-inch perch stool with back support, manual pencil sharpener, two pencils with carbon lead.

*Work Sample*

TOWER test 5, repeat of geometric forms, 1 hour 27 minutes. Circles and half-circles, 59 minutes. Floor plan office space 1, 1 hour 27 minutes.

*Results*

The client complained of a "tired back last night." She was given "Back" booklet.

The client alternated standing and sitting at standard drafting table 29¾ inches high and 42" × 29½". The table tilts from 25 to 65 degrees. The chair height was at 22 inches. The client stated that if the board was "too flat" her back was affected, but if the table was tilted too high her right arm had to be raised and she felt a "rubber band pull" at the outside of her shoulder and along the top of her forearm. A good position appears to be a chair height of 2 feet with the table tilted 30 degrees.

*Time*

9:00 A.M. to 3:30 P.M., with 1 hour 20 minutes for lunch and two 10-minute breaks.

MAY 5, A.M.

Client and therapist went to the Mission College campus where the client tried out CAD

*Equipment*

Computer table height 29 inches
Keyboard 31½ × 15" × 10"
Screen height 47 inches to center of monitor
Total screen height 50 inches
Monitor 18" × 7½"
Eye to screen 21½ inches
Digitizer 28 inches to the right of the client
Pad 17" × 14"

WORK DESCRIPTION

The stylus is positioned with the right hand. It is necessary periodically to press a button on the stylus with the right index finger. Very light pressure is required.

The client looks forward at screen while using the cursor with the right hand. The full arm is stretched 36 inches forward and to the right approximately 45 degrees.

The client uses two hands, one on the digitizer and one on the Hipad with the cursor. Her head is to the right momentarily then returns straight ahead to monitor screen.

*Results*

The client did not complain of pain, fatigue, or discomfort during the evaluation period.

MAY 5, P.M.

The client continued using a traditional drafting board, model 3042-ST, alternately standing and sitting on perch chair at 22 inches. She continued working on Office Floor Plan 2 for two hours. Her complaints remained the same.

MAY 6

*Equipment*

Drafting table model 3042-ST, Vemco drafting machine elbow; 0.5-mm Pentel P205 lead pencil; electric eraser (1¼ lbs); erasing shield; lead sharpener; masking tape; drafting paper; templates—circles, architecture, and electric; perch chair.

*Mixed Drawing and Printing*

Work Sample. The client alternated standing and sitting with the table at full 65-degree tilt and chair at 2 feet. The left hand constantly pulls up the elbow, which weighs 2 pounds, from 1 to 1¼ inches. This motion positions the verticle and horizontal 18- and 12-inch scale. While the left hand controls the elbow, the right hand draws the required line. The thumb and first finger are in constant pinch position. In addition to constant pinch, the drafter must twirl the pencil continually so that the lead will not flatten. These motions are necessary for all drafting requirements, including lettering. The client stated that product bill of parts on the job is 12 pages long with a minimum of two pages of printing lines ½ inch apart.

RESULTS

The client worked 90 minutes without complaints of discomfort. At the end of that time, she complained of pain in her right thumb and left wrist. She rested and then worked for another 30 minutes before she stopped and changed jobs.

The therapist tried a larger-diameter pencil to relieve constant pinch. This was ungainly and unacceptable to the client. The client worked on lettering with the chair at 2 feet and the table at a 25-degree tilt for approximately one hour. She complained of discomfort as described, both left and right hand.

ATTITUDE AND HISTORY

The client was cooperative and knowledgeable in all areas of her job. She worked last on November 22, 1981.

The client first noticed arthritis in her hands in the 1960s. She presently sees her physician every three weeks. She has received therapy twice weekly for two months. Therapy was discontinued as of May 6, 1983.

The client had a right carpal tunnel in 1967 with surgery in June 1980, and a left carpal tunnel in 1970 with surgery in August 1980.

The client stated she has had scoliosis since 14 years of age. This causes tension across her back. She was in a body cast for two years but had no surgery. She was followed by St. Mary's Hospital, San Francisco.

The client stated that her right eye is normal but since five years ago she has been unable to read with the left with correction.

The client has arthritis in C5 and C6.

The client started drafting in junior high school. She has had two years of college. She started drafting with Bell in 1948. In 1951 she worked as a cartographer for Rand McNally for three months and then started drafting with EIMAC. She continued with EIMAC when Varian bought out EIMAC.

The client stated that her interest is computers in addition to various hobbies that she pursues when her hands permit.

The client has looked into a Masters School course in CAD and took a minicourse with them in 1977 for six weeks. She learned how to do tape-ups. She has taken two Saturday courses at Radio Shack on computers.

The client said she would like to take a 20-week CAD course offered by the Masters School. The school requires a 20-week computer-aided manufacture (CAM) course as a prerequisite. She states that she already knows the CAM material and does not want to take this course, but Masters will not allow her to take the CAD course without first taking the prerequisite.

ASSESSMENT SUMMARY

1. The client has pain in left wrist, right palm, base of right and left thumb, and lower back. She is able to control the pain while working on traditional drafting by changing positions and tasks.
2. Range of motion loss in right hand is minimal and does not interfere with traditional drafting or CAD.
3. Grip strength loss below the tenth percentile on the right and at the fiftieth percentile on the left does not interfere with traditional drafting or CAD.
4. Pinch strength loss does not interfere with traditional drafting or CAD.
5. Muscle strength in both extremities is within normal limits.
6. Sensation is normal in both hands.
7. Swelling in both hands, which increased during the course of the five-day evaluation, does not interfere with traditional drafting or CAD.
8. Traditional drafting causes constant discomfort to the client. The client suffers the least discomfort in the hands and lower back when the drafting table has a 30-degree tilt, her chair with back support is in the 22-to 24-inch range, and she alternates standing and sitting and changes tasks frequently. Traditional drafting will continue to cause the client discomfort and pain in both hands.
9. CAD is best performed by the client in a support chair at the 22-to 24- inch range from seat to floor. If the Hipad with cursor position becomes a problem to the client, the pad should be moved from the right to the left of the computer keyboard. CAD is not as physically demanding to the client and does not appear to cause constant discomfort and pain.
10. The client's attitude is excellent, and she is motivated to learn CAD.

RECOMMENDATIONS

1. If the client is to pursue traditional drafting, the best position for the drafting table is a 30-degree tilt with a 29¾ inches table height. The chair should have a support back and the seat should be between 22 and 24 inches from the floor. The client should be able to change positions and tasks frequently.
2. If the client is to pursue CAD, the best chair height is 22 to 24 inches, and the chair should have a back support.
3. A short course of training in CAD and placement are recommended.

## HAND REHABILITATION SPECIALISTS

Another example of a private occupational therapy practice that specializes in hand rehabilitation is Hand Rehabilitation Specialists, located in Santa Monica, California. This practice, which is owned and staffed by Karen S. Schultz and Robert E. Dorer, Jr., provides consultations to a vocational rehabilitation equipment company, evaluations of upper-extremity function for a private rehabilitation firm, and a comprehensive acute hand rehabilitation service.

The professional relationship with the work evaluation equipment manufacturer and the private rehabilitation firm grew out of personal contact at workshops and conferences with people who are enthusiastic about occupational therapy's contribution to vocational rehabilitation efforts. Both industry and vocational rehabilitation providers have identified occupational therapy as the ideal profession to help translate the medical model into a vocationally relevant one.

The board of directors of WEST (Work Evaluation Systems Technology) targeted occupational therapists as a professional group in need of a sophisticated yet simple system of work evaluation equipment. In their efforts to educate occupational therapists about the equipment, they chose to utilize other occupational therapists who were skilled with the equipment. They assembled a group of therapists to participate as professional development consultants (PDCs). Each PDC had as an area of specialty such as cardiac or upper-extremity rehabilitation. Interested occupational therapists can contact PDCs at national conferences and in the PDC's home clinic. PDCs provide consultation to help a therapist or a facility decide whether the WEST equipment will meet their needs and will integrate with the occupational therapy program. The PDC also provides information regarding the ways the equipment can be used and can demonstrate the various functions of the equipment. The PDC also provides feedback to the manufacturer as ideas for new products present themselves and as product revision or adaptation is required.

Hand Rehabilitation Specialists also perform upper-extremity evaluation for private vocational rehabilitation firms. In this area an occupational therapist who is familiar with the various systems involved—worker compensation, personal injury, social security, disability—and with the continuum of rehabilitation services can make a valuable contribution. The therapist is able to understand in fine detail the sometimes voluminous medical reports and can translate these reports to the vocational counselor. The upper-extremity occupational therapy specialist can perform a physical status evaluation of the upper extremities (range of motion, strength, sensibility) and translate the findings into vocationally relevant information. Without these objective, hands-on data, the ability to interpret observed phenomena accurately is severely impaired. The occupational therapist is trained to observe carefully and identify a client's abilities (e.g., dexterity) and then describe the client's ability to *apply* those abilities in a functional manner.

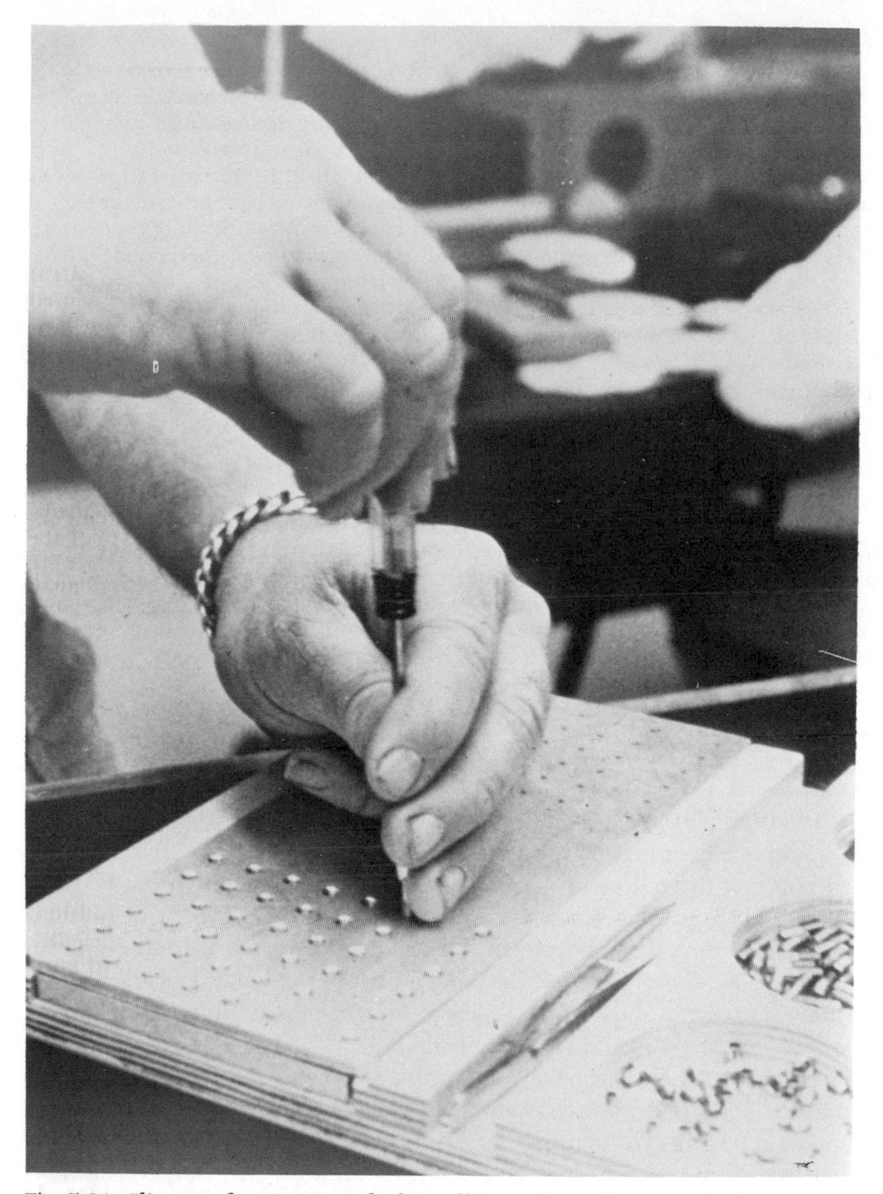

*Fig. 5-31. Client performing Crawford Small Parts Dexterity Test, which assesses fine manipulation, small tool use, and endurance. (Courtesy Hand Rehabilitation Specialists.)*

*Case Study**

An interesting client referred for an upper-extremity work tolerance screening (WTS) test was Winston, a 26-year-old right-dominant Guyanese man who had been employed as a wrapping machine operator at the time of his injury. He sustained two injuries to his hands while operating this machine. In 1981 the right middle and ring fingers were amputated through the distal interphalangeal joints. He returned to his usual and customary work 2½ months after that injury. Eight months after his return to work, he sustained a left index finger distal phalanx crush with an open fracture. When he recovered from the second injury, his treating physician questioned whether or not the client had adequate coordination to perform his work on such a machine.

Although assessment of upper-extremity coordination and dexterity was the stated purpose of the WTS, another problem surfaced as a major reason for the client's decreased ability to perform his work safely. During the sensory evaluation of the hand, it was found that the tips of the right middle and ring finger stumps were hypersensitive. The client jerked his hand away when the stumps were stimulated. In a further interview the client stated that he had not been able to perform his work in the usual manner since his first injury because of his need to protect the hypersensitive fingertips of his right hand. On a standardized test such as the Crawford Small Parts Dexterity Test (Fig. 5-31) and a standardized apparatus such as the WEST 2, the client demonstrated excellent hand coordination, dexterity, and attentiveness to detail as long as the right amputation stumps were not involved or inadvertently touched. Right hand skill deteriorated in the presence of stimulation of the right stumps. This information was summarized and presented to the referring counselor. The occupational therapist recommended a program of desensitization.

## School for the Developmentally Delayed

### WALTER E. FERNALD STATE SCHOOL

The Walter E. Fernald State School, founded in 1848, was the first publicly supported residential training facility for the mentally retarded. Historically, at Fernald occupational therapy has played an important role in client care, particularly with respect to work-related programming. In the early 1970s occupational therapists were actively involved in the development of Fernald's vocational training workshops. The introduction of vocational rehabilitation services to the school provided the catalyst for the occupational therapy department to redirect some of its resources from vocational training workshops to prevocational skills and behavior training.

Prevocational skills and behavior training is viewed as a fundamental part of a total habilitative plan to reach work skills, behaviors, and attitudes. As formulated by Carolyn Austin and John Basile [19], "An idealized long-term goal of prevocational training is competitive employment. However, a more realistic goal is the development of the client's work-related skills to their fullest potential with an increased sense of self-identity and accomplishment achieved through purposeful and meaningful activity." The prevocational programming is conceptualized on a continuum of increasing difficulty and includes prevocational training, a comprehensive training center, sheltered workshops, and on-the-job training. The transition from lower to higher levels

*This case study was provided by Karen S. Schultz, M.S., OTR, Hand Rehabilitation Specialists, Santa Monica, California.

of training is governed by the client's meeting specific predetermined admissions criteria.

*Prevocational Training*
Presented in a classroom designed to simulate a work environment, prevocational training is typically a component of the comprehensive day activity program coordinated by division staff. There are six day program divisions in which clients are grouped homogeneously by ability. Division 1 comprises the lowest-functioning clients; division 6, the highest-functioning clients.

The occupational therapist may work on a one-to-one basis with clients or in a group setting using treatment modalities such as sensory stimulation, motor development, prevocational skills development, fine motor training, and activities of daily living (ADL) training. The therapist also provides consultation to the division staff and clinical supervision of direct staff. The *comprehensive training center* specializes in the acquisition of prevocational skills by means of simulated and real work in a more realistic worklike environment. The therapist plays a role similar to that described for prevocational training.

*Sheltered Workshops*
The philosophy inherent in the sheltered workshop program at Fernald is to assist each client to maximize his or her abilities and acquire feelings of self-worth. This is accomplished by focusing on the client's *ability* rather than disability and by providing realistic work experiences in a sheltered workshop. The occupational therapist is available on a consulting basis to the workshop staff, providing evaluations of clients with perceptual difficulties, making recommendations on task analysis and work simplification, and designing and constructing jigs for clients with physical handicaps (Fig. 5-32) [35].

There are three workshop levels, each with its own admissions criteria (Table 5-6). Placement in each level may be long-term or short-term, depending on the individual client's needs and progress.

The entry-level workshops are the first stage in a continuum of experience with contract work (when available) in a real full-time work environment. For many clients these workshops represent their first experience in full-time work. The emphasis in this level is on the further development of basic work skills.

In the *intermediate-level workshop* clients have had some work experience that has increased their familiarity with the expectations of a full-time work adjustment program. Emphasis here is placed on the development of more advanced work behaviors and attitudes such as production levels, cooperation, and independence.

The *transitional programs* represent the final stage of the sheltered workshop continuum. These clients have had work experience and have successfully mastered a variety of work situations and tasks. The goal of complete work-related independence is consistently reinforced, and worker production and

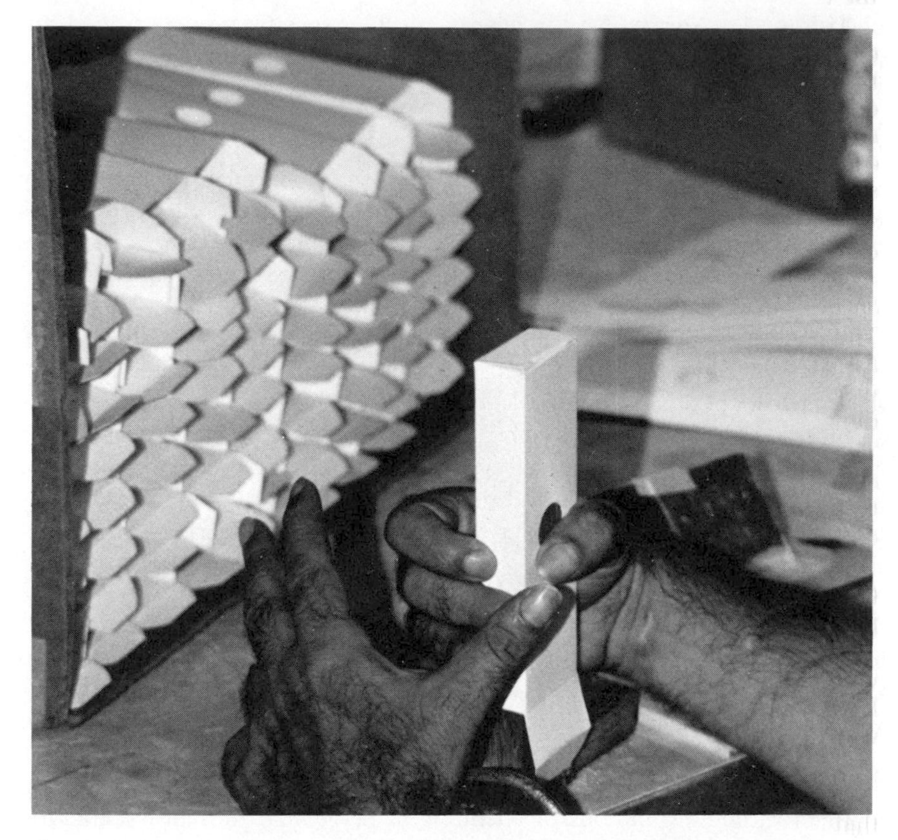

A

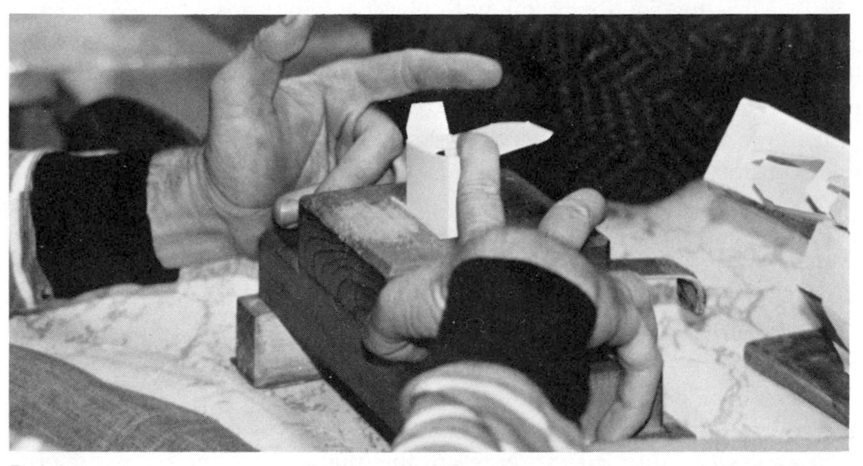

B

*Fig. 5-32. Jigs developed by therapists at Fernald State School to assist clients in performing sheltered workshop subcontract tasks of (A) assembling box and (B) stuffing and closing box. (Photos courtesy of Matthew Gold.)*

*Table 5-6. Workshop Entry Criteria*

I. Entry-level workshops
   A. Able to attend work daily
   B. Independent in basic ADL* skills
   C. Ability to make basic needs known through signs, gestures, or words
   D. Able to understand three-step tasks either verbally, visually, manually, or in combination
   E. Sitting tolerance of 50 minutes
   F. Ability to work independently for approximately 5 minutes
   G. Ability to work at least 2 hours per day 5 days per week
   H. Ability to participate in small, structured social groups

II. Intermediate workshops
   A. Ability to work in cooperative group setting
   B. Reinforced by money or verbal praise
   C. Ability to produce at approximately 10–12% NPA* on most tasks
   D. Ability to work for approximately 15 minutes with minimal supervision
   E. Demonstrated ability to acquire additional work skills
   F. Functionally understands such concepts as larger, smaller, front of, behind, between, before, after
   G. Ability to attend to task for 30–50 minutes with supervision and prompts
   H. Ability to accept changes in routine

III. Transitional programs
   A. Ability to work 6 hours per day, 5 days per week with appropriate breaks
   B. Production between 20 and 30% NPA on most tasks
   C. Ability to use leisure time such as breaks appropriately
   D. Funtional understanding of the supervisor-worker relationship
   E. Functional understanding of quality control as related to work
   F. Functional understanding of money as related to production
   G. Ability to work consistently for approximately 2½ hours with supervision
   H. Ability to pariticipate in a realistic way in the development of vocational goals and objectives

* ADL = activities of daily living; NPA = normal production average.

peer socialization are emphasized. At this level clients have evolved a fundamental understanding of work attitudes and behavior.

*On-the-Job Training*

Concurrent with the sheltered workshop program is on-the-job training (OJT). The OJT program offers the client the opportunity to learn a wide variety of meaningful activities and tasks in a normalized setting. Many OJT tasks offer an alternative for clients unable to tolerate assembly line tasks such as are offered in the sheltered workshops. Approximately 45 clients from divisions 2 through 6 participate in OJT. This program, like the sheltered workshops, has specific entry criteria (Table 5-7). Depending on the clients' needs, they may simultaneously participate in a sheltered workshop.

Both the sheltered workshop and OJT are certified under the Massachusetts Department of Labor and the Central Office of the Department of Mental Health. These agencies help to guarantee that clients are paid for their productivity.

*Table 5-7. Entry Criteria for On-the-Job Training*

| *Skill Area* | *Criteria* |
|---|---|
| Attending to task | Ability to attend to a learned task for up to 10 minutes |
| Cooperation | Ability to follow directions for secondary and delayed reinforcement such as weekly pay; response to money as a secondary reinforcer |
| Work tolerance | Ability to stay in work environment up to 2 hours; experience with day activity programming preferred |
| Communication skills | Ability to communicate basic needs and follow up to four-step instructions |
| Cognitive skills | Ability to discriminate by size and shape and to match items if sorted by color; one-to-one correspondence skills |
| Motor skills | Ability to perform jobs in program (types of work are dependent on training site) |

On-the-job training areas include a greenhouse, the North Café, the manual porter crew, the Polaroid porter crew, the clerical pool, the marketable crafts program, and individualized placements. The *greenhouse program*, in operation since 1975, uses horticultural therapy to provide prevocational and vocational skills training and leisure activity development. At present 15 clients work at the greenhouse approximately 4½ hours per day five days per week. Throughout the year these clients participate in seasonal horticultural activities. In the spring, for example, clients learn to replant seedlings, plant seed flats, and maintain the greenhouse; in the summer the focus shifts to vegetable and flower gardening, basic landscaping, and replenishing house plants for the greenhouse.

The sale of greenhouse products to the public facilitates a businesslike atmosphere and affords the clients the opportunity to interact with the community in a positive milieu of an exchange of labor for product. The community garden program provides clients with an additional opportunity to interact with the community. Garden plots on Fernald's ground are available to community members, as well as staff and clients. The success of this project with respect to positive public relations with the community has been expressed in the following way: "This project provides a positive setting for the community to become involved with Fernald and to learn more about mental retardation through a positive experience. Since the community gardens began many citizens have expressed positive feelings about Fernald and increased concern for its residents" [19].

The *North Café* is a structured restaurant training program in which 11 clients, under staff supervision, provide a variety of daily luncheon specials for staff and clients. Through restaurant-style experiences clients learn about hygiene, service skills, table setting, and clean-up procedures. The restaurant is also used to help other clients learn how to order a meal, wait appropriately for the meal to be served, and pay for items.

The clients in the *manual porter crew program* are trained in custodial work to maintain three buildings on the school grounds. Approximately six clients work four hours per day five days per week on tasks that typically allow them to channel their energy into physical activity. Team cooperation is greatly emphasized throughout the program.

The emphasis of the *Polaroid porter crew program* which is carried on at the nearby Polaroid plant, is on social adaptation in a community work setting and on developing and evaluating independent work skills. The program provides janitorial training; the work involves cleaning 18 bathrooms daily. Tasks include emptying trash, replenishing supplies, sweeping, mopping, and cleaning toilets, sinks, and shelves. This offers a work experience in a normal environment with normal work expectations. The skills that the clients acquire are assumed to be marketable.

The *clerical pool* consists of five clients who perform various clerical tasks (stapling, folding) for departments at the school.

The *marketable crafts program* provides the client with a creative outlet in the production of salable handcrafted items such as patchwork pillows, draft stoppers, and Christmas wreaths, while reinforcing general work skills and behaviors. At present clients sell their items to local shops, to craft fairs (the Little People's School annual arts and crafts fair—see Chap. 4) and to the Fernald staff. For those clients who are able to perform work duties independently, jobs are available through *individual placement* with the school's boiler house, farm, and grounds department.

*Conceptual Framework of Prevocational Program*

Austin and Basile have classified work-related skills into a four-category developmental framework: (1) basic work behavior skills, (2) work performance skills, (3) refined work behavior skills, and (4) refined work concepts.

*Basic work behavior skills* make up the foundation of task-related skill development and refined work behaviors. Such basic skills include attending to the task, sitting tolerance, work tolerance, independent working, compliance, and cooperation. The acquisition of these skills is a prerequisite for the development of more advanced prevocational skills such as performance, refined work behaviors, and work concepts.

*Work performance skills* are the physical, cognitive, sensory, sensorimotor, and communication skills necessary to perform tasks.

| *Skills* | *Examples* |
|---|---|
| Physical | Strength, endurance, range of motion, dexterity |
| Sensory | Body schema, position in space |
| Sensorimotor | Coordination of sensory and physical skills |
| Cognitive | Concept of task completion; concept of "one"; discrimination by shape, size, color, weight; sequencing ability |

Communication — Receptive language (ability to follow two- or three-step directions), expressive language (ability to express basic and work-related needs)

*Refined work behavior skills* are the advanced prevocational skills derived from well-developed basic work behavior skills. Examples of refined skills are work attendance, punctuality, initiative (working independently), frustration tolerance, adaptability to change, cooperation, appearance and hygiene, organizational ability, and appropriate communication.

*Refined work concepts* include such aspects of successful employment as liking one's job and understanding the relationship between productivity, employment, and success.

Austin and Basile have also identified a continuum of work behaviors from basic to refined (Fig. 5-33).

*Case Study**

Jane is a 24-year-old visually handicapped yet functionally sighted resident of Fernald. Primary care and service delivery within the institution have been augmented by federal funding for the past six years.

Jane was admitted to the institution at age 4 with the diagnosis of Down's syndrome. Her functional abilities are limited owing to both her organic disorder and subsequent developmental retardation resulting from extended institutionalization. During the first 14 years of Jane's residency in the institution, anomalies developed in her behavior partially because of her syndrome and partially because of extremely limited service delivery other than custodial care before ancillary funding made available by the federal government.

Jane has been receiving daily structured educational services in her residential building for the past four years. The emphasis has been on the development of self-care, communication, refined motor, cognitive, and work-related skills. Consistent behavioral interventions have been in effect for the last six years.

The residence interdisciplinary treatment team noted that Jane had made considerble progress in all skill areas. The incidence of inappropriate behavior was minimal and almost nonexistent in a structured setting. She was able to communicate basic needs and was receptive to elementary forms of expressive communication. She demonstrated a potential for independence in self-care and a marked ability to learn work-related tasks and to maintain appropriate behavior in a work-related setting.

Prompted by Jane's noted progress, the treatment team recommended her admission to First Step, a comprehensive out-of-building day activity program designed to address all need areas with an emphasis on teaching clients to generalize learned skills and incorporate them throughout their day.

Skill evaluations were conducted by the First Step treatment team, who agreed with the residence treatment team that Jane met the admission criteria to the program and that service delivery from the program would most appropriately meet her needs at that time.

Two years after her admission to First Step, Jane was nearly independent in self-care skills such as dressing, toileting, washing, and grooming, although she did require limited assistance in most of these areas. Her motor planning, strength, and range of motion were within normal limits. Her communication skills had improved enough

*This case study was provided by John Basile, Walter E. Fernald State School, Belmont, Massachusetts.

to greatly facilitate skill development in other areas; the incidence of inapproprate behavior continued to be minimal; and her cognitive, physical, and perceptual abilities had enabled her to learn new work-related tasks, some of which were fairly complex, quickly. Jane appeared to enjoy work and to understand the value of reward for work well done. Staff noted her ability to tolerate sitting and working for extended periods; to tolerate supervision and change in routine; and to work continuously, consistently, and cooperatively in a simulated work setting.

Jane's progress and skills were recognized by the residence and program treatment teams whose combined efforts had given Jane a continuous opportunity to learn. Her admission to Advance was recommended.

Advance is a comprehensive training center that specializes in the development and refinement of basic work behavior skills and work performance skills by means of a wide variety of prevocational tasks including multiple-step assembly and packaging, sorting, cooperative work, and housekeeping. Self-care, communication, and behavior continue to be addressed with an increased emphasis on the development of monetary skills, frustration tolerance, and other more complex prerequisites for vocational placement.

Jane met Advance admission criteria, and the treatment team agreed that her placement in the program would meet her needs.

During the 18 months after her admission to Advance, staff continued to note her consistent progress in communication, behavior, self-care, and other skill areas relevant to work. Her independent travel from residence to program site was monitored by staff. The residence treatment team continued to receive positive reports from the Advance program staff concerning Jane's responsiveness, cooperation, flexibility, and ability to learn in a work setting. After recommendation from Advance staff, the treatment team agreed to screen Jane for placement in an entry-level workshop. Observations and evaluations by workshop staff were completed; eight months after Jane was placed on a waiting list, she was admitted to Work Place, an entry-level workshop program providing services to fifteen clients, four of whom live in the same residential building as Jane. The workshop appeared to be the most appropriate environment to facilitate Jane's advancement toward ultimate normalization and independence.

Using both simulated and contract work (when available), Work Place focuses on increased tolerance to work-related frustrations produced by such features as a supervisor-employee, as opposed to a teacher-student, relationship. Work Place emphasizes the development of more advanced work behaviors, skills, and attitudes leading towards increaed work-related independence. The objectives include regular attendance, punctuality, cooperation, appropriate appearance, appropriate communication, and increased tolerance to change, or lack of change, in routine.

Work Place has offered Jane her first experience in a full-time work adjustment situation. Her placement in the workshop may be long-term or short-term, depending on her needs. In this setting, Jane is assisted in developing more advanced work-related skills and an increased sense of self-worth and accomplishment achieved through purposeful and meaningful activity. Now, as at any level in the continuum of prevocational training, Jane has the opportunity, if appropriate for her, to advance to any one of the higher levels of prevocational or vocational training or vocational placement. The options available to Jane include placement in another sheltered workshop (intermediate or transitional level), an on-the-job training program, or both, depending on her needs. Ultimately, if Jane is able to perform work duties independently, certain full-time employment positions within the institution can be made available to her. Moreover, concurrent with the potential for residential placement in the community, a wide variety of enriching employment experiences are available to Jane outside the institution.

*Fig. 5-33. Continuum of work-related behaviors.*

**Flow Chart of Work Behaviors**

| *Work Behavior Categories:* | *Basic* | | *Intermediate* | | *Refined* | | |
|---|---|---|---|---|---|---|---|
| Work tolerance | Ability to discriminate between home and work environment as measured by going to and from work. | Ability to remain in the work environment for up to one hour a day. | Ability to remain in work environment for up to two hours a day. | Ability to remain in work environment for 2–4 consecutive hours. | Ability to remain at work for up to 6 consecutive hrs. | Ability to remain at work for up to 8 hours daily. | Ability to utilize vacation and sick time appropriately. |
| Staying on the job<br>Sitting tolerance | Ability to sit in designated seat for immediate effective reinforcer. | Ability to sit in designated seat up to 45 minutes with intermittent effective reinforcer. | Ability to stay in designated seat up to 45 minutes for social reinforcement and edible contingency up to 45 minutes. | Ability to stay in designated seat for 45-min. period over 4-hr. day. Social praise, workcard, money. | Ability to stay in designated work space with minimal prompts. | Ability to stay and leave and return to workspace independently. | Ability to work independent of supervisor. Report to supervisor when necessary. |

| | | | | | | | |
|---|---|---|---|---|---|---|---|
| Attending to task<br>Task completion<br>Quality | Ability to perform one subunit of a task for immediate effective reinforcer. | Ability to complete one simple task for immediate effective reinforcer. | Ability to complete a quota of simple tasks for immediate effective reinforcer. | Ability to complete quota of simple tasks for ✓ on workcard; social praise—delayed reinforcer. | Ability to complete task independent of quota for delayed reinforcer. | Ability to complete tasks accurately and fast for social praise and weekly pay. | Ability to complete work for self-esteem and weekly pay. |
| Following instructions | Ability to respond to one-step instructions: Sit down. Time to work. | Ability to respond to additional one- and two-step simple-task, specific instructions. | Ability to follow 3–4 task-specific instructions. | Ability to follow complex 4–10 task-specific instructions. | Ability to follow general work rules; ability to quality, control work. | Ability to receive corrective feedback and change accurately. | Ability to problem-solve complex tasks and work issues. |
| Flexibility | Inapplicable | Inapplicable | Ability to tolerate the same tasks weekly if contract determines this. | Ability to accept change of task. | Ability to accept change of task. | Ability to work cooperatively with co-workers and supervisors. | Ability to discuss changes with supervisors and co-workers. |

**Flow Chart of Work Behaviors**

| *Work Behavior Categories:* | *Basic* | | *Intermediate* | | *Refined* | | |
|---|---|---|---|---|---|---|---|
| Responsibility Attendance | Staff dependent | Staff dependent | Staff dependent | Ability to attend work daily for reinforcement and with staff prompts. | Ability to attend work daily and arrive on time with prompts. | Ability to attend work daily and arrive on time with minimal prompts. | Ability to accumulate and use sick time and vacation time appropriately. |
| Appearance | Must be dressed for work. | Ability to remain appropriately dressed with staff supervision. | Ability to dress for work appropriately with minimal supervision. | Ability to dress for work appropriately, independently. | Ability to wear work-related clothing, aprons, uniforms, protective glasses. | Same | Same |
| Initiative | Inapplicable | Inapplicable | Ability to get more work with prompts. | Ability to get more work with minimal prompts. | Ability to seek help from supervisor with minimal prompts. | Ability to recognize route to success. | Ability to seek promotion and gain peer acceptance. |

| Work Behavior Categories: | Basic | | Intermediate | | Refined | | |
|---|---|---|---|---|---|---|---|
| *Physical* Strength Endurance Dexterity | Ability to reach for and grab large tabletop objects with either hand. | Ability to manipulate large tabletop objects: Ring on ring stack; ability to repeat fine motor skills necessary to perform simple tabletop activities for up to 45 minutes. | Ability to manipulate smaller tabletop objects; ability to perform more refined finger movements, for example: 3 jaw chuck grasp. | Ability to manipulate one part of tabletop object with one hand while steadying matching part with other hand, e.g., large jar hand dominance, unilateral coordination. | Ability to use both hands together to manipulate objects of smaller size, e.g., some types of nuts and bolts. Bilateral coordination, ability to sustain 2–4 hrs of assembly work. | Ability to use tools to manipulate objects, e.g., screwdriver, scissors, hammer, holepunch; ability to sustain 4–6 hrs. of object manipulation. | Ability to use machines; e.g., heat-sealer, drills, riveter, factory jigs; ability to do piecework for 8 hrs. |
| *Cognitive* Discrimination Matching 1:1 correspondence Task completion | Ability to recognize a change in environment; ability to discriminate between two functional tabletop objects, e.g., cup and plate. | Ability to discriminate between basic 3-dimensional shapes □ and ○ then □△ Ability to complete a subunit of a task, e.g., put all the way down on stack. | Ability to discriminate between additional 3-dimensional shapes; ability to put one object in a container, ability to complete up to a 6 subunit of tasks, e.g., one peg in each pouch of egg carton. | Ability to discriminate objects by size, shape, color; ability to object-count up to 5; ability to complete 2–3-step tasks using concept of 1; e.g., putting 1 nut, 1 bolt, 1 washer together. | Ability to discriminate and match objects by length, weight, width, size, color, shape; ability to object-count to 10; ability to complete 3–6-step tasks; e.g., packaging print-coaters. | Ability to discriminate and match letters, codes, numbers, symbols; ability to object-count to 100; ability to sequence multistep tasks. | Ability to quality-control using discriminative and counting skills; problem solving, using simple addition and subtraction. |

Fig. 5-33 (continued)

**Flow Chart of Work Behaviors**

| *Work Behavior Categories:* | *Basic* | | *Intermediate* | | *Refined* | | |
|---|---|---|---|---|---|---|---|
| *Sensory and Perceptual* Body schema | Ability to recognize and locate environmental stimuli. | Ability to locate and recognize environmental stimuli. | Ability to locate and recognize environmental stimuli in relation to self. | Ability to locate position and relationship of objects between self and between objects. | Ability to recognize qualities of objects; e.g., size, shape, color, in relation to each other. | Ability to recognize and reconstruct complex contructions. | Ability to recognize and construct complex constructions. |
| *Sensory-Motor* | Ability to manipulate meaningful stimuli, e.g., sit on chair, open door, step over plank. | Ability to manipulate objects in relation to self; in front of, behind self; throw ball. | Ability to manipulate objects in relation to objects; put block on top of door. | Ability to manipulate objects correct distance from self in relation to each other. | Ability to manipulate and match objects using discrimination skills. | Ability to build block patterns; put screw, nut, and bolt together. | Ability to assemble complex constructions and follow directions. |

Fig. 5-33 (continued)

**Habilitation Program***

UNITED CEREBRAL PALSY DAY HABILITATION PROGRAM

I would like to conclude this section with a brief description of a day program and assessment for adults with cerebral palsy. The work skills development component of the United Cerebral Palsy Day Habilitation Program provides clients with the opportunity to develop and apply to their potential those work habits, behaviors, and skills that are considered basic to successful participation in the work world. This work-related program serves as the foundation experience for those who aspire to higher-level referral and placement within the vocational structure for the developmentally disabled. Most such workers are employed in sheltered workshops. Thus this work program is designed for experience with those types of jobs and subtasks. The client's appropriate work participation is reinforced by a token economy system; tokens can be used to purchase items at the program.

Shana Krell, therapist for the program, has designed an evaluation that she found useful in measuring work skill acquisition (Fig. 5-34).

*This section was written by Shana Krell, OTR, Day Habilitation Program, United Cerebral Palsy Association, Newton, Massachusetts.

*Fig. 5-34. Evaluation of work skill acquisition. (Courtesy Shana Krell, OTR.)*

PP = physical prompt, PG = gestural prompt, PV = verbal prompt, JS = structural jig, JA = adaptive jig, I = independent, NA = not applicable.

Name ______________________

| A. WORK BEHAVIOR | *Init* | *Semi* | *Ann* |
|---|---|---|---|
| 1. Type of reinforcer | | | |
| a. Primary (food, drink) | ☐ | ☐ | ☐ |
| b. Social (verbal praise, attention) | ☐ | ☐ | ☐ |
| c. Activity (appropriate and pleasurable) | ☐ | ☐ | ☐ |
| d. Token—specify | ☐ | ☐ | ☐ |
| e. Combination of above—specify | ☐ | ☐ | ☐ |
| f. No reinforcer found successful | ☐ | ☐ | ☐ |
| 2. Schedule of reinforcer | | | |
| a. Continuous (after each piece of work) | ☐ | ☐ | ☐ |
| b. Fixed ratio (after specific no. of pieces) | ☐ | ☐ | ☐ |
| c. Variable ratio (after unspecified no. of pieces) | ☐ | ☐ | ☐ |
| d. Fixed interval (after specific time period: end of work period, 2×/day, end of week) | ☐ | ☐ | ☐ |
| e. Variable interval (unspecified time period during task, day, week) | ☐ | ☐ | ☐ |
| 3. Remains at work station | | | |
| a. 0–5 min | ☐ | ☐ | ☐ |
| b. 6–10 min | ☐ | ☐ | ☐ |
| c. 11–15 min | ☐ | ☐ | ☐ |
| d. 16–20 min | ☐ | ☐ | ☐ |
| e. 21–30 min | ☐ | ☐ | ☐ |
| f. 31–45 min | ☐ | ☐ | ☐ |
| g. 45 min–1 hr | ☐ | ☐ | ☐ |
| h. 1 hr or more | ☐ | ☐ | ☐ |

(Continued)

4. Attendance—leaves job station inappropriately during work period
   a. More than 15 × ☐☐☐
   b. 9–15 × ☐☐☐
   c. 5–8 × ☐☐☐
   d. 1–4 × ☐☐☐
   e. 0 × ☐☐☐
5. Task focus—work effort without interruption
   a. 0–5 min ☐☐☐
   b. 6–10 min ☐☐☐
   c. 11–15 min ☐☐☐
   d. 16–20 min ☐☐☐
   e. 21–30 min ☐☐☐
   f. more than 30 min ☐☐☐
6. Work tolerance
   a. Acts out when encounters job difficulty ☐☐☐
   b. Continues work after unsuccessful attempts ☐☐☐
   c. Appropriately indicates need for assistance when encounters difficulty ☐☐☐
   d. Waits patiently if work is delayed or stopped ☐☐☐
   e. Continues to work through peer outbursts ☐☐☐
7. Adaptability
   a. Changes tasks successfully within work period ☐☐☐
   b. Adapts to changes in routines (does not overreact or lose control) ☐☐☐
   c. Accepts and adjusts to new tasks ☐☐☐
   d. Accepts more difficult tasks ☐☐☐
   e. Works without complaints ☐☐☐
   f. Responds positively after correction ☐☐☐
   g. Continues work when being observed ☐☐☐
   h. Performs task following change in instruction ☐☐☐

B. WORK HABITS
1. Punctuality
   a. Arrives at work site ready for work ☐☐☐
   b. Begins task promptly after instruction ☐☐☐
   c. Leaves work area at appropriate times for toileting ☐☐☐
   d. Returns to work after appropriate amount of time (5–10 minutes) ☐☐☐
   e. Proceeds punctually to break or lunch ☐☐☐
   f. Responds positively to cues for time management ☐☐☐
2. Neatness—keeps work station neat by
   a. Picking up materials that have fallen ☐☐☐
   b. Arranging disorganized work materials ☐☐☐
   c. Maintaining task in work space ☐☐☐
   d. Placing correct items in indicated places ☐☐☐
3. Task acquisition—learns best with which type of guidance
   a. hand-over-hand ☐☐☐
   b. faded manual (specify) ☐☐☐
   c. gestural (demonstrating task in front of client) ☐☐☐
   d. verbal ☐☐☐
   e. written (or drawn) ☐☐☐
   f. combination of above—specify ☐☐☐

Fig. 5-34 (continued)

4. Responds to an instruction that requires compliance after how many verbal prompts
   a. 5+ ☐☐☐
   b. 4 ☐☐☐
   c. 3 ☐☐☐
   d. 2 ☐☐☐
   e. 1 ☐☐☐
5. Responds to instruction with cue
   a. Immediately ☐☐☐
   b. Within 1–2 min ☐☐☐
   c. Within 2–3 min ☐☐☐
   d. Within 3–4 min ☐☐☐
   e. Within 4–5 min ☐☐☐
   f. After more than 5 min ☐☐☐
6. Memory—ability to remember and follow how many progressive task steps
   a. 1 ☐☐☐
   b. 2–4 ☐☐☐
   c. 5–6 ☐☐☐
   d. 7–10 ☐☐☐
7. Work style—works
   a. Impulsively; requires cues to wait for supervision ☐☐☐
   b. Tentatively; lacks initiative to begin when appropriate ☐☐☐
   c. Begins tasks promptly after instruction ☐☐☐
   d. Appropriately; indicates when finished or in need of new work ☐☐☐
8. Maintains production rate on tasks with (specify) 1, 2–4, 5–6, 7–10 steps
   a. Less than 25% of the time ☐☐☐
   b. 25–49% of the time ☐☐☐
   c. 50–74% of the time ☐☐☐
   d. 75–99% of the time ☐☐☐
   e. 100% of the time ☐☐☐
9. Job performance—maintains production rate of work on same tasks from
   a. Day to day ☐☐☐
   b. Week to week ☐☐☐
10. Completes tasks with (specify) 1, 2–4, 5–6, 7–10 repetitive steps with
   a. Less than 25% accuracy ☐☐☐
   b. 25–49% accuracy ☐☐☐
   c. 50–74% accuracy ☐☐☐
   d. 75–99% accuracy ☐☐☐
   e. 100% accuracy ☐☐☐

C. JOB SKILLS

1. Disassembles item (specify task) of
   a. 2 like parts ☐☐☐
   b. 3 like parts ☐☐☐
   c. 4+ like parts ☐☐☐
2. Disassembles item (specify task) of
   a. 2 unlike parts ☐☐☐
   b. 3 unlike parts ☐☐☐
   c. 4+ unlike parts ☐☐☐

3. Assembles product (specify task) of
   a. 2 like parts ☐☐☐
   b. 3 like parts ☐☐☐
   c. 4+ like parts ☐☐☐
4. Assembles product (specify task) of
   a. 2 unlike parts ☐☐☐
   b. 3 unlike parts ☐☐☐
   c. 4+ unlike parts ☐☐☐
5. Matches object (specify) by
   a. 1 variable—color, shape, letter, number, size ☐☐☐
   b. 2 variables—color and shape, color and size, shape and size ☐☐☐
   c. 3 variables—color, shape, and size; letter, color and size ☐☐☐
6. Sorts objects (specify) by
   a. 1 variable ☐☐☐
   b. 2 variables ☐☐☐
   c. 3 variables ☐☐☐
7. Sorts items (specify) by type
   a. Broken or whole ☐☐☐
   b. Working or nonfunctional ☐☐☐
8. Places into open container
   a. 2 like items ☐☐☐
   b. 3–10 like items ☐☐☐
   c. 11–20 like items ☐☐☐
   d. 2 different items ☐☐☐
   e. 3–10 different items ☐☐☐
   f. 11–20 different items ☐☐☐
9. Seals containers
   a. Box top—insert item into box ☐☐☐
   b. Box cover ☐☐☐
   c. Bottle with snap top ☐☐☐
   d. Bottle with screw top ☐☐☐
   e. Plastic bag by folding top under ☐☐☐
   f. Plastic bag by folding and taping ☐☐☐
   g. Ziploc bag ☐☐☐
   h. Tucking envelope flap ☐☐☐
   i. Clasping envelope flap (clip or pin) ☐☐☐
   j. Moistening and sealing envelope flap ☐☐☐
   k. Taping box closed
10. Envelope stuffing
   a. Unstuffs envelope ☐☐☐
   b. Inserts one piece of paper into envelope ☐☐☐
   c. Folds one 8½″ × 11″ piece of paper into
      • halves ☐☐☐
      • thirds ☐☐☐
   d. Folds paper (specify) and correctly inserts into envelope ☐☐☐
   e. Places 3″ × 5″ card into envelope ☐☐☐
   f. Inserts already collated and stacked papers into envelope ☐☐☐
11. Collating—collates and stack
   a. 2 sheets of paper ☐☐☐
   b. 3–5 sheets of paper ☐☐☐
   c. 6+ sheets of paper ☐☐☐
   d. the above crisscross stacked ☐☐☐

Fig. 5-34 (continued)

12. Collates and places in envelope ☐☐☐
    a. 2 items ☐☐☐
    b. 3–5 items ☐☐☐
    c. 6+ items ☐☐☐
13. Ties with rubber bands, twist ties, string (specify)
    a. 2 items ☐☐☐
    b. 3 items ☐☐☐
    c. 4+ items ☐☐☐
14. Staples paper together at upper left-hand corner evenly (specify no. of pieces) ☐☐☐
15. Labelling
    a. Removes self-sticking label from backing ☐☐☐
    b. Centers and places label correctly ☐☐☐
    c. Marks envelope with rubber stamp neatly in center ☐☐☐
16. Measuring—fills marked container with items or liquid to
    a. capacity ☐☐☐
    b. ½ volume ☐☐☐
    c. ¼ volume ☐☐☐
17. Measures objects less than one foot to nearest inch with ruler ☐☐☐

## Industry Programs

In the future we may observe a rise in the number of therapists entering nontraditional areas of practice. Presently the role of the occupational therapist in industry is evolving, with some therapists acting in a consultant's capacity and others directly on staff in industry. Most of these therapists have had to define their roles to meet the individual needs of their employer. Some general areas of responsibility for occupational therapists in industry are as follows:

1. Work-related assessments—to identify difficulties or problems specific to the worker (e.g., recurrent injuries to an individual worker) or work environment (e.g. injuries indicating ergonomic problems) [20]
2. Application of work simplification and energy conservation techniques
3. Individual counseling, health maintenance programs, or both for employees
4. Liaison between management, employees, and adminstration
5. Application of ergonomics
6. Correlation of the demands of the work place with the needs and abilities of the worker

### Health Promotion Program*

UNITED HOSPITALS OF ST. PAUL

Occupational therapy has a unique contribution to make in industry although this has not been widely acknowledged or accepted. The therapist who wants to venture into this area typically must actively promote an awareness of the role he or she can play in industry.

*Most of this section was written by Barbara J. Johnson, OTR, United Hospitals, St. Paul, Minnesota.

Applying this approach, Barbara J. Johnson has become health extension director of United Hospitals of St. Paul, Minnesota. In this capacity she is responsible for designing a health promotion program for the medical center and its surrounding business community. Before this appointment Johnson established herself in this area of care by approaching a physician involved in occupational medicine with her desire to design a preventive approach to injury and illness. The physician responded with a challenge: One of the businesses with which he had a contract was experiencing an increasing number of tendonitis and carpal tunnel problems among employees working on an assembly line. What could be done? Johnson accepted this challenge and arranged for herself and another therapist to tour the work site and meet with the safety director. After that visit Johnson was able to devise a preliminary plan that entailed modifying an inefficient work layout and required work tasks. This plan was well received, and Johnson's role became defined as present as Health Extension Director. Continued assessment ensued in the areas of work process, work layout, and equipment. In addition employees were interviewed to obtain their suggestions for a more efficient and less stressful work process or layout. From their suggestions and the therapists' expertise in work simplification, specific recommendations were submitted and implemented. This first program has led to a continued working relationship with this physician.

United Hospitals, observing these successful endeavors, approached Johnson to head up their health promotion program. The hospitals' objectives for pursuing health promotion were to improve the hospitals' image in the community as a health resource, increase the use of their health resources, and position themselves in other markets.

For Johnson this new project posed questions such as How do the hospitals handle ill or injured employees? What particular trends in illness and injury are the hospitals experiencing? How are these handled?

At meetings with the medical director and nurse manager of the hospital's employee health service, Johnson learned that they were very concerned about the rise in neck and back strains among employees on one particular nursing unit. Johnson conducted a survey of these employees to ascertain their views of the problem. A task group was formed, and a questionnaire was developed to identify flexibility limitations of the staff, types of shoes worn at work, stressors associated with the work day, pain occurring at night or during the day, site of the pain, methods used to control the pain, the staff's understanding of body mechanics, and obstacles to practicing proper body mechanics. From the results of this survey, physical therapists designed flexibility exercises that the nurses could perform daily and before each work shift. Classes on stress management and aerobic exercise were given to the staff. Since this project started, there has been a statistically significant drop in the frequency and severity of neck and back strains on that unit.

Johnson has had many other challenging projects: performing a market study to ascertain where the hospitals should focus their health promotion efforts for the business community, proposal of a hospitals-wide employee health promotion program, and the development of a health promotion program at a small rural hospital affiliated with the United Hospitals. Johnson continues to ask questions that lead to new directions and new opportunities. Her creative and assertive method of practice should be an inspiration to all of us.

**Back Education Program**

CANADIAN BACK EDUCATION UNITS

Approximately 80 percent of the population will experience lower back pain sometime in their lives [16]. Research has found that the vast majority of this pain is of a chronic, mechanical nature; education of affected persons in proper body mechanics and back care could provide a solution to this problem.

The Canadian Back Education Units (CBEU) were developed in 1974 as a hospital-based program to address this issue. The program consisted of a series of four lectures designed to encourage the patient with chronic mechanical back pain to accept and successfully manage his or her own back problems. One of the keys to the success of the program was its team approach involving such individuals as psychiatrists, occupational therapists, orthopedic surgeons, physiatrists, and physical therapists.

The role to be played by occupational therapists in such programs is an important one:

> By virtue of the unique educational background in both the medical aspects of the programme and the vocational milieu, the occupational therapist is particularly suited to coordinate this or any industrial programme. It is the depth of knowledge in vocational assessment and rehabilitation that gives the occupational therapist special skills in evaluation of the workplace and in determining the areas of need which require emphasis in the lectures. The understanding of human relations enables the occupational therapist to effectively deal with various professional and lay people. [6]

Since the original inception of the CBEU, 15 other hospital-based programs have been established throughout Ontario, Canada. In addition there is one in Grand Rapids, Michigan, and others are planned throughout Canada.

The success of the hospital-based program gave the impetus for the establishment in 1977 of a modified version of the program in a community setting in Toronto. The program was established as a night school course in which persons such as housewives, businessmen, and laborers could enroll without a physician's referral to hear lectures by an occupational therapist, an orthopedic surgeon, and a physical therapist. This series of lectures is longer than the hospital-based program; the additional time allows the occupational therapist to emphasize back care techniques in relation to activities of daily living (ADL).

The industrial sector, observing the success of this group education approach to back problems, requested programs by the CBEU. In 1979 six firms had purchased CBEU programs for their employees. Each program is modified to meet the individual needs of the industry, with an occupational therapist as the coordinator of the program for the CBEU. The therapist "makes the arrangements with each industry in setting up a programme. Prior to each lecture series [the therapist] visits the workplace to carry out an ergonomic analysis and to take pictures of the employees at work. These are incorporated into the specific lecture series to add interest and a sense of relevance for the workers" [6].

The occupational therapists lecture on proper posture and techniques of back care in ADL at work, at home, and in leisure environments. Relaxation methods are discussed and practiced to convey an understanding of the psychosocial aspects of back pain. During another lecture the employees analyze themselves as they do numerous physical tasks required on their job; they also practice bending, lifting, and carrying techniques.

Clements and Dixon [6] challenge us with our role in industry: "There is a need for formalization of the consulting capacity of occupational therapists in industry either autonomously or under the umbrella of programmes such as CBEU."

The success of the CBEU programs indeed shows that our profession can make a valuable contribution to community and industrial health education programs. The expanding role of occupational therapy in industry was noted in a recent New York Times article [18]: "Industrial clinics are expected to hire more therapists in the decade ahead because employers want to get the injured back to work." We need to prepare for this role and accept the challenge.

## Geriatric Program

### Sheltered Workshop

JEWISH REHABILITATION CENTER FOR AGED

In the United States there are more than 24 million persons over age 65 (11% of the total population); by 2030, 18 percent of the population will be 65 or over [9]. As a nation we can ill afford to support the growing older population with tax dollars. Returning older persons to the work force or keeping them in it appears to be a viable solution.

The Jewish Rehabilitation Center (JRC) for Aged of the North Shore in Swampscott, Massachusetts, provides an on-site state-licensed sheltered workshop for its residents. Occupational therapy consultation has assisted in this workshop development.

JRC is a nonprofit institution established to provide complete health, nursing, and social care for the elderly residents of the North Shore communities of Massachusetts. The center has a 167-bed capacity. Late in 1982 the center expanded to include the Jewish Rehabilitation Adult Day Care Center, which offers structured activity within a therapeutic environment for elderly persons living independently in the community.

I have been a consultant to the center since 1981, providing restorative

Time Study Worksheet

Company ______________________ Date Run: ______________________

Job Description: ______________________ Space Requried:

______________________ Incoming Material __________ Sq ft

______________________ Production Area __________ Sq ft

______________________ Insp & Pack Area __________ Sq ft

______________________ Finished Outgoing __________ Sq ft

______________________ Total __________ Sq ft

Sketch

A. Nonhandicapped Time Data

| Name | No. of Pieces | Time Min | Time Sec |
| --- | --- | --- | --- |
| | | | |
| | | | |
| | | | |
| | | | |
| | | | |
| Total: | __________ Ⓐ | | Minutes Ⓑ |

B. Production Norm

$\frac{\text{50-min hr}}{Ⓑ} \times Ⓐ = Ⓓ$ number of pieces produced per 50-min hr.

$\frac{\text{50-min hr}}{\text{\_\_\_min}} \times \_\_\_ = \_\_\_\_\_\_$ Ⓓ (standard hourly production).

C. Piece Rate Computation

Prevailing hourly wage = PHW = $______

Piece rate per unit $= \frac{PHW}{Ⓓ} = \$\_\_\_\_\_\_ = \$\_\_\_\_\_\_$ per unit

Checked by ______________________

*Fig. 5-35. Time study worksheet used to determine piecework rates for contract or consignment work.*

care by means of direct service to residents and in-service training and consultation to staff and administration. In this capacity I consulted with the activity department of the JRC during the development of its sheltered workshop, offering activity analysis, time studies, and suggestions for jobs.

The JRC sheltered workshop was designed to provide employment opportunities for its residents. The rationale for establishing the workshop was that the "work ethic" is a strong motivating factor for this generation. The

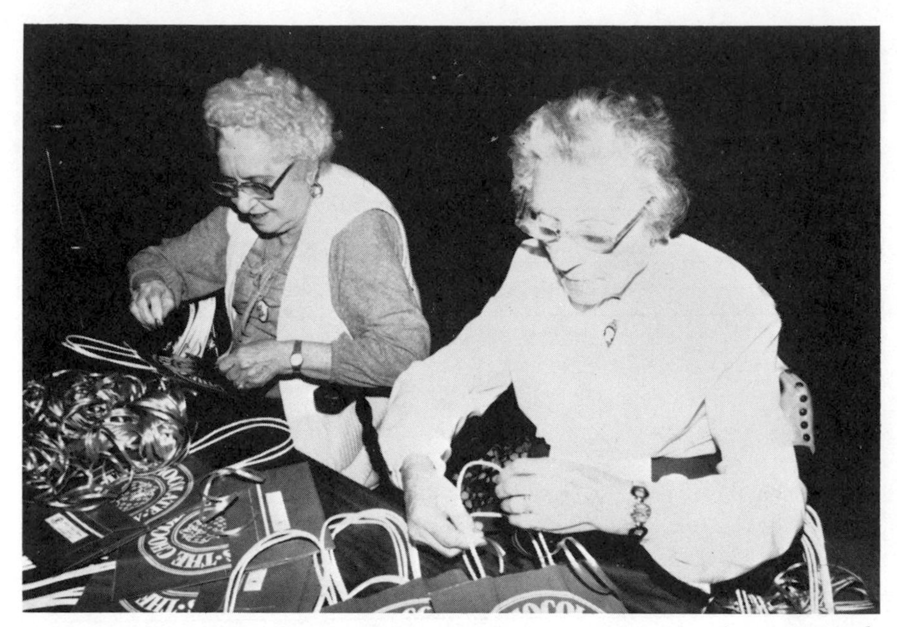

*Fig. 5-36. Members of sheltered workshop for the aged completing subcontract work.*

development of productive, useful roles in the community for the residents reestablishes their feelings of pride and self-esteem. Residents are able to socialize with others while performing their jobs, which helps to develop a group identification and sense of belonging. In addition it encourages the residents to work to their capacity in an environment that is best suited to their needs.

Work is performed on a contract or consignment basis at piecework rates based on current minimum wage standards. A time study of a sample of the job is done to establish these rates. When the resident feels efficient at a job he or she does it for 10 minutes. This figure in turn is multiplied by 5 to equal a 50-minute hour. The result is then divided by the minimum wage to come up with a piece rate. In my capacity as consultant, I provided the activity department with these procedures for performing time studies (Fig. 5-35).

The residents therefore do piece work and are paid according to their ability. This extra money allows them to purchase items they might not otherwise be able to afford on their fixed incomes.

This workshop has provided a reliable labor pool for local businesses. An example of an ongoing job is the tying of pink and red ribbons on bright red shopping bags for a local candy store (Fig. 5-36). Other jobs include addressing letters, collating, stamping, sewing, packaging, stapling, and sanding and finishing prefabricated wooden toys for a local children's store. These kits were made by the students at the Learning Prep School (see Chap. 4).

## References


1. Allen, Claudia. Independence through activity: The practice of occupational therapy (psychiatry) *Am. J. Occup. Ther.* 36: 731, 1982.
2. Barth, Tina. *The Barth Time Construction* (© 1978). Available from Health Related Consulting Services, 130 West Twenty-eighth Street, New York, New York 10001.
3. Beard, J. H. Psychiatric Rehabilitation at Fountain House. In Maislin, J. (ed.). *Rehabilitation Medicine and Psychiatry*. Springfield, Ill.: Charles C Thomas, 1976.
4. Blackmore, J. Community corrections. *Corrections Magazine*, October 1980, pp. 4–15.
5. Brayman, S.J., Kirby, T. F., and Misenheimer, A. M. Comprehensive occupational therapy evaluation scale. *AJOT*. 30: 94, 1976.
6. Clements, L., and Dixon, M. A model role of occupational therapy in back education. *Can. J. Occup. Ther.* 46: 161, 1979.
7. Community Service Department of the Queen Elizabeth Hospital. 1202 Old Port Road, Royal Park, Australia 5014. *Alfreda Rehabilitation Unit Fitness for Work and Living* (brochure).
8. Community Service Department of the Queen Elizabeth Hospital. 1202 Old Port Road, Royal Park, Australia 5014. Western Domiciliary Care and Rehabilitation Service The Alfreda Unit . . . (in-house handout).
9. Crispin, Marjorie L. *Braintree Council on Aging News* 4:2, September 1982. Available from the Braintree Council on Aging, 71 Cleveland Avenue, Braintree, Massachusetts 02184.
10. Daub, Mary Margaret. "The Human Development Process." In Hopkins, Helen L., and Smith, Helen D. (eds.). *Willard and Spackman's Occupational Therapy* (6th ed.). Philadelphia: Lippincott, 1983.
11. Day, S. R., and McCane, M. R. *Vocational Education in Corrections*. Columbus, Ohio: Ohio State University National Center for Research in Vocational Education, 1982.
12. Dean, P., Cox, R., and Aurich, R. *The Role of Occupational Therapist in the Alfreda Rehabilitation Unit* (in-house handout). 1982.
13. Gatti, D. *Open Door Thrift Shop* (handout for patients). Belmont, Massachusetts: McLean Hospital, 1982.
14. Goldenberg, E. P. *Special Technology for Special Children*. Baltimore: University Park Press, 1979.
15. Gross, D. Personal communication, 1982.
16. Hall, H., and Iceton, J. Back school: An overview with specific reference to the Canadian back education unit. Unpublished, 1983.
17. Harris, P. The Role of Occupational Therapy in Cognitive Remediation and Prevocational Rehabilitation (Conference.) Presented at New England Rehabilitation Hospital, Woburn, Massachusetts, November 1983.
18. Johnson, S. Physical rehabilitation market in fine shape. *The New York Times*. October 16, 1983.
19. Jones, P. D. *Walter E. Fernald State School. A Photo Essay*. Belmont, Massachusetts: Office of Communications, Walter E. Fernald State School (P.O. Box 158, Belmont, Massachusetts 02158), 1983.
20. Lewchuk, S. The occupational therapist in industry: A developing challenge *Can. J. Occup. Ther.* 47: 159, 1980.
21. Lewis, Sandra. *The Mature Years: A Geriatric Occupational Therapy Text*. Thorofare, N.J.: Charles B. Slack, 1979.
22. LIFT, Inc., 714 Woodland Avenue, Westfield, NJ 07090; tel. (201) 789-2443.
23. Matheson, L. N. *Work Capacity Evaluation: A Training Manual for Occupational Therapists*. Trabuco Canyon, California (16400 Pacific Coast Highway, Suite 211, Huntington Beach, California 92649): Rehabilitation Institute of Southern California, 1982.

24. Matheson, L. N., and Ogden, L. D. *Work Tolerance Screening.* Trabuco Canyon, California (16400 Pacific Coast Highway, Suite 211, Huntington Beach, California 92649): Rehabilitation Institute of Southern California, 1983.
25. *The Occupational Therapy Microcomputer Club Journal*, 1 (2): 10 November, 1982.
26. *The Occupational Therapy Microcomputer Club Journal*, 2 (1): 4 January, 1983.
27. Palmer, F., and Gatti, D. Transitional employment project. *Occupational Therapy in Mental Health.* 2:23, 1982.
28. Palmer, S. Personal communication, 1983.
29. Penner, D. A. Correctional institutions: An overview. *AJOT.* 32:517, 1978.
30. Platt, N. P., Martell, D. L., and Clements, P. A. Level I field placement at a Federal correctional institution. *AJOT.* 31:385, 1977.
31. Potter, J. Will work release ever fulfill its promise? *Corrections Magazine*, June 1979, page 60.
32. *Rehabilitation of the Mental Patient in the Community* (application form and handout). New York: Fountain House National Training Program (47 West Forty-seventh Street, New York 10036).
33. Schneider, Robert. *Workshop Description and Proposal for Workshop Contract and Orientation Program.* Calgary, Alberta, Canada: Calgary General Hospital, 1983.
34. Tiffany, Elizabeth G. "Psychiatry and Mental Health," in Hopkins, H. L. and Smith, H. D. (eds.). *Willard and Spackman's Occupational Therapy* (6th ed.) Philadelphia: Lippincott, 1983.
35. Jageman, L. W. *Adaptive Fixtures for Handicapped Workers.* Menomonie, Wisc.: Materials Development Center, Stout Vocational Rehabilitation Institute, University of Wisconsin—Stout, 1984.

# 6. Future Considerations

Work is an important aspect of most people's lives. Occupational therapists are challenged to examine their knowledge, skills, and attitudes in the area of work-related programs and assessments for the individuals they treat. Examples of innovative, futuristic programs have been presented throughout this text in the hope that they will stimulate an increased interest in work-related programming. Using our expertise to promote research and development in this area will open up new vistas for us.

Already, beginning research has shown us the need for work-related intervention at an early age for special needs children [1]. Occupational therapists could develop, coordinate, or perform direct service in such programs in the schools and at home.

Many opportunities await us in the future.

Labor researchers have shown us a view of the future that includes a shift of the labor economy out of assembly-intensive industries into technological and service industries. The researchers have also shown us robotization of the workplace and the accompanying disappearance of semiskilled and unskilled jobs in the labor market. Labor researchers have also found a growth area in the services industry [2].

Occupational therapists need to respond to these changes by exploring the growth area of services and alternative training for those who have been displaced by technology.

The personal computer revolution has widened the potential for meaningful employment of the disabled, in both information services and industrial jobs. Imagine, for instance, a quadriplegic supervising an automated factory with televised views of key areas and a computer keyboard through which he or she can regulate the automated processes as needed.(The Appendix to this chapter is a guide to the use of computers in occupational therapy.)

For occupational therapists industry is another wide-open sector. We need to define more clearly the contribution we can make to industry and then actively promote our participation.

The key for us is anticipation of changes in society, so that we and our clients will be ready to meet the demands of the future.

*Fig. 6-1. Form used in evaluating computer software. (Courtesy Nancy Wall, OTR.)*

SOFTWARE EVALUATION

Name: Date:

*Preliminary Information*

Name:
Producer/Publisher:
Date:
General Category:
Objectives of Program:
Age/Cognitive Level:
Cost:

*Technical Information*

Hardware Needed:
Peripherals Needed:
Quality:
Color:
Graphics:
Print:
Sound:
Documentation:
Written:
Within software:
Packaging:

*Consumer Information Policies*

Copyright:
Backup copies or policies:
Trial period:
Return policies:
Human Factors:
Ease of initial use by noncomputer person:
Error-free:
Options to restart, end, grade level of difficulty, exit, get help, review instructions, etc.
User-friendly:

*General Content*

Organized, Complete, Accurate:
Unbiased:

*Therapeutic/Educational Content*

Goals and Objectives Identified:
Promotes Motivation and Creativity:
Content Suitable for Identified User:
Feedback Appropriate, Timely, Informative:
Color, Sound, Graphics Appropriate for Therapeutic Goal:

*Program Applications*
Suggested Uses in Rehab:
Client population and needs
Goals and objectives of program
Special procedures for use
Appropriate Use of Computer:

*Suggestions for Adapting Program for Special User*

*Additional Comments*

*Fig. 6-2. Computer program developed to reinforce appropriate work behavior.*

WORK BEHAVIORS

Using correct work behaviors is a good way of being successful on a job. Sometimes we take these work behaviors for granted or forget to use them.

This program has been developed to reacquaint you with some of these behaviors. Six short stories about workers will be presented, followed by a question pertaining to the story. You are to select from the three choices presented the one correct answer to the question.

Do you understand?

Type Y for yes or N for no and then press the Return key.

Work behaviors are those behaviors such as coming to work neat, clean, and appropriately dressed; this is called good personal appearance.

Please press any key to continue.

Cooperative behavior, or getting along with other workers, is another example of good work behavior.

Punctuality is an important work behavior. Punctuality means arriving at work on time and adhering to your work schedule. An example of being punctual is returning from lunch break on time.

Please press any key to continue.

This program has been developed to reacquaint you with these behaviors. Six short stories about workers will be presented, followed by a question pertaining to the story. You are to select from the three choices presented the one correct answer to the question.

Please press any key to continue.

Here is an example story and its question, three possible answers, and the correct answer.

John works at a gas station and is responsible for opening the station each morning. Today he is one hour late because he was fooling around with his friends. When he arrives at the station, he finds angry co-workers and customers in their cars on line at the pumps. What should John do?

Please press any key to continue.

A. John should apologize to his co-workers and customers and assure them this will never happen again.
B. John should ignore them and act as if he did nothing wrong.
C. John should make the excuse that his car broke down as the reason for being late.

The correct answer is A. When a person has a job he should always be punctual. Most businesses, like the gas station, are open for certain hours. When John was late, it caused the station not to be opened at its scheduled time. Those people who depend on the station to be opened were right to be angry with John.

John made the right decision by apologizing rather than making up an excuse or ignoring the situation. John should be punctual in the future.

Please press Return to continue.

Name? Karen.

Male or female? Female.

Please read the following paragraph and then choose the correct answer.

Karen works at a fast-food place. Her hair is rather long and after an evening over the hot grill looks dirty, stringy, and unappealing. Which approach would you use if you were the boss?

Please press Return to continue.

A. You look like a slob with your hair that long. Did you ever think about cutting and washing it?
B. Karen, in any place where food is served a person has to be a little more careful of personal appearance. I'd like you to get your hair cut or tie it back while you're working—okay?
C. Don't come to work again until you get your hair cut!

After reading choices A to C, which answer do you think is correct? Please type in the answer A, B. or C and then press the Return key to continue.

Great! You have selected the correct answer. Although Karen's personal appearance was poor, her boss told her in a way that did not make Karen feel bad. Karen should always come to work neat, clean, and appropriately dressed. If Karen has long hair, she should remember to tie it back or wear a hair net. Press any key to continue.

Question 2. Karen works the early morning shift at a local supermarket. Last night she stayed out late dancing and was so tired the next morning that she overslept and was late for work. What should Karen do?

Please press any key to continue.

A. Karen should apologize to her boss, tell him this will never happen again, and offer to work overtime.
B. Karen should act as if she were due to work the late shift today.
C. Karen should sneak in the back door of the supermarket and pretend she has been there all morning.

After reading choices A to C, which answer do you think is correct? Please type in the answer A, B, or C and then press the Return key to continue.

C is not the correct answer. It is your responsibility to be punctual, or on time to work. Pretending that you did nothing wrong is not acting responsibly. You should not stay out late the night before you are on the morning shift if you have a hard time getting up and out to work on time.

Please review the answers again and select the one that is correct. Press any key to continue.

A. Karen should apologize to her boss, tell him this will never happen again, and offer to work overtime.
B. Karen should act as if she were due to work the late shift today.
C. Karen should sneak in the back door of the supermarket and pretend she has been there all morning.

Fig. 6-2 (continued)

After reading choices A to C, which answer do you think is correct?
Please type in the answer A, B, or C and then press the Return key to continue.
A? Karen, your're right. You know that it is your responsibility to be punctual to work. Oversleeping for work because you stayed out late the night before is no excuse for not being on time for work the next day.
Press any key to continue.
Question 3. You are working as a bagger at a supermarket. It is a very busy afternoon. One of your fellow baggers asks if you would help her lift a very heavy bag. What should you do?
Please press any key to continue.

A. Ask your boss if it is all right to help your fellow bagger. If he says it's OK, then help the bagger. After you finish, continue with your own job.
B. Tell the other bagger she should do her work by herself—that's why she's getting paid!
C. Tell her to "bug off." You've worked hard today and don't feel like helping her!

After reading choices A to C, Karen, which answer do you think is correct? Please type in the answer A, B, or C and then press the Return key to continue.
A? You're right! Working cooperatively with co-workers is an important work behavior. Asking your boss before helping the other bagger was the right procedure to follow. Please press any key to continue.

Fig. 6-2 (continued)

## References

1. Lynch, Kevin. "Analysis of Mentally Retarded Subjects' Acquisition and Production Behavior in Synthetic Prevocational Training Environments—Observational Report." In Lynch, K.P., Kiernan, W.E., and Stark, J.A. (eds.). *Prevocational and Vocational Education for Special Needs Youth: A Blueprint for the 1980s*. Baltimore: Paul H. Brookes Publishing Co., Inc., 1982.
2. Stout Vocational Rehabilitation Institute. *Materials Development Center Newsletter*, Winter 1983–84. Menomonie, Wisc: University of Wisconsin–Stout, 1983.

# Appendix

*While the revolution in information and technology is changing all facets of society, one of its most profound impacts lies in its potential to free handicapped citizens to pursue new fields and opportunities both at work and at home.*

*Terrel H. Bell*
Former Secretary, U.S. Department of Education

**Work-Related Programs, the Microcomputer, and Occupational Therapy***

Occupational therapists are in an excellent and unique position to use microcomputers in work-related programs. Occupational therapists work with the whole person, and they understand disorders and how they interfere with functioning. They also know how to identify a person's assets and capitalize on them. They can formulate realistic and functional goals for the client and determine priorities among needs and goals. In addition, they know how to integrate activities into a therapeutic program and assess and reassess progress. Their ability to break down an activity into component parts is an essential skill for therapeutically applying activity. This skill is particularly useful in using computer activities and in first learning about computers.

The computer has become another modality that occupational therapists can use. This modality happens to be very powerful, versatile, and excitingly progressive. It will be an integral part of our society and of work and something with which every person will have to interact in some capacity.

Does the microcomputer have a place in practice? A way to answer this question before making a commitment is to perform a needs assessment. Three important areas should be addressed: yourself (the therapist), your environment (setting and facility), and your client population.

*Yourself.* What is your attitude as therapist toward microcomputers—positive, negative, ambivalent? If it is negative or ambivalent, analyze why. What skills and knowledge do you have in the field of microcomputers? If the answer is none, are you willing to learn? What type of training is available, and how large a time commitment can you make? What is the cost of the training, and will your facility reimburse you?

*Nancy Wall, OTR, co-authored this appendix.

*Your environment.* Is your facility using a microcomputer? Do you have access to it for your own use? For use with a patient? If there is limited access, would integrating the computer into occupational therapy programming be feasible? If there is no microcomputer, what is the facility's attitude or philosophy regarding them? Would the facility support your using one? Is there funding in your budget for the purchase of a computer, software, and peripherals? Is there sufficient space for a computer?

*Your client population.* What are the interests of your clients? Do these include the computer? Have your clients had any experience with computers? Was this a positive or negative experience? What goals are being addressed in therapy? Are some of these goals easily achievable by computer activities? For example, goals involving cognition, academic skills, fine motor coordination, and social skills can be attained directly through computer activity, while activities of daily living—feeding, for example—can not. Will computer use lend itself to a realistic job choice?

If after analyzing and weighing the pros and cons of these three categories you have decided that the use of a microcomputer would be an asset in therapy, it is beneficial to become familiar with computer terminology. The microcomputer is really a system made up of two primary components: hardware and software. The hardware is the actual machine—the electronics, metal, and plastic that make up the computer itself, the monitor, the disk drive, and the printer. It is analogous, in simplified terms, to the record player with its turntable, amplifier, and speakers. The software consists of the programs, instructions, and activities that the computer works with. Software is analogous to the music, words, or stories on the records that the record player plays. The hardware and software are generally mutually dependent: The activity or program on the disk or cassette cannot happen without the computer, and the computer is limited in its capabilities without a program from the disk or cassette.

Peripherals, a third component of microcomputer systems, are especially useful in occupational therapy and rehabilitation. Peripherals are basically special devices or methods of putting information into and getting information out of the computer, aside from the standard keyboard, monitor, and printer. Special input methods include single switch control, voice recognition, joystick, game paddles, electromyographs, adapted keyboards, and graphic tablets. Special output devices include robots and robotic arms, environmental controls, and synthesized speech. The variety of adaptive peripherals that can be integrated with a microcomputer provides the opportunity to customize computer access for most special needs users.

How do you decide which computer and software to use? This decision involves three primary steps:

1. Identify all the potential uses for the computer in the clinic or therapy setting. Anticipate needs that may arise in the future. Include clients'

needs and goals and nonclient needs in administration, research, management, and education.

2. Become familar with and assess the commercially available software to determine which programs will best meet your clients' needs. (Fig. 6-1). In making this selection, certain client characteristics must be considered. Programs must be age appropriate, that is, matched to the client's developmental age, chronological age, and educational age. Your clients' computer-related interests—video games, word processing, data base management—should be taken into account. The activity should have value and usefulness to the client it should be tied to some work-related role(s) the client plays in society. Client involvement in the choice of the activity is essential and facilitates a greater commitment. You should also plan the amount of time at the computer so that it is within the client's task focus ability. For example, if the client has had a head injury that has resulted in a task focus of 10 minutes, the length of the activity should be within this time limitation. In addition to considering your clients' needs, you may find it helpful to ask other therapists what software they have found useful or to read journals that critique software. Finally, go to a local vendor and try out some of the programs that you think may be useful. Many vendors will allow you to sit down in the store and try out the program. Others will lend you a program on a 30-day trial basis for your clinical use. On the basis of all this research, develop a list of software that you have determined would be useful.
3. Now, knowing your specific needs and the specific software programs that will be useful in meeting these needs, look at computers. Most people seem to agree that the computer is only as good as the software. If you know the programs you want to use, then your choice of computers will be narrowed down to a few.

The following are some examples of the role of microcomputers in work-related programming:

1. Evaluation
2. Job placement
3. Communication aid
4. Work simulation
5. Problem solving
6. Educational skills
   a. Drill and practice in mathematics
   b. Grammar practice
7. Community skills
   a. Budgeting
   b. Banking

8. Cognitive skills
   a. Attention span
   b. Initiation and follow-through
   c. Perceptual activities and challenges
9. Physical skills
   a. Motor control
   b. Sitting posture and endurance
   c. Adaptive use of hardware
10. Social skills
    a. Group interaction
    b. Leadership
11. Learning a vocational skill
    a. Word processing
    b. Programming
    c. Financial management
    d. Data base management

Microcomputers can be used to evaluate realistic job-related skills. Two clinical programs may serve as examples. In Iowa occupational and physical therapists are using computers in the schools with physically and developmentally handicapped children, some of whom are taught beginning programming as a prevocational assessment [4]. With an adult physically disabled population, the Institute of Rehabilitation Medicine, New York University Medical Center, (discussed in greater detail in Chap. 5, Section 2) has used a microcomputer since 1981 in its prevocational evaluation unit. As noted by Dorothy Millner [3], "These patients saw the benefits of the computer directly related to their former jobs . . . One of these patients, a C6 quadriplegic and bank auditor, was specifically told by his employer that if he could learn computer programming, his job at the bank was assured. Another patient, a right hemiplegic with mild aphasia, had been a systems analyst. . . . He saw the computer as a means of regaining those skills he felt had been lost as a result of his CVA."

What about realistic job placement in this area? At present the outlook is optimistic. For example, a non-profit corporation, LIFT, Inc., trains and hires those with severe physical disabilities who are cognitively intact for computer programming. Founded in 1975, LIFT operates out of Chicago, New York, Los Angeles, Phoenix, Denver, and Boston, serving over 50 major corporations and disabled computer programmers. LIFT matches the disabled client with a corporate client before training begins, which allows the training program to be geared to specific employment needs and helps to establish worker-employer rapport. After training has been completed, each programmer is hired by LIFT and is assigned to full-time projects for the corporate client. When a year of contract employment has been satisfactorily completed, the programmer is hired directly by the corporate client[1].

However, "even among those who live with the computer for the rest of their lives and must become their own personal programmers, not all will be able, or want, to be programmers vocationally" [2]. For some clients, the computer represents only a temporary aid to education. For example, in special needs educational programs such as the Learning Prep School (see Chap. 4), software that reinforces appropriate work behaviors and skills has been purchased or developed. One such program uses case simulations to facilitate problem solving ability in relation to appropriate cooperative behavior, attendance, punctuality, and personal appearance (Fig. 6-2). These programs are used in therapy either individually or in groups. For the brain-damaged adult software on budgeting and banking, as a reinforcer to hands-on training, may facilitate reentry into the community. For the nonverbal, word processing may represent a life-long communication aid that enables them to obtain gainful employment.

Sources of information on computers for the handicapped are listed below, as are manufacturers of computer hardware.

**Resources**

1. Computers to Help People, Inc.
   1221 West Johnson St.
   Madison, WI 53715
   *Software*

2. Hammett Microcomputer Division
   P. O. Box 545
   Braintree, MA 02184
   *Software and hardware*

3. Opportunities for Learning, Inc.
   8950 Lurline Ave.
   Chatsworth, CA 91311
   *Software*

4. Plato
   Computer Based Education
   Control Data Publishing Co.
   P. O. Box 261127
   San Diego, CA 92126
   *Software*

5. Prentke Romich Company
   8769 Township Rd.
   Shreve, OH 44676
   *Hardware and adaptations*

6. Random House School Division
   Dept. 9062
   400 Hahn Rd.
   Westminster, MD 21157
   *Software*

7. Trace Research and Development Center for the Severely Communicatively Handicapped
   314 Waisman Center
   1500 Highland Ave.
   Madison, WI 53706
   *Excellent general resource*

8. Tufts University
   Boston School of Occupational Therapy
   Medford, MA 02155
   *General resource and microcomputer course for occupational therapists*

9. Zygo Industries, Inc.
   P. O. Box 1008
   Portland, OR 97207
   *Hardware and adaptations*

**Hardware Manufacturers**

1. Apple Computer, Inc.
   10260 Bandley Dr.
   Cupertino, CA 95014
   (408) 996-1010

2. Atari
   1265 Borregas Ave.
   Sunnyvale, CA 94086
   (408) 745-2038

3. Compaq Computer Corp.
   12337 Jones Rd.
   Houston, TX 77070
   (800) 231-9966

4. CompuPro
   3506 Breakwater Ct.
   Hayward, CA 94545
   (415) 786-0909

5. Commodore Business Machines, Inc.
   1200 Wilson Dr.
   West Chester, PA 19380
   (215) 431-9100

6. Cromemco, Inc.
   280 Bernardo Ave.
   Mountain View, CA 94040
   (415) 964-7400

7. Digital Equipment Corp.
   2 Mt. Royal Ave.
   Marlboro, MA 01752
   (617) 480-4111

8. Epson America, Inc.
   Computer Products Division
   3415 Kashiwa St.
   Torrance, CA 90505
   (213) 539-9140

9. Heath Co.
   Benton Harbor, MI 49022
   (800) 253-0570

10. IBM
    P. O. Box 1328
    Boca Raton, FL 33432
    (305) 998-2000

11. Radio Shack/Tandy Corp.
    1600 One Tandy Center
    Fort Worth, TX 76102
    (817) 390-3111

12. Texas Instruments
    P. O. Box 202146
    Dallas, TX 75220
    (214) 995-2011

13. Wang Laboratories, Inc.
    One Industrial Ave.
    Lowell, MA 01851
    (617) 459-5000

## References

1. *A Description of the Operations of LIFT, Inc.—Computer Programming by the Severely Disabled*, June 1, 1983. Available from LIFT, 350 Pfingsten, Suite 103, Northbrook, Illinois 60062 (publisher's address for Eastern Region: 714 Woodland Avenue, Westfield, New Jersey 07090).
2. Goldenberg, E. Paul. *Special Technology for Special Children.* Baltimore: University Park Press, 1979.
3. Milner, D., and Dickey, R. "Use of Microcomputers at the Institute of Rehabilitation Medicine, New York Medical Center." *Occupational Therapy Microcomputer Club Journal*, Vol. 1, No. 2, November 1982, pp. 10–13.

   For more information on the *Occupational Therapy Microcomputer Club Journal*, write to Nelson Clark, OTR, 1833 Jolliff Road, Chesapeake, Virginia 23321.
4. Stulak, Jane. *Occupational Therapy Microcomputer Club Journal*, Vol. 2, No. 1, January 1983, p. 4.

   For more information on the *Occupational Therapy Microcomputer Club Journal*, write to Nelson Clark, OTR, 1833 Jolliff Road, Chesapeake, Virginia 23321.

# Index